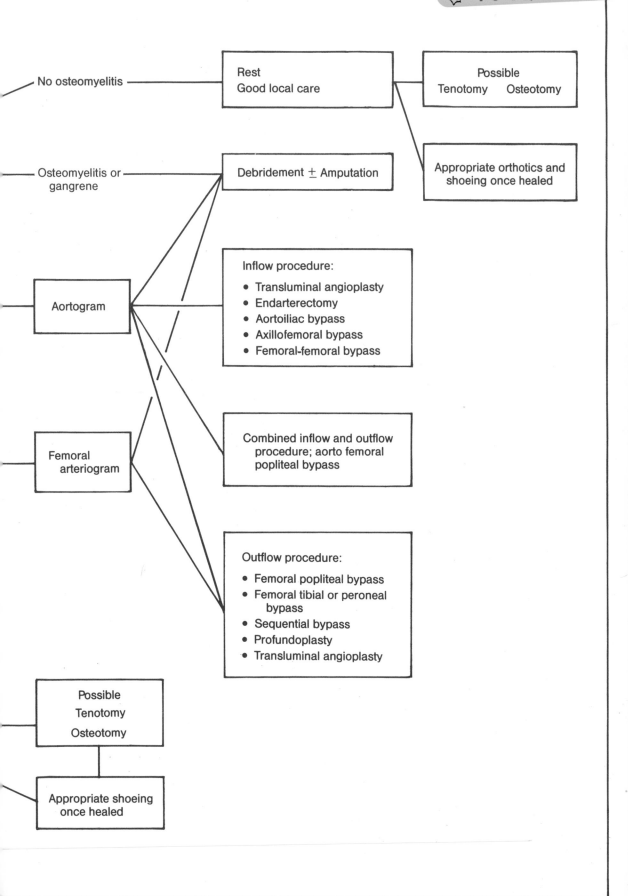

No osteomyelitis ——— Rest
Good local care

Possible
Tenotomy    Osteotomy

Osteomyelitis or ——— Debridement ± Amputation
gangrene

Appropriate orthotics and
shoeing once healed

Aortogram

Inflow procedure:

- Transluminal angioplasty
- Endarterectomy
- Aortoiliac bypass
- Axillofemoral bypass
- Femoral-femoral bypass

Femoral
arteriogram

Combined inflow and outflow
procedure; aorto femoral
popliteal bypass

Outflow procedure:

- Femoral popliteal bypass
- Femoral tibial or peroneal
bypass
- Sequential bypass
- Profundoplasty
- Transluminal angioplasty

Possible
Tenotomy
Osteotomy

Appropriate shoeing
once healed

# MANAGEMENT
OF
# DIABETIC
# FOOT
# PROBLEMS

# MANAGEMENT OF

# DIABETIC FOOT PROBLEMS

*Second Edition*

## GEORGE P. KOZAK, MD

Associate Clinical Professor of Medicine
Harvard Medical School
Boston, Massachusetts

## DAVID R. CAMPBELL, MD

Assistant Clinical Professor of Surgery
Harvard Medical School
Boston, Massachusetts

## ROBERT G. FRYKBERG, DPM, MPH

Attending Podiatrist, Department of Surgery
New England Deaconess Hospital
Boston, Massachusetts

## GEOFFREY M. HABERSHAW, DPM

Clinical Instructor of Surgery (Podiatry)
Harvard Medical School
Boston, Massachusetts

**W.B. SAUNDERS COMPANY** · Philadelphia · London · Toronto · Montreal · Sydney · Tokyo
*A Division of Harcourt Brace & Company*

**W.B. SAUNDERS COMPANY**
*A Division of Harcourt Brace & Company*

The Curtis Center
Independence Square West
Philadelphia, Pennsylvania 19106

**Library of Congress Cataloging-in-Publication Data**

Management of diabetic foot problems / George P. Kozak . . . [et al.].—2nd ed.

p.    cm.

ISBN 0–7216–3284–X

1. Foot—Surgery.    2. Diabetes—Surgery.    3. Diabetes—Complications.    I. Kozak,George P.

[DNLM:   1. Diabetes Mellitus—complications. 2. Foot Diseases—etiology.   3. Foot Diseases—therapy.   WK 835 M266   1994]

RD563.M35   1995

617.5′85—dc20

DNLM/DLC                                                                                          93-37401

MANAGEMENT OF DIABETIC FOOT PROBLEMS                    ISBN 0–7216–3284–X

Printed in the United States of America.

Last digit is the print number:      9     8     7     6     5     4     3     2     1

*Dedicated to diabetic patients with foot problems.*

*'Tis not knowing much, but
what is useful that makes a man wise.*

Thomas Fuller   1732

# CONTRIBUTORS

**HARRY BAILEY, M.D.**
Chairman Emeritus, Department of Radiology, Naval Hospital, San Diego, California; Former Radiologist, New England Deaconess Hospital, Boston, Massachusetts.
*Radiology in the Diabetic Foot*

**E. JAMES BUSICK, M.D.**
Instructor, Harvard Medical School; Attending Physician, New England Deaconess Hospital, Boston, and Waltham-Weston Hospital and Medical Center, Waltham, Massachusetts
*Management of Diabetes During Surgery*

**DAVID R. CAMPBELL, M.D.**
Assistant Clinical Professor of Surgery, Harvard Medical School; Attending Surgeon, New England Deaconess Hospital, Boston, Massachusetts.
*Guidelines in the Examination of the Diabetic Leg and Foot; Aortoiliac Reconstruction; Amputations*

**JAMES S. CHRZAN, D.P.M.**
Clinical Instructor in Surgery, Harvard Medical School; Director, Podiatric Residency Training, New England Deaconess Hospital, Boston, Massachusetts.
*Biomechanical Considerations of the Diabetic Foot; Reconstructive Foot Surgery for the Diabetic*

**LEONARD CONNOLLY, M.D.**
Instructor, Harvard Medical School; Radiologist, New England Deaconess Hospital, Boston, Massachusetts.
*Radiology in the Diabetic Foot*

**GEORGE M. ELIOPOULOS, M.D.**
Associate Professor of Medicine, Harvard Medical School; Infectious Diseases Division, New England Deaconess Hospital, Boston, Massachusetts.
*Infection of the Diabetic Foot: Medical and Surgical Management*

**DONALD W. FOSTER, M.D.**
Clinical Instructor of Anaesthesia, Harvard Medical School; Staff Physician, Department of Anaesthesia, New England Deaconess Hospital, Boston, Massachusetts.
*Anesthesia in Diabetic Patients*

**JANE C. FRASCA, R.N.**

Vascular Nurse Coordinator, New England Deaconess Hospital, Boston, Massachusetts.

*Local Treatment of the Diabetic Foot*


**DOROTHY V. FREEMAN, M.D.**

Clinical Instructor of Surgery, Harvard Medical School; Attending Surgeon, Vascular Surgery, and Surgical Director, Introduction to Clinical Medicine, and Co-Director, Vascular Noninvasive Laboratory, New England Deaconess Hospital, Boston, Massachusetts.

*Guidelines in the Examination of the Diabetic Leg and Foot; Aortoiliac Reconstruction*


**ROBERT G. FRYKBERG, D.P.M.**

Attending Podiatrist, Department of Surgery, New England Deaconess Hospital, Boston, Massachusetts.

*Podiatric Problems in Diabetes; The Diabetic Charcot Foot*


**GARY W. GIBBONS, M.D.**

Associate Clinical Professor of Surgery, Harvard Medical School; Clinical Chief, Division of Vascular Surgery and Assistant Chairman, Quality Assessment for Surgery, New England Deaconess Hospital, Boston, Massachusetts.

*Diabetic Foot Disease: A Major Problem; Infection of the Diabetic Foot: Medical and Surgical Management; Local Treatment of the Diabetic Foot; Arterial Reconstruction: Femoral to Popliteal, Tibial, Peritoneal, and Pedal; Amputations*


**JOHN M. GIURINI, D.P.M.**

Clinical Instructor of Surgery, Harvard Medical School; Director, Podiatric Education and Research, New England Deaconess Hospital; Consultant, Joslin Diabetes Center, Boston, Massachusetts.

*Diabetic Neuropathies: Lower Extremities; Reconstructive Foot Surgery for the Diabetic*


**HERBERT F. GRAMM, M.D.**

Assistant Professor, Harvard Medical School; Vice Chairman, Department of Radiology, New England Deaconess Hospital, Boston, Massachusetts.

*Radiology in the Diabetic Foot*


**ANTONIO GRANFONE, M.D.**

Assistant Clinical Professor of Medicine, Tufts University School of Medicine and Boston University School of Medicine; Attending Physician, Department of Medicine, New England Deaconess Hospital, Boston, Massachusetts; Chief, Endocrinology Section, Whidden Memorial Hospital, Everett, Massachusetts.

*Hyperlipidemia in the Diabetic: Accelerated Atherosclerosis*


**MICHELE GRAY, R.N.**

Special Dressing Nurse (inactive), New England Deaconess Hospital, Boston, Massachusetts.

*Local Treatment of the Diabetic Foot*

## GEOFFREY M. HABERSHAW, D.P.M.

Clinical Instructor of Surgery (Podiatry), Harvard Medical School; Chief, Division of Podiatry, New England Deaconess Hospital; Chief of Podiatry, Joslin Diabetes Center, Boston, Massachusetts.

*Biomechanical Considerations of the Diabetic Foot; Reconstructive Foot Surgery for the Diabetic*

## DANA BENNETT KARBASSI, M.S.P.T.

Assistant Director of Physical Therapy and Physical Therapy Liaison to the Arnold Pain Center, New England Deaconess Hospital, Boston, Massachusetts.

*Physical Rehabilitation of the Diabetic Foot*

## URMILA KHETTRY, M.D.

Assistant Professor of Pathology, Harvard Medical School; Pathologist, New England Deaconess and New England Baptist Hospitals, Boston, Massachusetts.

*Pathology of the Diabetic Foot*

## GEORGE P. KOZAK, M.D.

Associate Clinical Professor of Medicine, Harvard Medical School; Physician, New England Deaconess Hospital and New England Baptist Hospital; Former Physician, Joslin Diabetes Center, Boston, Massachusetts.

*Diabetic Foot Disease: A Major Problem; Guidelines in the Examination of the Diabetic Leg and Foot; Diabetic Neuropathies: Lower Extremities; The Diabetic Charcot Foot; Management of Diabetes During Surgery*

## ISTRATI A. KUPELI, M.D.

Clinical Instructor in Anaesthesia, Harvard Medical School; Staff Physician, Department of Anaesthesia, New England Deaconess Hospital, Boston, Massachusetts.

*Anesthesia in Diabetic Patients*

## O. STEVENS LELAND, M.D., F.A.C.C.

Assistant Clinical Professor of Medicine, Harvard Medical School, Boston, Massachusetts.

*Preoperative Evaluation of the Diabetic Patient*

## STANLEY M. LEWIS, M.D., F.A.C.C.

Assistant Professor of Medicine, Harvard Medical School; Director of Clinical Cardiology, New England Deaconess Hospital, Boston, Massachusetts.

*Preoperative Evaluation of the Diabetic Patient*

## FRANK W. LoGERFO, M.D.

Professor of Surgery, Harvard Medical School; Chief, Division of Vascular Surgery, New England Deaconess Hospital, Boston, Massachusetts.

*Diabetic Vascular Disease; Arterial Reconstruction: Femoral to Popliteal, Tibial, Peritoneal, and Pedal*

## H. ESTERBROOK LONGMAID, M.D.

Assistant Professor of Radiology, Harvard Medical School; Staff Radiologist and Director of Education and Training, Department of Radiological Sciences, New England Deaconess Hospital, Boston, Massachusetts.

*Arteriography; Transluminal Angioplasty and Laser Treatment*

## ROBERT C. MELLORS, Jr., M.D.

Clinical Assistant, Professor of Medicine, Boston University School of Medicine; Staff Physician, Braintree Medical Associates, Braintree, Massachusetts.

*Other Arthritic Disorders in the Diabetic Foot*

## LEONARD B. MILLER, M.D., F.A.C.S.

Clinical Instructor in Surgery, Harvard Medical School; Active Staff, New England Deaconess Hospital, Boston, Massachusetts.

*Plastic Surgical Reconstruction of Difficult Diabetic Foot Wounds*

## ELLISON C. PIERCE, Jr., M.D.

Associate Clinical Professor of Anaesthesia, Harvard Medical School; Chairman, Department of Anaesthesia, New England Deaconess Hospital, Boston, Massachusetts.

*Anesthesia in Diabetic Patients*

## FRANK B. POMPOSELLI, Jr., M.D.

Assistant Professor of Surgery, Harvard Medical School; Vascular Surgeon, New England Deaconess Hospital, Boston, Massachusetts.

*Diabetic Vascular Disease; Noninvasive Evaluation of the Arterial System in the Diabetic Lower Extremity; Arteriography; Arterial Reconstruction: Femoral to Popliteal, Tibial, Peritoneal, and Pedal; Transluminal Angioplasty and Laser Treatment*

## BARRY I. ROSENBLUM, D.P.M.

Clinical Instructor of Surgery, Harvard Medical School; Division of Podiatry, New England Deaconess Hospital, Boston, Massachusetts.

*Plastic Surgical Reconstruction of Difficult Diabetic Foot Wounds*

## JOHN L. ROWBOTHAM, M.D.

Assistant Clinical Professor of Surgery, Harvard Medical School; Surgeon and Honorary Staff, New England Deaconess Hospital, Boston, Massachusetts.

*Diabetic Foot Disease: A Major Problem; Local Treatment of the Diabetic Foot*

## MICHAEL A. SASSOWER, M.D.

Clinical Fellow in Medicine, Harvard Medical School; Cardiology Fellow, New England Deaconess Hospital, Boston, Massachusetts.

*Preoperative Evaluation of the Diabetic Patient*

## KENNETH R. STOKES, M.D.

Assistant Professor, Harvard Medical School; Vascular and Interventional Radiology, New England Deaconess Hospital, Boston, Massachusetts.

*Arteriography; Transluminal Angioplasty and Laser Treatment*

**FRANK C. WHEELOCK, Jr., M.D.**

Associate Professor of Surgery (Retired), Harvard Medical School; Formerly Chief of Vascular Surgery, New England Deaconess Hospital; Visiting Surgeon, Massachusetts General Hospital, Boston, Massachusetts.

*Amputations*


**STUART W. ZARICH, M.D., F.A.C.C.**

Clinical Instructor in Medicine, Harvard Medical School; Director of the Coronary Care Unit, New England Deaconess Hospital, Boston, Massachusetts.

*Preoperative Evaluation of the Diabetic Patient*

# PREFACE

Time marches on . . . since the First Edition, three of the associate editors have departed to the happy world of retirement. Carl Hoar has retired to Cape Cod and is working on his metal-crafting hobby; John Rowbotham is a country squire living in the White Mountains of New Hampshire, and Captain Frank Wheelock is sailing his ship off the coast of Maine. We all express our deep thanks to our former teachers, colleagues, and dear friends. Their initial interests and contributions will always be felt and have made this second edition possible.

The goal of the book remains as before to provide comprehensive and practical clinical coverage from patient evaluation to therapeutic management and surgical techniques. A practical team approach in diagnosis and therapy is stressed.

Five completely new chapters have been added and four chapters have been completely revised. Five new chapters include Diabetic Vascular Disease, Diabetic Neuropathies, Transluminal Treatment: Angioplasty and Laser Treatment, Reconstructive Foot Surgery, and Plastic Reconstructive Procedures of the Foot. The completely revised chapters are Hyperlipidemia in the Diabetic, Noninvasive Diagnostic Studies, Arteriography, and Physical Rehabilitation. The remaining chapters have all been revised as needed.

Great strides have been made over the past ten years, but certainly continued improvements in medical surgical treatment still need to be found. Improvements in radiologic techniques have made it possible to visualize the pedal arteries. Arterial bypasses to pedal vessels have decreased the frequency of major limb amputations.

Since 1980 a number of advances have occurred to significantly reduce the number of patients requiring major leg or partial foot amputations. First, with improved understanding of the way in which neuropathy leads to tissue loss, our podiatric group is straightening toes and performing metatarsal osteotomies to prevent the consequences of the claw foot. This has dramatically reduced the number of toe amputations that we now perform. Second, with chronic infection involving the metatarsal heads, it is now possible to remove the metatarsal heads and leave the toes. In the right situation this produces a better cosmetic and functional result than the transmetatarsal amputation (TMA). Finally, the introduction of the in situ technique and arterial digital subtraction arteriography has allowed us to revascularize many patients with isolated tibial arterial occlusion who, in the past, would not even have been candidates for arteriography. It can certainly be said that the popliteal to dorsalis pedis artery bypass graft has replaced the TMA as the "diabetic operation."

A great deal of thanks is owed to the many secretaries who worked on numerous revisions of the manuscripts. Our secretaries include Kathleen Pratt, Beverly Hadley, Sheila Janus, Angela Grassa, Mary Ann Baker, Lynn Blalock, Heather Frykberg, and Ann Marie McCarthy. For the hospital statistics, we are indebted to Mr. Gerald Galuardi.

Despite the delay in preparation of manuscripts, the staff at W.B. Saunders Company was always most encouraging and cooperative. We are especially indebted to our Senior Editor Raymond Kersey, Senior Supervising Editor Edna Dick, Team Manager and Designer Lorraine B. Kilmer, and Production Manager Frank Polizzano. They all made the task of preparing this text a most stimulating and pleasant experience.

GEORGE P. KOZAK, M.D.
DAVID R. CAMPBELL, M.D.
ROBERT G. FRYKBERG, D.P.M.
GEOFFREY M. HABERSHAW, D.P.M.

# CONTENTS

# Chapter 1

# DIABETIC FOOT DISEASE: A MAJOR PROBLEM

GEORGE P. KOZAK, M.D.,
JOHN L. ROWBOTHAM, M.D., and
GARY W. GIBBONS, M.D.

Since diabetes mellitus is a chronic disorder and affects a large segment of the population, it is a major public health problem. Diabetes affects approximately 5 per cent of the United States population (approximately 12 million people). In the United States, diabetes and its complications is the third leading cause of death. Diabetes is the leading cause of new blindness. In contrast to nondiabetics, diabetic patients are 25 times more likely to develop blindness, 17 times more likely to develop gangrene, and twice as likely to develop heart disease. Five of six major limb amputations occur in diabetic patients. In view of the multiple complications and debilitating nature of diabetes, 14 per cent of the diabetic population (usually older patients) are hospitalized yearly for an average of six weeks per stay. Diabetic foot problems account for many hospital days per year. It is a strange paradox that in spite of great advances in the knowledge and treatment of diabetes, more than 70 years after the discovery of insulin, the diabetic foot is still and continues to be a major problem.

Why is this so? As the population grows older and increases, so does the number of diabetic patients. Before the availability of insulin treatment, many insulin-dependent diabetics either died young or barely survived. Now they live longer and have families, passing on genetic traits to their offspring. As they age, they may have an increased likelihood of developing diminished sensation, decreased peripheral circulation, and increased chance of infection, especially with poorly regulated diabetes. These developments make diabetic patients particularly vulnerable to severe foot and leg problems.

With these basic facts, it is understandable why diabetic foot lesions create a major medical, hospital, and economic problem. Therefore, diabetic foot disease must be both recognized and properly treated. All efforts must be made to prevent it and to rehabilitate the patients.

Diabetes and foot problems are almost synonymous. That diabetics are prone to foot disease has been known for many years, and the fear of gangrene is ever-present in the minds of diabetics who are striving to maintain their health and protect their lives. It is a common misconception that all diabetics have poor circulation. Indeed, some do—but a large proportion, over 20 per cent, have exceedingly good circulation. However, they are vulnerable to foot problems because they have neuropathy and associated loss of acute sensation of pain. They are vulnerable to trauma by being unaware of it. Thus diabetes mellitus can lead to foot problems because it may dispose a patient to peripheral vascular atherosclerosis with associated ischemia, or may cause peripheral neuropathy with altered proprioception, touch or pain sensation, and secondary atrophy of skeletal muscles in the legs and feet.

The metabolic effects of diabetes are profound and insidious, affecting all parts of the body (Table 1–1). It causes premature aging of all parts of the body. The peripheral vascular system commonly develops arteriosclerosis obliterans and the nervous system deteriorates.

There is considerable overlap between diabetic patients with ischemia and those with neuropathy, because each person may develop one or the other or a combination of both. However, ischemic foot lesions are usually seen in older patients whose diabetes began in adult years. The diabetic with neuropathy, on the other hand, is one who had juvenile or early-onset (insulin-dependent) diabetes and whose symptoms are associated with nephropathy and retinopathy. Whether a patient has ischemic- or neuropathic-related foot problems, the general statement must be made that while careful personal attention to daily management of diabetes through diet, insulin (oral agent), and exercise may postpone the development of foot problems, it will probably not prevent them.

One seldom sees neuropathy developing in the ischemic foot, yet it is not unusual to see the neuropathic foot develop ischemic changes. When this happens, it is in later years when the patient might be expected to show atherosclerosis. The ischemia becomes

the dominant disease and the neuropathic traits seem to diminish.

In 1969 at the New England Deaconess Hospital in Boston, in which approximately 5000 patients are treated yearly at the Joslin Clinic, 417 patients with a variety of foot lesions required hospitalization and occupied a total of 10,742 patient days (Table 1–2). Yearly hospital cost, not including surgical and medical fees, was more than $1,000,000 for the diabetic foot patients. During the last few years, hospital costs have escalated at an incredible rate. The economic burden of diabetic foot problems is even more striking (Tables 1–3 and 1–4).

Although the number of hospitalized diabetic foot patients increased by 50 in 1980 at New England Deaconess, the number of patient days in the hospital was essentially the same. The daily hospital cost had increased fivefold to approximately $500 per day. In

## TABLE 1–1.   TYPES OF DIABETES AND CHARACTERISTICS

|  | TYPE I—INSULIN-DEPENDENT DIABETES (JUVENILE ONSET, JOD) | TYPE II—NON-INSULIN-DEPENDENT DIABETES (MATURITY ONSET, MOD) |
|---|---|---|
| Age at onset | <30 years | >40 years |
| Body weight | Normal or underweight | Overweight (80 per cent) |
| Prevalence | 0.5 per cent | 5 per cent |
| Etiology | Unknown<br>*Heredity:* associated with specific HLA types but only 50 per cent concordance in twins<br>*Autoimmune Disease:* 70 per cent circulating islet cell antibodies<br>? *Viral Infections:* as trigger | Unknown<br>*Heredity:* not associated with specific HLA types but 95 per cent concordance in twins<br>*Autoimmune Disease:* 10 per cent circulating islet cell antibodies<br>No evidence for viral infections |
| Insulin | Early in disease, insulin secretion is impaired; late in disease, insulin secretion may be totally absent | Insulin deficiency and/or insulin resistance<br>*Deficiency:* Insulin secretion insufficient to meet demands created by the obese state; possible impairment in the glucose receptor of the β-cell<br>*Resistance:* In nonobese patients, there is hyperinsulinemia and defect in tissue responsiveness to insulin; insulin resistance may be mediated by a decreased number of insulin receptors |
| Ketosis | Common | Rare |
| **COMPLICATIONS** | **Frequent**<br>Microangiopathies<br>Neuropathies<br>Accelerated atherosclerosis | **Frequent**<br>Accelerated atherosclerosis<br>Microangiopathies<br>Neuropathies |
| Leading cause of death | Microangiopathies, i.e., renal failure secondary to diabetic nephropathy | Accelerated atherosclerosis, i.e., myocardial infarction |
| Treatment | Diet and insulin | 1. Diet (reduction)<br>2. Diet and oral hypoglycemia<br>3. Diet and insulin |

## TABLE 1-2. DIABETIC FOOT ADMISSIONS, NEW ENGLAND DEACONESS HOSPITAL, 1969

| CONDITION | NO. CASES | PATIENT DAYS |
|---|---|---|
| Gangrene | 142 | 4719 |
| Infection | 32 | 724 |
| Ulcer | 159 | 3391 |
| Charcot foot | 6 | 64 |
| Abscesses; cellulitis | 33 | 580 |
| Osteomyelitis | 45 | 1264 |
| Total | 417 | 10,752 |

Total hospital admissions, 10,321 (including diabetics).
Total patient days, 119,870.
Average total cost per hospital day, $101.08.
Yearly hospital cost (not including medical fees) was more than $1,000,000 for care of patients with severe foot lesions and complications in this one hospital alone.

1980 the hospital costs for these patients, not including surgical and medical fees at the New England Deaconess, were more than $5,200,000. In 1992, total charges for care of diabetic foot patients exceeded $243,000,000 at the New England Deaconess.

Finally, the economic costs associated with diabetic foot complications and amputations are astronomical. Direct hospital costs alone in the United States exceeded $200 million a year in 1980. This figure does not include other direct medical expenses or indirect costs due to disability pay, unemployment, and loss of productivity. No recent cost estimates are available for diabetic foot care in the United States, but obviously these are staggering in view of 1992 total charges at the New England Deaconess.

## CLASSIFICATION OF DIABETIC FOOT DISEASE

Diabetic foot disease may be caused by infection alone, may be neuropathic in origin,

## TABLE 1-3. DIABETIC FOOT ADMISSIONS, NEW ENGLAND DEACONESS HOSPITAL, 1980

| CONDITION | NO. CASES | PATIENT DAYS |
|---|---|---|
| Gangrene | 199 | 5074 |
| Infection, cellulitis, abscess | 46 | 902 |
| Ulcer | 138 | 2544 |
| Charcot foot | 23 | 328 |
| Osteomyelitis | 61 | 2255 |
| Total | 467 | 10,475 |

or may be caused by ischemic problems (Plates 1 to 3 and 6 to 8).

Anyone may develop a foot infection, but diabetics are likely, by virtue of associated traits of disease, to be more susceptible than others. The cause is not, as some believe, that hyperglycemia causes bacteria to thrive; rather, it is because poorly oxygenated tissues in the ischemic foot are less able to muster a vigorous immune response. The neuropathic patient is less aware of the existing problem and therefore may not institute protective measures. The neuropathic foot with ischemic changes is particularly vulnerable because most of the protective defenses are stripped, leaving it prey to any harmful agent, be it trauma or bacterial invasion.

The common foot problems are:
• Blisters, corns, and calluses caused by poorly fitting shoes
• Plantar warts
• Fissures
• Interdigital fungal infection
• Paronychia
• Ingrowing toenails
• Accidents associated with nail trimming

Depending upon factors affecting diabetics already mentioned, any of these problems may be corrected or the lesions may be healed or may evolve into serious infection with ultimate development of abscess and cellulitis that may progress to gangrene. This in turn could necessitate surgery with incision and drainage, removal of a toe or toes, or even leg amputation.

The foot conditions to which anyone is susceptible are blisters, fungal infection, plantar warts, and improperly cut toenails. Each of these may progress to a local or generalized infection.

The neuropathic foot is characteristically healthy. It is well nourished, has hair, maintains good dorsalis pedis and posterior tibial pulses, has a high arch, and may have cocked-up hammer toes. Callus formation is common on pressure points of the soles or toes, and there may be sweating. This indicates lumbar sympathetic nerve activity. It is the pressure points that cause problems. On the soles, thick calluses can act as foreign bodies and cause bruising of the subcutaneous tissues with extravasation of blood and serum from the capillaries. This leaves a culture medium pool for local bacteria to grow and cause an abscess. The condition may be unsuspected because of the anesthesia con-

**TABLE 1–4.   DIABETIC FOOT ADMISSION, NEW-ENGLAND DEACONESS HOSPITAL, 1992**

| CONDITION | NO. CASES | NO. PATIENT DAYS | TOTAL CHARGES |
|---|---|---|---|
| Gangrene | 166 | 2936 | 6,016,950 |
| Osteomyelitis | 89 | 1043 | 1,450,456 |
| Ulcer | 446 | 4970 | 9,977,364 |
| Charcot's foot | 48 | 595 | 820,212 |
| Infection, abscess, cellulitis | 35 | 321 | 422,518 |
| TOTAL | 784 | 9865 | 18,687,500 |
| Total hospital 1992 | 12,822 | 106,491 | 243,455,031 |

ferred by the neuropathy, and it can expand without being detected until the patient develops generalized infection or the process is detected by its foul odor or its invasion of less anesthetic areas of the same foot. At times the overlying callus is so hard that the infection can more easily invade the underlying joint capsule and metatarsal head than the callus itself. Thus, osteomyelitis associated with calluses can be explained and easily understood. The same disease process may occur on the top of hammer toes or in relation to deformed and collapsed bones and joints associated with neuro-osteoarthropathy (Charcot foot) (see Chapter 9).

The ischemic foot is characteristically dry, atrophic, scaly, hairless, and undernourished. It is cool to touch. The nails are apt to be thick and overgrown with dry scales piled up under the nail itself. The dorsalis pedis and posterior tibial pulses are diminished or absent, and there are often fissures on the heel or beside the prominent metatarsal heads. Such ischemic feet often have a small infection beside or behind a nail or in the depth of a fissure. These feet hurt when walked on, and the infected spots are very painful to touch or pressure. The ischemic foot may show small, flat, dry, atrophic ulcers with full-thickness skin necrosis in the center and with a rim of erythema surrounding the ulcer as a crimson corona. From such ulcers or spots of gangrene there may be a spreading area of cellulitis or a red streak of lymphangitis leading up to the foot or leg to tender lymph nodes in the groin. Seldom is osteomyelitis seen with ischemic ulcers, and seldom is a true abscess found, but pus lurks behind the gangrenous plaque and is unroofed only by cutting away the necrotic tissue by sharp dissection.

The patient with a black toe or toes fre-quently has an antecedent history of pain and a small sore near a toenail. Cellulitis has developed and dry gangrene has occurred because the infection itself has caused occlusion or thrombosis of the small digital vessels. Wet gangrene of ischemia is seen when a higher vessel, one in the thigh or calf, becomes suddenly occluded, leaving much or all of the foot without enough blood to survive. The tissues are still "wet," and the ensuing gangrene is manifested first by pallor, then rubor, and finally the unmistakable blistered skin with underlying blue-black tissue shining through. This is accompanied by the characteristic odor of dying tissue intermingled with the unmistakable essence of *Pseudomonas.*

Only the ischemic foot has these characteristics, and often the destruction of tissues is so great that even mechanical restoration of blood flow into the patent major vessels is not sufficient or not in time to revive the injured tissues or to restore them. Therefore, higher amputations are necessary.

## SOLVING THE PROBLEM

In this introductory chapter, an overview of management is given; the reader should refer to individual chapters for detailed discussion.

Bed rest is the key to managing diabetics with foot disease (Table 1–5). No matter how much effort is put into treating the local lesions by giving antibiotics and regulating diabetes, the foot with a lesion must be put to rest if it is to heal. Crutch walking or walking "on the heel" is in most cases no alternative. Bearing weight on an ulcer or a healing incision breaks down the fibroblast network or barriers and slows healing by squeezing bacteria into the surrounding healthy tissues. Every step is a moment of ischemia to the

## TABLE 1-5.  MANAGING THE ACUTE PROBLEM OF THE DIABETIC FOOT

1. Appraise problem
   a. Careful inspection with emphasis on web spaces and backs of heels
   b. Record pulses, venous filling time, and rubor
   c. Record sensation
2. Describe lesion
3. Debride necrotic tissue, probe sinuses with sterile probe to determine extent of disease
4. Culture pus for aerobic and anaerobic organisms
5. Begin a broad-spectrum antibiotic until appropriate antibiotics can be given according to drug sensitivity data; use caution with renal insufficiency
6. Determine state of diabetes control
7. X-ray both feet (uninvolved one for comparison)
8. No weight bearing
   a. Hospitalize with absolute bed rest when indicated
   b. Crutches or walker when feasible
9. Surgical management of problem
   a. No soaks
   b. Antibiotics
   c. Medical management of diabetes
   d. Dressing changes at least once daily
   e. Surgical debridement, frequently if necessary
   f. Consideration for possible arterial reconstruction
   g. Drainage or open amputation
10. Rehabilitation
   a. Podiatrist for patient education, preventive maintenance, orthotics, healing sandals, and special shoes
   b. Physiatrist for return to normal activity, gait training to prepare for a prosthesis, and prophylactic exercises to maintain body tone
   c. Nutritionist to advise on diet needs
   d. Surgeon to ensure proper wound healing and proper prosthetics
   e. Physician to make final decision about diabetes management

damaged area. Therefore, bed rest is the first order of treatment.

## INFECTION

Infection affects diabetic control, and uncontrolled diabetes affects infection. An abscess or cellulitis may cause hyperglycemia. Conversely, hyperglycemia may interfere with the healing of an abscess. The usual means of maintaining normal blood sugar levels may have to be changed. Patients who usually take oral agents may temporarily need insulin during the course of the infection, and often those who take insulin have to change the dose, i.e. increased amounts of insulin, one to two injections, and supplements of regular insulin. In other words, the diabetes must be carefully monitored and the infec-

tion must be carefully treated. Each affects the other, and if a clinical response or improvement is not evident in a few days, it is an indication of undrained pus, uncontrolled infection, or inadequate diabetic treatment. It is interesting to note that a healing infection often permits a reduced insulin dosage or changing to an oral agent.

Local wound care is next. Draining areas must be cultured to determine the organisms growing and to find their specific antibiotic sensitivities. Encrusted lesions must be unroofed, and obvious deep abscesses must be opened to obtain accurate culture. Surface bacteria over crusts may give misleading information. Foot infections in diabetics usually have multiple types of bacteria, and often unsuspected anaerobic organisms cause the greatest tissue damage.

It is imperative that the cardinal principles of treating infection be closely adhered to in the management of the infected diabetic extremity. The importance of aerobic gram-positive and enteric gram-negative bacilli in diabetic foot ulcers cannot be overemphasized. A high frequency of anaerobes can also be seen. The mixed infections tend generally to have a poor response to therapy.

Since diabetic patients tolerate infection poorly, it is imperative that treatment protocols for moderately and severely infected foot ulcer begin immediately after diagnosis. Ulcers with a fetid odor or crepitance or subcutaneous gas should be particularly suspected of harboring anaerobic organisms. Our experience with patients with severely infected ulcers indicates that a single antibiotic is seldom sufficient at the onset. Because aerobic gram-positive and gram-negative organisms and anaerobic bacteria are frequently isolated and because there is a major threat to limb survival, initial intravenous antibiotic coverage for all of these bacteria is indicated as soon as adequate wound and blood cultures are obtained.

Reasonable initial antibiotics for mild to moderate infections include cefazolin, ampicillin plus sulbactam, and ticarcillin plus clavulanate. Antibiotic allergy precludes use of the antibiotic, and careful monitoring for signs of antibiotic toxicity is mandatory. A reasonable initial combination of antibiotics for severe infections might include an aminoglycoside plus ticarcillin or mezlocillin plus clindamycin. (Antibiotic use is discussed further in Chapter 12.) As soon as the bacterial sensitivity studies become available, appropriate changes should be made in these medications.

Particular attention should be paid to a culture that is positive for *Pseudomonas*. We have found this organism to be responsible for continuing and extensive tissue destruction. The most effective treatment at this time for *Pseudomonas* appears to be a combination of an aminoglycoside plus ticarcillin or mezlocillin. Similarly, ulcers whose cultures grow *Enterococcus* plus *Proteus* species (50 per cent of patients) demand aggressive antibiotic therapy, as do those ulcers found to contain anaerobic organisms. With the continuing introduction of newer antibiotics with specific antimicrobial action, carefully designed clinical trials are needed to determine the most effective regimen of antibiotics for moderate and severe diabetic foot infection.

It goes without saying that the better the circulation in the foot, the better the possibility of saving it, even though an amputation of a toe, a toe and metatarsal head, or the forefoot (transmetatarsal) might be necessary. Deep foot necrosis in the presence of ischemia has usually been the forerunner of major leg amputation unless a reversal of the septic spread can be effected by the aforementioned measures coupled with possible arterial reconstruction (see Chapters 19 and 20). Table 1–6 shows the type and number of arterial reconstruction procedures done from October 1980 to October 1982 at the New England Deaconess Hospital, and Table 1–7 shows those for 1990 to 1992. Thus bac-

### TABLE 1–6.  ARTERIAL VASCULAR SURGERY PROCEDURES AT NEW ENGLAND DEACONESS HOSPITAL, OCT. 1980 TO OCT. 1982

| | | |
|---|---|---|
| INFLOW | Aorto-iliac-femoral bypass | 66 |
| | Endarterectomy | 7 |
| | Axillo-femoral bypass | 8 |
| | Femoral-femoral | 14 |
| | | 95 (29%) |
| OUTFLOW | Femoral-popliteal bypass | 184 |
| | Femoral-tibial | 23 |
| | Femoral-peroneal | 10 |
| | Endartectomy | 14 |
| | | 231 (71%) |
| | Total | 326 |

Compiled by D. R. Campbell, M.D.

### TABLE 1–7.  ARTERIAL VASCULAR SURGERY PROCEDURES AT NEW ENGLAND DEACONESS HOSPITAL, OCT. 1990 TO OCT. 1992

| | | |
|---|---|---|
| INFLOW | Aorto-iliac-femoral bypass | 201 |
| | Axillo-femoral bypass | 10 |
| | Femoral-femoral | 19 |
| OUTFLOW | Femoral-popliteal bypass | 168 |
| | Femoral/popliteal to tibial | 186 |
| | Femoral/popliteal to peroneal | 66 |
| | Femoral/popliteal to dorsalis pedis | 154 |
| | Local endarterectomy | 23 |

Compiled by D. R. Campbell, M.D. and F. W. LoGerfo, M.D.

terial cultures and sensitivity studies are necessary to indicate the antibiotics to be used. However, the physician must institute antibiotic therapy promptly and not wait several days for specific culture and sensitivity results. A Gram stain of the bacteria is often helpful, but clinical judgment is usually just as good. Intravenous administration of antibiotics is imperative if there is clinical evidence of cellulitis, lymphangitis, tender lymphadenopathy, fluctuant tender areas, or uncontrolled diabetes. Any or all of these should suggest a need for a combination of broad-spectrum antibiotics administered, at least initially, intravenously. If after 48 hours of therapy there is still evidence of active infection, the antibiotics might be empirically changed despite the culture reports. Moreover, surgical drainage should be considered, if it has not already been done, because pockets of expanding necrosis can often respond to treatment only by being laid open to the air with appropriate and adequate incisions—both to remove necrotic material and to give adequate dependent drainage to a wound.

Concomitantly, local wound debridement and dressing done at least once daily are a necessary part of the care. Debridement means sharp trimming of all obvious necrotic tissue with a knife or scissors and forceps, as well as seeking out and opening up sinuses and channels that harbor pus and foster bacterial growth. Proteolytic enzymes or debriding ointments or solutions are costly and in most cases are not as effective as the act of cutting; therefore, they are infrequently used at the New England Deaconess Hospital. The drained wounds and those treated surgically are managed with a liquid or ointment with a pH near 7.4, which serves either to assist natural debridement or to kill surface bacteria. One quarter strength Dakin's solution (Chlorazene) does the former, and one quarter strength povidone-iodine (Betadine) or 1 per cent neomycin solution does the latter. These solutions are best used on open granulating or septic wounds, whereas antibiotic ointments are used on dry, scaly, fissured, or callused areas.

There is nothing magic about dressings, but changing them, in addition to affording the physician or nurse an opportunity to remove a dirty pus-laden dressing, allows inspection and appraisal of the state of the wound, and verification that the dressing both protects the wound and prevents contamination of the bed and general environment. Although changing a dressing once a day is adequate and proper in many cases, multiple daily dressing changes should be made whenever wounds are very septic. Such frequent dressing change in a hospital setting with many "foot patients" may be more efficiently managed by having a designated hospital floor or area on a floor. Another method would be a team of "foot nurses" who do such dressing changes for these patients (Chapter 13).

*Foot soaks should never be done.* Soaking macerates the skin and spreads infection. The heat of the water may burn and literally cook the vulnerable ischemic foot or be too hot for the insensitive neuropathic foot. Foot soaks lead to more complications in diabetics than any other common form of treatment. Foot soaks contribute to the development of gangrene with ultimate amputation more than any other home remedy. Feet should be washed with tepid water and gentle hand soap, but washing feet is not soaking them.

Elevation of an infected part is a sound general surgical principle; however, the diabetic foot with ischemia should be elevated only to the horizontal position. Raising the legs above horizontal reduces the flow of blood to toes already ischemic and therefore should not be done. Edema and cellulitis in patients with congestive heart failure can be adequately managed with the patient flat in bed and does not put at risk those patients whose legs might be harmed by prolonged elevation to a high level.

Chronic illness and malnutrition go hand in hand, and the infected diabetic is no exception. The often-painful disease with associated anorexia contributes to patient debility. The nutritional needs of each patient must be assessed and all efforts made to assure proper daily balanced food intake. For those unable to take an adequate diet, parenteral supplements or total intravenous hyperalimentation must be considered—especially in those who face peripheral arterial reconstruction and major limb amputation. Without proper nutritional support, the patient is deprived of a major building block for adequate healing.

## NEUROPATHIC DISEASE

The neuropathic foot has poor sensation and good circulation. All specific problems related to it are based on these two facts. Loss of sensation in the feet makes them vulnerable to trauma, yet good circulation makes them more able to recover from or heal wounds or infections. The diabetic with a neuropathic foot usually has an antecedent history of paresthesias and pains in the feet or legs.

The usual findings in the neuropathic foot are:

1. Well-nourished tissue
2. Good dorsalis pedis and posterior tibial pulses
3. Sensation, vibration sense, and Achilles tendon reflex diminished or absent
4. Tendency for hammer toes and high foot arch
5. Calluses at pressure points
6. Charcot deformities
7. Foot drop (advanced cases)
8. Superimposed infections: ulcers, osteomyelitis

The neuropathic foot is healthy, often has hair, and may have moisture between the toes. The pulses are present, indicating good gross circulation, but there may be microvascular disease, leaving the skin and other tissues more vulnerable than usual to infection or injury. Furthermore, it must be remembered that the neuropathic foot has diminished pain sensation—at times it cannot detect a pinprick. In addition, the vibration sense of the foot and leg, as well as the Achilles tendon reflexes, may be diminished or absent. In short, the patient may be unaware of the position of his foot.

The peripheral neuropathy directly affects the muscle receptors, causing atrophy of some muscle groups in the leg and foot. This results in a disproportionate muscle tone in the feet, causing the cavus deformity as well as foot drop in advanced cases.

As though to protect itself, the foot develops calluses on pressure points. The trauma to the underlying tissues from the calluses causes, at times, abscesses and ulcers deep within the calluses. These may extend into joints and bones, causing osteomyelitis.

There is a type of neuro-osteoarthropathy that develops in the neuropathic foot. It is characterized by joint swelling, bone disruption and absorption with fractures, and eventual healing with bone deposits, leaving joints disrupted, arches collapsed, and toes shortened. The resultant wide, deformed foot is subject to calluses and ulcers too, because of its irregular contour. This is Charcot disease (see Chapter 9).

Beyond the physical examination, the usual diagnostic aids are x-ray studies and nerve conduction studies. X-rays help differentiate between osteomyelitis and osteoarthritis, and nerve conduction studies can confirm a clinical diagnosis of neuropathy. The clinical picture is so distinct that nerve conduction studies are rarely needed.

## PREVENTION OF NEUROPATHIC PROBLEMS

Good hygiene is the single most important step in preventing problems in the anesthetic foot. Next, heat must be avoided. Hot soaks, heating pads, and electric blankets must never be used. Sitting too close to a fire or an electric heater may cause skin burns. Chemical corn or hair removers may harm insensitive skin and likewise should be avoided.

"Bathroom surgery" should never be done! Cutting of toenails, corns, and calluses should be done by a podiatrist or physician who will be able to recognize and treat problem areas and to advise when surgical consultation is indicated. A podiatrist will also be able to make and provide inner soles and prosthetics as well as recommend the proper type of shoe.

Walking barefoot is dangerous and must not be done by diabetics with peripheral vascular disease or neuropathy or both. It goes without saying that any surface can be too hot or too cold or have sharp objects that can penetrate skin and inoculate virulent bacteria. Diabetics must inspect their own feet daily. The blind diabetic must have a sighted person inspect his feet once a day.

Because of adequate circulation, the prognosis for diabetic neuropathic foot problems is good. Injuries will heal and infections can be controlled. When foot surgery such as drainage or amputation of a toe or toes must be done, the likelihood is that the incision will heal. For the foot problems of diabetics to be minimal, they must protect their feet with good hygiene, wear proper shoes, avoid objects or situations that cause injury, and maintain good daily control of their disease.

## ISCHEMIC VASCULAR DISEASE

The diabetic foot with ischemia has poor circulation and very acute sensation. As in the case of neuropathic problems, all specific problems related to it are based on these two facts. Because of ischemia, the foot is vulnerable to trauma and diseases that endanger the very life of the foot and that cause much pain. Ischemia makes the foot hypersensitive, and any lesion such as an infected fissure or inflammation around a nail is more painful than one might normally expect. Furthermore, ischemia itself makes any lesion a serious condition that can quickly develop to a limb- or life-endangering problem.

Historically, the ischemic foot is associated with intermittent claudication in the calf, usually caused by a narrowing or blockage of the superficial femoral artery in the adductor canal. With severe atherosclerosis obliterans, pains can be noted in the feet even at rest. Other pains, stabbing in nature, occur in the feet, legs, and thighs, and following no specific nerve distribution are the paresthesias of ischemia. They resemble neuropathy and may be a form of it, but may be related to ischemia alone. It is often difficult to determine the predominating agent, ischemia or neuropathy, that is causing the pain.

Signs of foot ischemia are:

1. Dry, scaly skin (dyshidrosis)
2. Atrophy of soft tissues
3. Absence of hair
4. Tendency to fissures on heels and prominences
5. Diminished or absent dorsalis pedis and posterior tibial pulses

6. Prolonged venous filling time (over 20 seconds)
7. Rubor of toes or foot on dependency
8. Blanching of foot on elevation

The ischemic foot is thin and grossly malnourished. The skin is thin, dry, and scaly, and there are usually no hairs. Fissures are present on the heels and the ends of the toes or near the prominent knuckles. There may be significant rubor of the foot when it is dependent. Elevation causes the rubor to vanish, leaving a blanched appearance to the foot. No posterior tibial or dorsalis pedis pulses are felt, and there may be no popliteal or femoral pulse as well; however, the ischemic foot is alive. A bruit may be detected over the femoral artery in the fossa ovalis or in the adductor canal.

Muscle atrophy of the entire lower leg and foot may be evident and is based on general ischemia of the entire limb rather than on selected muscle bundle atrophy with neuropathy. Infections in the ischemic foot heal slowly, whether they be fungus between the toes, tiny ulcers in fissures, or cellulitis in a toe or in the foot.

Much can be done to help some patients with ischemia. Reconstruction of major vessels of the leg may restore circulation to a poorly nourished part. Therefore, several studies can be done to evaluate patency of the vessels. Arterial angiography, which outlines the aorta, iliac, femoral, and distal leg and foot arteries, is the most direct approach and usually the most helpful test to perform. Noninvasive studies employing oscillometry, pulse volume recordings, and ultrasonic (Doppler) flow meter measurements all contribute to an understanding of the status of circulation in any limb. Thermography, on the other hand, has no significant role in assessment in these cases. A simple clinical evaluation of skin temperature may help determine the best site for a limb amputation. For example, a below-knee amputation is never done on a leg that is cold above the ankle malleoli.

Further detailed discussions of pathogenesis, evaluation, management, and treatment of diabetic foot problems are covered in the following chapters.

# Chapter 2

# GUIDELINES IN THE EXAMINATION OF THE DIABETIC LEG AND FOOT

DAVID R. CAMPBELL, M.D., DOROTHY V. FREEMAN, M.D., and GEORGE P. KOZAK, M.D.

In the last 20 years there has been tremendous improvement in the management of the diabetic foot, resulting in saving many legs that otherwise would have been amputated. It has come about because of better understanding of the factors that make the diabetic patients different from the nondiabetic. As will be discussed in detail in subsequent chapters, diabetic patients are more prone to infection, often suffer from peripheral polyneuropathy, and have a higher incidence of arterial insufficiency. Each patient may have one or more of these processes going on at the same time. After completion of the history and physical examination, it is important for the examiner to ask himself or herself how much of the observed pathology is due to infection, how much to neuropathy, and how much to arterial insufficiency. Unless this is done, it is not possible to design a rational treatment plan for the patient.

## HISTORY

### General

The initial patient interview is extremely important in the subsequent management of the patient. The physician needs to get a complete picture of the patient's general condition as well as a good understanding of the current problem. Patients with diabetic foot problems are usually terrified of losing their legs. Many have known relatives who were diabetics and seemed to be doing well until they developed a foot problem. They were admitted to the hospital and underwent toe amputations, forefoot amputations, and major leg amputations before they died of a heart attack. It is no wonder that they regard the development of a foot lesion as the beginning of the end. It is often helpful to reassure the patient that, at this time, feet are rarely lost because of infection and neuropathy and up to 90 per cent of legs with arterial insufficiency can be salvaged. Once the patient is reassured, a more complete history can usually be obtained.

It is important to start by checking the patient's diabetic history. A long history of insulin-dependent diabetes is associated with a higher incidence of neuropathy, retinopathy, and nephropathy (diabetic "triopathy"). Conversely, an older patient with diet-controlled diabetes is more likely to have purely ischemic problems as seen in the nondiabetic. Poorly controlled diabetes with increased blood glucose is associated with increased thrombogenicity and the complications that may result from this. Severe triopathy is thought to be secondary to basement membrane thickening, and in patients who have this, wound healing appears to be delayed. This is particularly true of those patients with renal failure. Consideration of patients' renal function is also important in deciding if they are candidates for arteriography for further evaluation of their arterial insufficiency.

Hypertension, tobacco consumption, and hypercholesterolemia are also factors in the development of arterial insufficiency, and a careful history should be obtained. Heart disease is the major source of mortality in diabetic patients, and it is often asymptomatic. Severe cardiac disease may be a contraindication for aggressive management of a diabetic foot problem. Review of patients' medications may reveal a large dose of diuretics, which may be indicative of a low ejection fraction. These patients are particularly prone to perioperative myocardial events, and this may encourage more conservative management. Other important features to be elicited from the general history include a history of allergy to contrast material and previous saphenous vein stripping.

## Specific

Once the patient's general status has been recorded, the patient's presenting problem can be discussed in detail. Again, it is useful to think in terms of infection, neuropathy, and arterial insufficiency. If the patient describes a rapidly enlarging lesion associated with drainage or swelling, perhaps with red lines extending up the leg and fever or shaking chills, then infection would seem very likely. Loss of control of the patient's blood glucose may be an early sign of infection. Unexplained elevation of the blood glucose level may therefore be an indication to look for occult sepsis.

The classic distal polyneuropathy seen in diabetics may not only cause lesions on its own but may mask the symptoms of infection and arterial insufficiency. In its mildest form, the patient may simply notice that there is less feeling in the feet and perhaps be more likely to develop blisters or other traumatic injuries. As increasing motor neuropathy with intrinsic muscle paralysis develops, the metatarsal heads become more prominent. This causes calluses to develop over the pressure points. Hyperglycemia causes glycosylation of collagen so these calluses may become rigid and inflexible and a potent source of injury to the foot. Thus the classic neuropathic lesion is a painless ulcer occurring over a pressure point, often under a metatarsal head.

Pain in the diabetic limb is extremely difficult to evaluate because of the variable effects of neuropathy. First, the foot may lose pain sensation and therefore is more likely to become injured. Second, this may modify the pain normally noted in infection and arterial insufficiency. It is not an all-or-none phenomenon, but there is a broad spectrum from minor to complete sensory loss. As well as sensory loss, diabetic neuropathy may also result in pains that may be chronic and disabling for the patient. The patient may complain of a burning sensation in the feet, that the feet feel cold or as if encased in concrete or of the sensation of walking on glass. Sometimes the patient describes knife-like shooting pains running up the legs, often on the anterior surface. The pain tends to be intermittent and not related to anything. Usually both legs are equally involved, and this may be helpful in distinguishing neuropathic from ischemic pain, although patients not uncommonly have both types of pain. Pain at night is often prominent in patients with neuropathic pain and may be difficult to distinguish from ischemic pain. The patient with neuropathic pain will awaken at night with pain and rub the legs or elevate them, but usually the pain will go away by itself. Although getting up because of the pain is unusual, some patients will get up to take a pain pill or occasionally to walk off leg cramps. The fact that the pain does not come on every night is markedly different from ischemic rest pain. The development of sudden painless deformity of the foot is characteristic of diabetic neuropathic arthropathy (Charcot foot). Painless swelling and increase in temperature, perhaps with erythema, does not necessarily mean infection, because it is also noted with an acute Charcot injury. It may be difficult to distinguish between these two.

The history of ischemia is frequent in patients with diabetic foot lesion, although again these symptoms may be masked by the presence of neuropathy. A history of cardiac or carotid disease would certainly make the presence of peripheral vascular disease more likely. Claudication or pain in muscle groups on exercise is the usual presenting symptom of peripheral vascular insufficiency. In the diabetic, outflow disease, or obstruction of the vessels below the groin, is more common, and therefore calf claudication is more frequent. This pain comes on on walking and is immediately relieved by stopping for a minute or so. It tends to be a cramping or ache in the calf muscles. Usually the patient can then continue to walk for a similar distance before the pain comes on again. The pain comes on sooner when going up hill, when walking faster, or when it is cold, or when the patient has just eaten a heavy meal. A prominent feature that helps distinguish claudication from neuritic pain is the consistency of the ischemic symptoms. Neuropathy, however, may make a significant difference to ischemic symptoms. Claudication may be described as tiredness on walking rather than pain, although often the patient denies even this. On specific questioning, however, the patient is found to have adapted his life-style to involve almost no walking at all.

Occasionally, particularly in smokers, inflow disease is responsible for the ischemia, and then buttock and thigh claudication may be the presenting symptoms. This is the Leriche syndrome, as described by René Leriche, which is due to obstruction of the aortoiliac vessels. This may be associated with impotence in men. Low back problems such as disc compression may cause similar symptoms, and this is known as the *cauda equina syndrome.* So many diabetic men suffer impotence because of their neuropathy that this symptom is often difficult to evaluate when taking the history.

Once the ischemia progresses, the patient may go on to develop rest pain. This is because, without the help of gravity, not enough blood reaches the feet. Thus, once he goes to bed and elevates the feet, he develops pain in the toes that wakes him and that is relieved by getting up. The patient may start sleeping in a chair to avoid getting the pain. Characteristically, the pain is consistent, coming on every night, in contradistinction to neuropathic pain, which tends to be intermittent. Many diabetics with profound neuropathy, however, may never get rest pain but may develop gangrene directly. In the patient without neuropathy the tissue loss is at the most distal part of the extremity and associated with severe pain. The patient with neuropathy, however, may have painless gangrene of the extremities or, alternatively, a neuropathic lesion on the weight-bearing portion of the foot that fails to heal because of ischemia.

## PHYSICAL EXAMINATION

Once the history has been taken the examiner may have a good indication of the pathological processes taking place, and these can now be confirmed by a careful physical examination. The examination of the feet and legs must be done on an examining table on which the patient can lie supine, can elevate both legs freely, and can sit with both legs dangling. The patient must be disrobed to allow complete inspection of the feet and legs and to allow easy examination of all peripheral pulses. A good light is essential, and a percussion hammer and a pin for touching the skin may be helpful. The most important piece of equipment is a sterile debridement set, consisting of a scissor, a forceps, and a probe (Fig. 2–1). Without this, the wound cannot be assessed truly, nor can it be determined whether the patient can be managed as an outpatient or needs to be admitted to the hospital. A pocket Doppler and sphygmomanometer are useful but not essential in the evaluation of arterial insufficiency.

As the patient moves into the examining room, it is useful to note whether he is limping or in pain when the foot hits the ground. Patients with severe neuropathy may be unsteady getting up on the table because of their lack of proprioception. If the patient is short of breath getting up onto the table, that may be a sign of cardiac or respiratory insufficiency. It is helpful to start the examination away from the area of interest as this may otherwise be forgotten. The carotids should be checked for bruits and the presence of pulses in arms confirmed to detect possible obstruction. Atrial fibrillation, as a possible source of embolization, can also be noted. The abdomen should be carefully examined for an abdominal aortic aneurysm, which also may be a source of distal emboli.

### Specific

It is useful to start the examination of the extremity by checking all of the pulses. Dia-

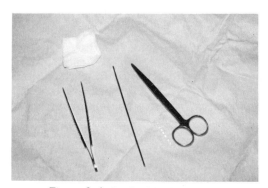

**Figure 2-1.** Sterile debridement set.

betic patients can be divided into those with good pulses and those without. Those with good pulses are more likely to have problems secondary to neuropathy, whereas those without good pulses often have an ischemic component. If the patient has classic claudication symptoms and yet good pulses distally, it may be necessary to briefly exercise him and then re-examine them. If the symptoms are still present, then he may have a cauda equina syndrome secondary to a back problem. Examination of the back and checking his straight-leg raising ability would then be appropriate. Weakness or absence of femoral pulses would suggest inflow disease. Good femoral but absence of popliteal pulses suggests superficial femoral artery occlusion. Good femoral and popliteal pulses but absence of distal pulses may be indicative of the isolated tibial disease so prominent in the diabetic. It is helpful to carefully document the status of the pulses at the initial examination by grading them on a scale of 1 to 4, with 1 the weakest and 4 the strongest. One instrument that has become increasingly popular for office examination of the circulation is the pocket Doppler instrument (Fig. 2–2). This works on the principle that the ultrasound emitted by a piezoelectric crystal is shifted in frequency by moving blood, and this is recorded by the same crystal, which then converts this change to an audible sound. Thus, by listening to the patient's distal pulses the examiner can hear a sound that is triphasic like the heartbeat. When a patient has significant proximal obstruction, the sound becomes monophasic. With a little practice, the quality of the pulses can be readily assessed. It should be remembered, however, that a loud signal reflects the speed of the blood, not the volume. Thus, a small amount of blood traveling through a stenosis may produce a loud monophasic sound. By means of a Doppler and a sphygmomanometer, it is possible to measure the pressure in the arm and compare it to the pressure in the dorsalis pedis or posterior tibial artery. An ankle-brachial ratio of 0.75 is associated with mild claudication. Below 0.5, the limb is usually severely ischemic. In diabetics there is often calcification of the media of the artery, rendering it relatively incompressible, and so the pressure measurements are often artifactually high and therefore less useful. The degree of arterial calcification has been shown to correlate best with the extent of the neuropathy and has nothing to do with atherosclerosis. Thus the young patient with marked triopathy is particularly likely to have incompressible vessels.

## The Ischemic Foot

The ischemic leg, besides absence of or reduced pulses, also has other characteristic features. The skin may be thin or atrophied and there is usually loss of hair on the foot and ankle. Purely ischemic lesions tend not to be on the weight-bearing part of the foot but rather are on the most distal part of the foot. Thus the patients have gangrenous toes or areas of gangrene around the forefoot. Fissures or necrotic areas on the heel are also common. In the patient without neuropathy, these lesions are usually extremely painful, but many diabetics are also neuropathic and so the lesions are not painful. The skin next to these lesions may be deeply erythematous. This is because the tissue is critically ischemic, and therefore the capillaries are maximally vasodilated and filled with relatively desaturated blood. This erythema can be distinguished from cellulitis by the fact that it disappears when the foot is elevated and reappears when the foot is again made dependent. Even when there are no lesions on the foot, it is important to determine the venous filling time and look for the presence of dependent rubor. This is done by first elevating the foot for 20 seconds. At this point the ischemic foot develops a characteristic pallor secondary to the difficulty in perfusing the foot against the force of gravity. The foot is then made dependent and carefully watched. The time is noted that it takes for the veins on the dorsum of the foot to fill.

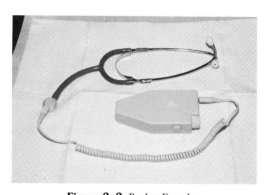

**Figure 2–2.** Pocket Doppler.

Anything over 20 seconds is characteristic of ischemia. As gravity allows the foot to fill with blood, the vasodilated capillaries fill with blood and the foot develops the characteristic dependent rubor associated with ischemia. The slower it takes for this rubor to develop the worse the ischemia.

## The Neuropathic Foot

The neuropathic foot also has some very characteristic features. The feet tend to be warm and dry, secondary to loss of the autonomic system resulting in the characteristic "autosympathectomy." The foot is relatively insensitive, with loss of pinprick and vibration sensation. Some centers have stressed the importance of quantifying the degree of sensory loss. We have not found this to be helpful, preferring instead to assess the lesion that it causes. Profound sensory loss that does not cause lesions to develop on the feet is less significant than a case in which sensation is better but breakdown occurs with less trauma. There is also a motor component to the neuropathy that results in paralysis of the intrinsic muscles of the foot. This causes clawing of the foot. The protective fat pads overlying the metatarsal heads are pulled forward, leaving the skin over the metatarsal heads exposed to the trauma of weight bearing. These areas respond with callus formation. This callus, because of glycosylation of collagen that occurs with hyperglycemia, is particularly hard and rigid and may contribute to the injury to the foot. Besides the structural changes that result from this paralysis, there is also wasting of the intrinsic muscles that can easily be identified by loss of muscle mass in the middle of the foot.

The lesions associated with neuropathy are numerous. The most characteristic is the skin breakdown over the exposed metatarsal head. This is called a mal perforans ulcer; it may penetrate to the underlying bone. The cocked-up toes caused by the clawing of the foot require more room in the toe box of the shoe. Lack of room may result in callus formation and ulceration of the dorsal surface of the toe that may also penetrate deeply. Lack of sensation may result in pressure from inappropriate shoeing. Occasionally an object left inadvertently in the shoe, such as a sock, may result in gangrene of the toes secondary to pressure necrosis. Decubitus ul-

ceration of the heel or calf may also occur in patients who are immobilized.

Diabetic osteoarthropathy or Charcot's disease may be responsible for acute or chronic changes to the foot. Acute Charcot's disease is associated with swelling, erythema, and increased temperature in the injured part of the foot. It may be distinguished from infection by the fact that there is usually no break in the skin and that it quickly responds to non–weight bearing. Progression of the disease because of continued weight bearing before the foot has healed may result in dislocation of the bones of the foot with consequent deformity. The classic deformity is the one in which the arch drops to become weight bearing, the so-called rocker-bottom foot. While the acute Charcot process occurs only in patients with good circulation, it is possible to see chronic Charcot deformity in patients with ischemia.

## Infection

Both ischemic and neuropathic lesions are commonly complicated by infection. Since extensive tissue loss may occur very quickly as a result of unrecognized sepsis, it is critically important to accurately identify infection during the initial examination. In severe cases the patient may complain of fevers, shaking chills, or loss of glucose control. Red streaks running from an ischemic or neuropathic lesion secondary to lymphangitis or regional lymphadenopathy are clear-cut signs of sepsis. For more localized lesions, purulent drainage or localized cellulitis may be indicative of sepsis. Unlike dependent rubor, the erythema of cellulitis does not disappear when the foot is elevated. When one is examining an ulcer, it is important to debride any callus or necrotic tissue and probe the wound extensively. If the probe goes directly into the bone, it is safe to assume that the patient has osteomyelitis and should be admitted directly to the hospital. It is not uncommon to find a small ulcer that, when debrided, reveals extensive underlying necrosis.

## Combined Lesions

It is common for a patient to have all three processes occurring at the same time. Thus an infected neuropathic lesion in a patient with poor circulation is not unusual. Significantly, neuropathy may hide the signs and symptoms of ischemia, and the resultant failure to diagnose the underlying ischemia may result in mistreatment. Severe neuropathy may result in a pain-free foot that is autosympathectomized and, thus, warm, but, at the same time, severely ischemic. A minor podiatric procedure on such a foot could result in gangrene. In such a case the presence of dependent rubor or weak monophasic pulses by Doppler may make the correct diagnosis.

## TREATMENT

One of the most important aspects of the initial evaluation is to explain to the patient what is going on. Reassurance will go a long way toward calming the patient, but at the same time it is important to emphasize the need for compliance on the part of the patient. The physician must decide whether the case can be managed on an outpatient basis or whether the patient needs to be admitted to the hospital.

All patients with significant and deep infections need to be admitted for intravenous antibiotic treatment. It is therefore important to probe all ulcers to determine the extent of any infection. Superficial lesions can be initially managed by non–weight bearing and oral antibiotics, but if on follow-up they are not improving, admission should be advised. Patients with severe acute Charcot's disease should be admitted for stabilization and to be taught how to live in a non–weight-bearing manner. Chronic deformity may require special shoeing, and this, together with routine callus and nail care, can be provided in the podiatry clinic. Polyneuropathy requires careful explanation of what may be expected and reassurance that it will not result in loss of limb. For many patients, medication is not required, but when it is, various regimens are available. The patient with intermittent claudication should also be reassured and encouraged to stop smoking and to exercise; in some cases, pentoxifylline (Trental) is indicated. If claudication becomes truly disabling or the patient develops rest pain or an ischemic lesion, arrangements need to be made for arteriography. Increasingly this is being done on an outpatient basis, and then the patient is admitted for a definitive procedure.

# Chapter 3

# DIABETIC VASCULAR DISEASE

FRANK W. LoGERFO, M.D., and
FRANK B. POMPOSELLI, JR., M.D.

In recent years there has been considerable progress in our understanding of the nature and management of peripheral vascular disease associated with diabetes. In the past, clinical management has been impeded by a widespread and incorrect assumption that diabetes is associated with an occlusive lesion in the microcirculation. This misconception can be traced to an early uncontrolled study that indicated that amputation specimens from diabetics showed an increased incidence of arteriolar occlusion due to proliferation of endothelium and deposition of PAS-positive material. However, a subsequent prospective controlled study of amputation specimens from diabetics and nondiabetics failed to confirm the existence of either a small artery or arteriolar occlusive lesion associated with diabetes. A similar prospective study using a sophisticated arterial casting technique yielded identical results. In a study of patients undergoing femoropopliteal bypass, it was noted that the response to papaverine vasodilatation was the same in diabetics and nondiabetics, arguing against the idea that patients with diabetes have fixed, high arteriolar resistance. Arterial noninvasive studies, including toe plethysmography, have also failed to demonstrate the existence of a small vessel or microvascular occlusive lesion in diabetics with foot ulcers as compared with nondiabetics.

Thus a great deal of evidence has accumulated over several years from different investigators using a variety of techniques that there is no microvascular occlusive lesion associated with diabetes. This is a fundamental step toward the appropriate clinical management of diabetic foot problems. If, indeed, diabetics had a microvascular occlusive lesion leading to foot ulceration, the prognosis would be justifiably hopeless. Furthermore, the prognosis for vascular reconstruction would be poor, since there would be no runoff bed to sustain graft patency. Once the myth of small vessel occlusion is dispelled, the foundation for appropriate and optimistic clinical management can be laid.

While there are many studies that argue against the existence of an occlusive lesion in the microcirculation, there is also considerable evidence that abnormalities of a nonocclusive nature do exist. For example, the capillary basement membrane is thickened in diabetes. However, this is not an occlusive lesion. Studies of both neural and dermal capillaries in patients with diabetes have demonstrated that the capillary lumen is actually slightly larger than the capillary lumen in nondiabetics. The abnormal capillary basement membrane may alter the flux of molecules across the capillary wall. It has been argued that nonenzymatic glycosylation of the basement membrane proteins reduces sulfonation and the charge on the basement membrane. This may explain why highly charged molecules, such as albumin or pentetic acid, have been demonstrated to leak from the capillaries in diabetics. On the other hand, there does not appear to be any impairment of oxygen diffusion, since diabetics with foot ulceration actually have a higher transcutaneous $Po_2$ than nondiabetics with foot ulceration. Thus there is no physiological basis for considering diabetic foot ulceration to be amenable to hyperbaric oxygen therapy.

Although it has not been possible to draw a direct cause-and-effect relationship, it is certainly conceivable that a thickened capillary basement membrane contributes to compromised biological responses in the diabetic foot. This in combination with sensory and motor neuropathy sets the stage for ulceration. The diabetic foot is susceptible to ulceration, in the absence of ischemia or, more commonly, with moderate degrees of ischemia. For example, atherosclerotic occlusion of the superficial femoral artery might ordinarily result only in claudication. However, when combined with the compromised biology of the diabetic foot, ulceration often occurs. In other words, the diabetic foot is less tolerant of ischemia resulting from atherosclerosis.

When atherosclerosis occurs in the diabetic patient, the histological characteristics are no different from those in the nondiabetic. Based on noninvasive tests, there is a higher incidence of lower-extremity arterial occlusive disease in diabetics, it is more rapidly progressive, and there is a higher rate of cardiovascular mortality than in nondiabetics. It is most important to note that the specific location of the lesions tends to be different. Histological and angiographic studies and arterial casting have all demonstrated that patients with diabetes have a propensity to develop occlusive lesions in the infrageniculate arteries, i.e. the anterior tibial, posterior tibial, and peroneal arteries. It is a mistake to regard this as small vessel disease because, in fact, all of these studies demonstrated that diabetics actually have less occlusive disease in the foot vessels. Thus the atherosclerotic occlusion lesion tends to be confined to the leg segment with relative sparing of the foot arteries, especially the dorsalis pedis. With the advent of successful distal arterial reconstruction, this observation has opened up the possibility of limb salvage for many patients.

Because of the pattern of atherosclerotic occlusion, it is important that arteriography always demonstrate the status of the foot arteries even when all three infrageniculate arteries are occluded in the leg. A common mistake is to terminate arteriography when the infrageniculate obstruction is noted, on the assumption that all of the distal vessels must also be occluded. Such a case might be deemed "nonreconstructible" when, in fact, the possibility of a very successful arterial reconstruction is being overlooked. With diabetes, the most commonly patent vessel in the foot is the dorsalis pedis. Surprisingly, arterial reconstruction to the dorsalis pedis artery yields results that are as good as or better than those of standard femoropopliteal or tibial reconstruction. The technical details of these distal reconstructions and the outcome are described elsewhere in this book. The value of reconstruction to the dorsalis pedis artery is exemplified by the fact that nearly 30 per cent of our lower extremity arterial reconstructions in diabetics are grafts that terminate in the dorsalis pedis. The gradually increasing use of dorsalis pedis bypass on our vascular surgery service has correlated closely with a marked concomitant decrease in major amputation rates (Fig. 3–1). The excellent results with these extreme distal bypass grafts confirms in a different way the absence of any significant microvascular occlusive lesion in the diabetic patient. If such a lesion existed, it would be expected that patency rates in bypass grafts to the foot vessels would be very poor because there would be no runoff. In fact, the opposite is the case.

The details for evaluation of ischemia in the diabetic foot are presented elsewhere in this book. Suffice it to say here that all diabetic foot ulcers should be evaluated for ischemia. This is true even when neuropathy and/or infection is also present. As a rule, all patients with ischemia should be considered for arteriography and arterial reconstruction prior to any significant foot surgery. Severe infection, also discussed elsewhere, takes priority in the sense that adequate drainage must be established and systemic sepsis must be controlled. Once that has been accomplished, the foot should be assessed for ischemia. Prompt arteriography and arterial reconstruction will then maximize the possibility of limb salvage and minimize tissue loss.

In summary, when foot ulcerations occur in patients with diabetes, they should not be attributed to a microvascular occlusive lesion. As a priority, severe infections must be drained and sepsis controlled. All cases of ulceration should be evaluated for ischemia, and, if it is present, they should be evaluated by arteriography. It is important that arteriography always be carried out to demonstrate the status of the foot vessels even when all three infrageniculate arteries are occluded. Since the foot vessels are often spared, there is often the opportunity for arterial reconstruction, especially to the dorsalis pedis artery. Modern results with this bypass procedure have been excellent and have greatly reduced the major amputation rate.

In recent years, we have gradually adopted this management plan for ischemia in the

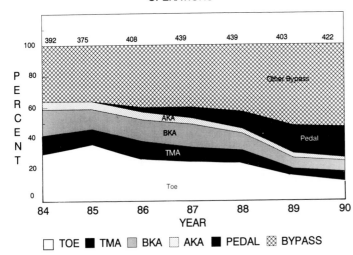

**Figure 3-1.** Summarization of the operative experience at the New England Deaconess Hospital in recent years. As we have increasingly adopted the management plan for ischemia described in this chapter, the major amputation rate has declined. The decrease in major amputation rates correlates almost precisely with the increasing use of bypass grafts to the dorsalis pedis artery. (From LoGerfo, F. W., Gibbons, G. W., Pomposelli, F. B., Jr., et al: Trends in the care of the diabetic foot: Expanded role for arterial reconstruction. Arch. Surg. 127:617–621, 1992.)

diabetic foot. As a result, there has been a marked decline in all amputations, including the amputations in patients with diabetes (Fig. 3–1). Revascularization makes it possible to apply innovative tissue-sparing procedures such as joint resection and osteotomy that were not previously possible in the diabetic foot with compromised perfusion. Improved understanding of the etiology and role of ischemia and the success of extreme distal revascularization procedures have provided the foundation for a new and optimistic era in the case of the diabetic foot. This should not be construed to mean that vascular surgery alone can solve these often complex problems. Skilled interdisciplinary care from a patient care team organized to focus on this challenging clinical problem is essential to maximizing success.

## SUGGESTED READING LIST

Barner, H. B., Kaiser, G. C., and Willman, V. L.: Blood flow in the diabetic leg. Circulation 43:391–394, 1971.

Beach K. W., Bedford, G. R., Bergelin, R. O., et al.: Progression of lower-extremity arterial occlusive disease in type II diabetes mellitus. Diabetes Care 11:464–472, 1988.

Britland S. T., Young R. J., Shurma, A. K., and Clark, B. E.: Relationship of endoneural capillary abnormalities to type and severity of diabetic polyneuropathy. Diabetes 39:909–913, 1990.

Brownlee, M., Cerami, A., and Vlassara, H.: Advanced glycosylation end products in tissue and the biochemical basis of diabetic complications. N. Engl. J. Med. 318:1315–1321, 1988.

Conrad, M. C.: Large and small artery occlusion in diabetics and nondiabetics with severe vascular disease. Circulation 36:83–91, 1967.

Irwin, S. T., Gilmore, J., McGrann, S., et al.: Blood flow in diabetics with foot lesions due to 'small vessel disease.' Br. J. Surg. 75:1201–1206, 1988.

Katz, M. A., McCuskey, P., Beggs, J. L., et al.: Relationships between microvascular function and capillary structure in diabetic and nondiabetic human skin. Diabetes 38:1245–1250, 1989.

LoGerfo, F. W., and Coffman, J. D.: Vascular and microvascular disease of the foot in diabetes: Implications for foot care. N. Engl. J. Med. 311:1615–1619, 1984.

LoGerfo, F. W., Gibbons, G. W., Pomposelli, F. B., Jr., et al.: Trends in the care of the diabetic foot: Expanded role for arterial reconstruction. Arch. Surg. 127:617–621, 1992.

Menzoian, J. O., LaMorte, W. W., Paniszyn, C. C., et al.: Symptomatology and anatomic patterns of peripheral vascular disease: Differing impact of smoking and diabetes. Ann. Vasc. Surg. 3:224–228, 1989.

Parving, H. H., and Rasmussen, S. M.: Transcapillary escape rate of albumin and plasma volume in short- and long-term juvenile diabetes. Scand. J. Clin. Lab. Invest. 32:81–87, 1973.

Pomposelli, F. B., Jepsen, S. J., Gibbons, G. W., et al.: Efficacy of the dorsalis pedis bypass for limb salvage in diabetic patients. J. Vasc. Surg. 11:745–752, 1990.

Pomposelli, F. B., Jr., Jepsen, S. J., Gibbons, G. W., et al.: A flexible approach to infra-popliteal vein grafts in patients with diabetes mellitus. Arch. Surg. 161:724–729, 1991.

Rosenblatt, M. S., Quist, W. C., Sidawy, A. N., et al.: Lower extremity vein graft reconstruction: Results in diabetic and non-diabetic patients. Surg. Gynecol. Obstet. 171:311–335, 1990.

Sidawy, A. N., Menzoian, J. O., Cantelmo, N. L., and LoGerfo, F. W.: Effect of inflow and outflow sites on the results of tibioperoneal vein grafts. Am. J. Surg. 152:211–214, 1986.

Siperstein, M.D., Unger, R. H., and Madison, L. L.: Studies of muscle capillary basement membrane in normal subjects, diabetic and prediabetic patients. J. Clin. Invest. 47:1973–1999, 1968.

Wyss, C. R., Matsen, F. A., Simmons, C. W., and Burgess, E. M.: Transcutaneous oxygen tension measurements on limbs of diabetic and nondiabetic peripheral vascular disease. Surgery 95:339–346, 1984.

# Chapter 4

# HYPERLIPIDEMIA IN THE DIABETIC: ACCELERATED ATHEROSCLEROSIS

ANTONIO GRANFONE, M.D.

Atherosclerosis is the process of thickening and hardening of the arterial wall secondary to deposition of lipid particles in the intimal layer. The three basic atherosclerotic lesions are fatty streaks, plaques, and complicated plaques. Formation of the atherosclerotic plaques is dependent upon multiple factors: hemodynamic, cellular, humoral. A large portion of this chapter will be dedicated to abnormalities of lipid metabolism and their treatment in diabetes mellitus.

## HEMODYNAMIC FACTORS

The importance of hemodynamic factors in the development of atherosclerosis is supported by the tendency of plaque formation in the areas of arterial division and curvatures. These are considered areas of low shear stress that might lead to modifications of local factors and accumulation of certain types of cells and particles, including platelets, mononuclear cells, and lipoproteins.

## ENDOTHELIAL DYSFUNCTION AND CELLULAR FACTORS

The endothelium of the arterial walls has to be viewed as an active tissue; its dysfunction may stimulate the initial phenomena leading to atheroma formation (Fig. 4–1). There is in vitro and in vivo evidence that damaged endothelium may respond by vasoconstriction to substances such as acetylcholine that in normal arteries would

cause vasodilatation. Damaged endothelium in susceptible areas of decreased shear stress is thought to favor adhesion of mononuclear cells to the endothelial surface; this is considered an important initial step in atherogenesis; the release of various substances follows, including interleukin-1 (IL-1). IL-1 is secreted in response to injury and inflammation. One of the functions of IL-1 is to stimulate the adhesion process. It also stimulates the secretion of monocyte chemotactic protein (MCP), which favors the migration of monocytes into the subendothelial space. Some of the cellular and endothelial abnormalities detected in diabetes mellitus are listed in Table 4–1.

## HUMORAL FACTORS

The major humoral factors implicated in atherosclerosis in diabetes mellitus include insulin and lipoprotein metabolism abnormalities.

### Insulin

Numerous studies have demonstrated an association between increased insulin levels and ischemic heart disease. In some of these studies, fasting insulin levels were similar in the various groups, but the post three-hour glucose tolerance test (GTT) insulin levels were higher in the patients than in the controls. Other studies have not demonstrated the same results. The majority of them,

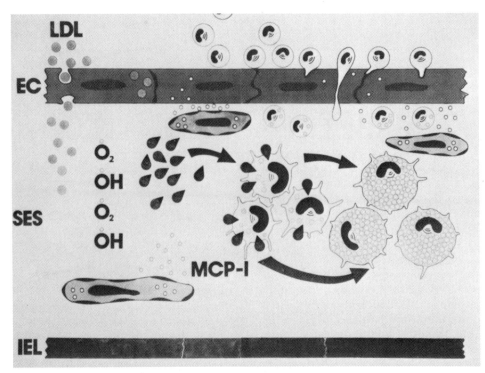

**Figure 4–1.** Schematic depiction of the basic mechanisms in arterial intimal foam cell formation and fatty streak development that occur preferentially in hemodynamically determined lesion-prone areas in the presence of elevated cholesterol (EC) and lipoprotein levels. LDL's and other lipoproteins (e.g., VLDL and Lp[a]) probably traverse the EC's principally by vesicular transport. Having entered the subendothelial space (SES), LDL molecules are oxidatively modified by ROS generated by macrophages, EC's, and SMC's. Ox-LDL particles augment the expression and synthesis of monocyte chemotactic protein (MCP)-1 by EC's and SMC's, thus facilitating further monocyte recruitment to the SES. Within the SES, monocytes undergo activation-differentiation, becoming the much larger macrophages. Through their non-down-regulating scavenger receptor pathway, they bind and internalize the Ox-LDL particles as shown, with CE accumulation and foam cell formation. $O_2$ = superoxide; OH = hydroxyl radical. (From Schwartz, C.J., et al.: Pathogenesis of the atherosclerotic lesion. Implications for diabetes mellitus. Diabetes Care 15:1156–1167, 1992.)

though, reveal an association between increased insulin levels and atherogenesis. Ethnic groups with a high incidence of non–insulin-dependent diabetes mellitus (NIDDM) and high fasting and post GTT insulin levels are at increased risk for cardiovascular disease, even if fasting plasma glucose does not differ from controls; this has been well demonstrated in the San Antonio Heart Study. Upper body obesity is another parameter as-

### TABLE 4–1.  CELLULAR AND ENDOTHELIAL ABNORMALITIES IN DIABETES MELLITUS

Increased interleukin-1 secretion
Abnormal response to acetylcholine
Endothelial cell basilar membrane thickening
AGE-BSA–induced increased endothelial permeability
Impaired phagocytosis and chemotaxis
Non-enzymatic protein glycosylation
Diminished endothelial thromboresistance
Impaired fibrinolysis
Increased platelet adhesiveness and aggregation
Increased thromboxane formation
Enhanced lipoprotein oxidation

### TABLE 4–2.  CARDIOVASCULAR RISK FACTORS ASSOCIATED WITH HYPERINSULINEMIA

Hypertension
Hypertriglyceridemia
Hypercholesterolemia
Hypoalphalipoproteinemia
Upper body obesity
Decreased physical activity
Male sex
Decreased plasminogen-activator inhibitor
Type A personality

From Stout, R. W.: Insulin and atheroma: 20 year perspective. Diabetes 13:631–654, 1990.

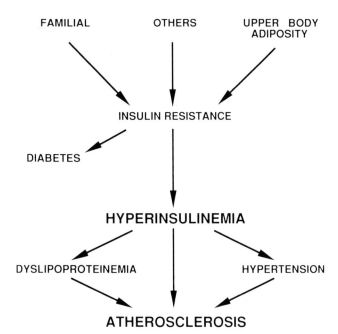

**Figure 4-2.** Schema linking hyperinsulinemia with atherosclerosis and some of its major risk factors. (From Stout, R.W.: Insulin and atheroma: 20 year perspective. Diabetes Care 13:631–654, 1990.)

sociated with increased insulin response and risk for cardiovascular disease (Table 4–2). A schematic representation of how hyperinsulinemia might be linked to atherosclerosis is outlined in Figure 4–2.

## Dyslipidemias

A number of studies have provided evidence that the treatment of some forms of dyslipidemias has been associated with a reduction of the risk for coronary artery disease (CAD). Some of the studies will be mentioned shortly. Early evidence linking hypercholesterolemia (total and LDL cholesterol) to increased risk for CAD came from the Framingham study, which began in 1948 and enrolled men and women; the study also provided evidence of an inverse correlation between the HDL cholesterol level and development of CAD (Fig. 4–3).

In the Multiple Risk Factor Intervention Trial (MRFIT) 356,222 individuals without a history of coronary disease were screened; CAD was found to be uncommon in individuals with a cholesterol level lower than 150 mg/dl. A subgroup of people was sent to special clinics for the treatment of hypercholesterolemia and hypertension; in this subgroup the mortality from CAD and from all causes

was 10.6 and 7.7 per cent lower, respectively, at 10½ years.

Diabetes mellitus is associated with a twofold to threefold increase in the risk for CAD, including type I and type II and in women. Lipoprotein abnormalities are common among diabetic patients and are accentuated when the diabetes is poorly controlled.

## Lipoprotein Physiology and Metabolism

Lipoproteins are macromolecules composed of a hydrophobic core of triglycerides and cholesteryl esters surrounded by a hydrophilic envelope of proteins (apolipoproteins) and phospholipids. There are five major lipo-

### TABLE 4-3.  PHYSICAL PROPERTIES OF LIPOPROTEIN

| | | LIPID CONTENT % | |
| LIPOPROTEIN | DENSITY | TG | C |
| --- | --- | --- | --- |
| Chylomicrons | 0.95 | 80–95 | 2–7 |
| VLDL | 0.95–1.006 | 30–80 | 55–80 |
| IDL | 1.006–1.019 | 25–35 | 20–50 |
| LDL | 1.019–1.063 | 18–25 | 5–15 |
| HDL | 1.063–1.21 | 5–12 | 15–25 |

TG = triglycerides; C = cholesterol.

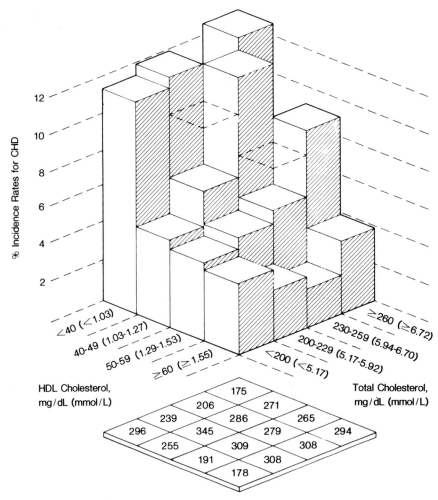

**Figure 4-3.** Incidence of coronary heart disease in four years by high-density lipoprotein cholesterol and total plasma cholesterol level for men and women free of cardiovascular disease. Dashed lines indicate two bars that are hidden from view: HDL cholesterol less than 40 mg/dl (< 1.03 mmol/L), total cholesterol 230 to 259 mg/dl (5.94 to 6.70 mmol/L), rate = 10.7%; HDL cholesterol 40 to 49 mg/dl (1.03 to 1.27 mmol/L), total cholesterol greater than or equal to 260 mg/dl (6.72 mmol/L), rate = 6.6%. Diagram at bottom shows number of observations from combined sample that fell into each cell and were therefore at risk for CHD. CHD = coronary heart disease. (From Castelli, W.P., et al.: Incidence of coronary heart disease and lipoprotein cholesterol levels. The Framingham Study. JAMA 256:2835–2838, 1986.)

## TABLE 4-4.    APOLIPOPROTEINS: PROPERTIES AND FUNCTIONS

| TYPE | MW | SYNTHESIS | LIPOPROTEIN | FUNCTION |
|---|---|---|---|---|
| Apo A-I | 28,000 | Liver, intestine | HDL, chylomicrons | LCAT activation, reverse cholesterol transport, structural function |
| Apo A-II | 16,000 | Same as for Apo A-I | Same as for Apo A-I | Structural function |
| Apo A-IV | 46,000 | Same as for Apo A-I | HDL, VLDL, chylomicrons | Unclear |
| Apo B-48 | 250,000 | Intestine | Chylomicrons | Chylomicron synthesis |
| Apo B-100 | 550,000 | Liver | VLDL, LDL | VLDL synthesis Binding to LDL receptor |
| Apo C-I | 6,000 | Liver | Chylomicrons, VLDL, HDL | LCAT activation |
| Apo C-II | 7,000 | Liver | Same as Apo A-I | LPL activation |
| Apo C-III | 7,000 | Liver | Same as Apo A-I | Unclear |
| Apo D | 21,000 | Liver | Chylomicrons, HDL | Cholesterol ester exchange |
| Apo E | 34,000 | Liver | Chylomicrons, VLDL, HDL | Binding to HL receptor |

proteins (Table 4–3). Very low-density lipoprotein (VLDL) and chylomycrons are rich in triglycerides and relatively poor in cholesterol; intermediate-density lipoprotein (IDL), low-density lipoprotein (LDL), and high-density lipoprotein (HDL) are rich in cholesterol and relatively poor in tryglycerides. Apolipoproteins are located on the lipoprotein surface. They represent important lipoprotein structural components and major determinants of their function and metabolism. A list of the major apolipoproteins and their functions is provided in Table 4–4. Some apolipoproteins merit special attention.

Apo A-I is the major apoprotein of HDL; it is synthesized in the liver and the intestine; it is important in activation of lecithin-cholesterol acyltransferase (LCAT), an enzyme that is needed for the maturation and function of HDL. Apo A-II is the second most important protein of HDL; it is also synthesized in the intestine and the liver. Apo A-IV is a small component of HDL and chylomycrons with unknown functions.

Apo B-100 is the major apoprotein of LDL and a major component of IDL and, to a lesser degree of VLDL; it is synthesized in the liver and plays an important role in the catabolism of LDL by promoting the binding of LDL to the LDL receptors in the peripheral tissues.

C apolipoproteins are synthesized in the liver. Apo C-II is an important coenzyme of lipoprotein lipase (LPL); its deficiency results in inability to clear triglycerides. Apo C-III is a component of VLDL and an inhibitor of hepatic uptake of chylomycrons and VLDL remnants.

Apo E, synthesized in the liver, is a major component of VLDL, IDL, chylomycron remnants, and HDL; it is important in the removal of lipoprotein remnants from the plasma. Several variants have been found; the normal isoform is E-3; E-2 and E-4 lead to increased VLDL and LDL cholesterol levels.

Apo a is the apoprotein of lipoprotein (a) [Lp(a)], an unusual lipoprotein that resembles LDL; apo a binds to apo B-100 and increases the density of Lp(a). Lp(a) has been found in atherosclerotic plaques, and elevated levels are associated with increased risk for CAD. Apo a is synthesized in the liver and is usually present in small amounts in normal individuals. Lp(a) is associated with increased incidence of stroke also; structurally it is very similar to plasminogen and may compete with plasminogen for binding to fibrinogen and fibrin, impairing its activity, and leading to increased propensity to thrombosis.

### Lipoprotein Metabolism in Nondiabetic Individuals (Fig. 4–4)

CHYLOMICRON METABOLISM. The fat contained in our meals is broken down by the intestinal enzymes and absorbed by the intestinal cells as fatty acids and cholesterol. Intracellularly they are re-esterified to triglycerides and cholesteryl esters and incorporated into nascent chylomicrons, which are synthesized in the intestinal cells and released into the lymphatic system and into the superior vena cava through the thoracic duct. Nascent chylomicrons gradually acquire apoproteins C-II, C-III, E and cholesterol from HDL by cholesteryl ester transfer protein (CETP). Apo C-II facilitates the interaction of chylomicron with LPL; the deficiency of apo C-II or LPL results in inability to clear chylomicron. LPL is found on the surface of the endothelial cells of the pulmonary, muscular, and adipose tissues. Chylomicron remnants are the resulting products of this enzymatic reaction; cholesterol, phospholipids, apo C-II, and apo C-III are retransferred to HDL, and the remnants are taken up by the liver through either the LDL receptors or the specific apo E receptor. A defect of apo E will result in the accumulation of chylomicron remnants in the plasma.

VLDL METABOLISM. VLDL's are synthesized in the hepatocyte; their synthesis appears to be regulated by the presence of cholesterol with an unclear mechanism. After their release into the plasma, VLDL particles are attacked by LPL and catabolized by hydrolysis to either IDL or VLDL remnants; IDL's are in turn catabolized by hepatic triglyceride lipase (HTGL) to LDL. The partially catabolized VLDL's are cleared by HTGL.

LDL METABOLISM. After their formation, some of the LDL's are transported back to the liver (about 50 per cent), where they are taken up by the hepatocytes via the hepatocyte LDL receptor; the remainder of LDL's are taken up by the other peripheral tissues, mostly via the LDL receptor and, to a lesser degree, nonreceptor-mediated mechanisms (i.e. pinocytosis). The interaction between LDL and the LDL receptor is promoted by

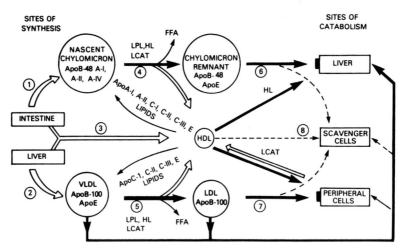

**Figure 4–4.** A conceptual overview of lipoprotein metabolism: LPL = lipoprotein lipase, HL = hepatic lipase, LCAT = lecithin:cholesterol acyltransferase, FFA = free fatty acid. *Open arrows* signify synthetic pathways and *closed arrows* catabolic pathways. (Reprinted with permission from Schaefer, E.J., et al.: Pathogenesis and management of lipoprotein disorders. N. Engl. J. Med. 312:1300–1310, 1985.

apo B-100. Once bound to the LDL receptor, LDL's are internalized and exposed to the cytoplasm and broken down by lysosomes; cholesterol is then freed and may exert a feedback regulation on the synthesis of the LDL receptor, uptake of LDL, and intracellular metabolism of cholesterol.

**HDL METABOLISM.** HDL's are synthesized in the liver and the intestine. The initial appearance of HDL is discoid (nascent HDL); by the subsequent addition of proteins (A-I, -II, -IV) and the action of LCAT they are transformed into a spherical form (mature HDL). HDL$_3$ particles are believed to be the major acceptors of free cholesterol from the cellular membrane of the peripheral tissue cells; this is the first step of the reverse cholesterol transport. Subsequently, free cholesterol is esterified by LCAT and transported into the lipoprotein core. The catabolism of HDL is complex and not completely clarified; it seems to be related to the catabolism of apo C-II, -III, and apo E by the liver and apo A-I principally by the liver and, to a lesser degree, by the kidneys.

## Lipoprotein Metabolism in Diabetes Mellitus (Fig. 4–5)

**CHYLOMICRON.** In type I diabetes there is a deficiency of LPL; this defect results in inability to clear chylomicrons and VLDL, with consequent accumulation of their remnants, and in an increase of triglycerides. LPL is sensitive to the presence of insulin. Insulin therapy will increase LPL with clearance of triglycerides. In type II diabetes the deficiency of LPL is less frequent and of minor degree. Chylomicron remnants are taken up by the liver; this process is stimulated by apo E. HDL might also play a role in this removal process.

**VLDL.** In type I diabetes VLDL triglycerides frequently are elevated. This is the result of increased production and decreased clearance of VLDL triglycerides; insulin will correct the abnormality. In type II diabetes there is excessive secretion of VLDL in the presence of hyperglycemia. Recent evidence suggests that VLDL particles in type II diabetes may be atherogenic because they appear to be enriched not only with triglycerides, but also with cholesteryl esters. The increased secretion of VLDL in type II diabetes is felt to be due to the partial removal of the inhibitory effect of insulin on VLDL secretion; in fact, type II diabetes is associated with relative insulin insufficiency despite elevation of absolute insulin levels. Syndrome X is a typical example of hyperglycemia and increased free fatty acids associated with increased synthesis of VLDL in a state of insulin resistance.

**LDL.** In type I diabetes, LDL synthesis is usually normal; in severe insulin deficiency the catabolism of LDL via the peripheral receptor may be slightly reduced. In type II diabetes, LDL tends to be enriched with triglycerides as well as with cholesterol; in addition, the rate of synthesis is increased in the

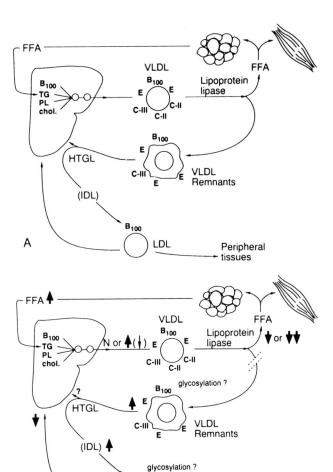

**Figure 4–5.** Lipoprotein physiology in nondiabetic *(A)* and diabetic *(B)* patients. See text for explanation. (From Ginsberg, H.N.: Lipoprotein physiology in nondiabetic and diabetic states: Relationship to atherogenesis. Diabetes Care 14:839–855, 1991.)

presence of hyperglycemia. The catabolism of LDL has been observed to be normal, increased, or decreased. LDL of diabetic patients might be more atherogenic than in normal individuals. In fact, LDL is subjected to glycosylation; such glycosylated LDL tends to be taken up by the macrophages present in the intima of the arterial wall with consequent formation of foam cells. Finally, it appears to be more intesively undergoing oxidation, one of the processes involved in atherogenesis.

**HDL.** In type I diabetes the concentration of HDL is usually normal. In type II diabetes, a low concentration of HDL is common; the reasons are unclear. There appears to be an increase in the clearance rate of HDL; hypertriglyceridemia may contribute to this.

## CLASSIFICATION OF HYPERLIPIDEMIAS

A phenotypic classification has been used for years; its usefulness has been questioned; reference to it will be made for some dyslipidemias discussed next (Table 4–5).

## DIFFERENTIAL DIAGNOSIS OF HYPERCHOLESTEROLEMIA

It is important to undertake a differential diagnosis of the various dyslipidemias before any consideration is given to the management. There are primary and secondary causes of hypercholesterolemia. The primary causes are polygenic hypercholesterolemia,

### TABLE 4–5. PHENOTYPIC CLASSIFICATION OF HYPERLIPIDEMIAS

| LIPOPROTEIN PHENOTYPE | ELEVATED LIPOPROTEIN |
|---|---|
| Type I | Chylomicrons |
| Type IIa | LDL |
| Type IIb | LDL and VLDL |
| Type III | IDL |
| Type IV | VLDL |
| Type V | VLDL and chylomicrons |

familial hypercholesterolemia, and combined hyperlipidemia.

POLYGENIC HYPERCHOLESTEROLEMIA. Polygenic hypercholesterolemia is present in about 25 per cent of the American population; the average concentration of total cholesterol is about 280 mg/dl and of LDL cholesterol about 190 mg/dl. The risk of CAD is increased two to four times. The condition is probably the result of a combination of underlying (possibly multiple) genetic abnormalities and superimposed environmental factors, such as poor dietary habits and lifestyle.

FAMILIAL HYPERCHOLESTEROLEMIA. This form of hyperlipidemia is caused by a genetic abnormality of the LDL receptor gene leading to total or partial absence of LDL receptor. In the heterozygous form only one gene is affected; it is relatively common (1/500); the total cholesterol level is usually between 400 and 600 mg/dl, and the LDL cholesterol between 200 and 400 mg/dl. In the rarer homozygous form (1/1,000,000) both genes are affected; the clearance of LDL is more profoundly affected; the total cholesterol may reach levels higher than 1000 mg/dl; the LDL cholesterol level is usually between 400 and 800 mg/dl. Both these forms of dyslipidemias are associated with premature CAD. Common clinical findings in familial hypercholesterolemia include corneal arcus, xanthelasmas, tendon xanthomas, premature CAD (before the age of 50 years in the heterozygous form and in childhood in the homozygous), and peripheral vascular disease.

FAMILIAL COMBINED HYPERLIPIDEMIAS. This type of dyslipidemia may be manifested by three phenotypes: hypercholesterolemia (1/3), hypertryglyceridemia (1/3), and hypercholesterolemia and hypertryglyceridemia combined (1/3). It is associated with in-creased risk for CAD; multiple genetic defects are considered responsible for this dyslipidemia; and family members may have different defects and phenotypic manifestations.

Common causes of secondary hypercholesterolemia include diabetes mellitus, drugs, hepatic disease secondary to biliary obstruction, and nephrotic syndrome. The major defect in hypothyroidism is a reduction in the clearance of LDL. In hepatic disease, multiple metabolic abnormalities of lipid metabolism occur. In nephrotic syndrome the loss of proteins stimulates secretion of lipoproteins. Both thiazide diuretics and glucocorticoids may increase the LDL cholesterol level. Progestins tend to increase LDL.

## DIFFERENTIAL DIAGNOSIS OF HYPERTRIGLYCERIDEMIA

Hypertriglyceridemia may also be primary or secondary.

Primary hypertriglyceridemia may be subdivided into familial hypertriglyceridemia, familial combined hyperlipidemia, and sporadic hypertriglyceridemia. All of these forms have elevated levels of VLDL and triglycerides except one of the phenotypes of familial combined hyperlipidemia, discussed earlier.

*Familial hypertriglyceridemia* can occur in two forms: type IV hyperlipidemia and type V hyperlipidemia. Type IV hyperlipidemia occurs in about 1 per cent of the population. It is caused by a genetic defect that leads to excessive secretion and probably decreased clearance of VLDL; often an autosomal dominant transmission is found in affected families. The triglyceride level is usually above 250 mg/dl. Levels of HDL tend to be low. This pattern is often associated with diabetes mellitus and hyperuricemia. Type V hyperlipidemia is characterized by elevation of VLDL and chylomicron; it occurs in 1 per cent of the population. The triglyceride level is very high, up to 5000 mg/dl; it is caused by excessive secretion of VLDL and decreased clearance of VLDL and chylomicron, leading to elevated levels of VLDL, chylomicron, and their remnants. The HDL level is almost invariably low. Patients with this dyslipidemia are predisposed to pancreatitis. Some secondary forms of hyperlipidemia may have similar features (see below).

*Combined hyperlipidemia* may present as

familial combined hyperlipidemia, dysbeta-lipoproteinemia, hypertriglyceridemia, or multiple genetic defect hyperlipoproteinemias. Dysbetalipoproteinemia is a relatively rare dyslipidemia characterized by abnormalities in apo E, resulting in decreased clearance of VLDL and chylomicron and accumulation of their remnants. Clinical features include tuberoeruptive xanthomas, planar xanthomas, and premature CAD and peripheral vascular disease. LDL levels are normal; the total cholesterol/triglyceride ratio is about 1:2. Lipoprotein should be analyzed by ultracentrifugation when this dyslipidemia is suspected. Hyperchylomicronemia syndrome is phenotypically classified as type I hyperlipoproteinemia, a rare dyslipidemia (1/1,000,000) appearing in childhood and caused by the absence of LPL or its coenzyme apo C-II. This leads to severe hypertriglyceridemia and hyperchylomicronemia, with triglycerides often exceeding 2000 mg/dl. Clinical features include lipemia retinalis, eruptive xanthomas, and hepatosplenomegaly.

Lipemia retinalis is easily appreciated by examining the ocular fundi; the retinal blood vessels are pinkish or whitish because of the milkiness of the circulating blood. Eruptive xanthomas are pruritic (sometimes painful) maculopapular skin lesions about 0.5 cm in diameter with a central slightly yellowish appearance, due to accumulation of macrophages engorged with fat. Patients often have abdominal pain, which may be caused by hepatic and splenic distention (the liver and the spleen are infiltrated with fat-filled macrophages), pancreatitis, and, more rarely, splenic infarct. The common causes of secondary hypertriglyceridemia include alcohol, diabetes mellitus, drugs, obesity, and renal diseases.

Alcohol is associated with increased secretion of VLDL. The effect of diabetes mellitus on the lipoprotein metabolism has been discussed at length earlier. Drugs such as estrogen, beta blockers, retinoids, and bile acid–binding resins also raise VLDL; in patients with underlying hypertriglyceridemia the use of these drugs could exacerbate their metabolic abnormalities; there are well-documented cases of massive hypertriglyceridemia associated with the use of estrogen. Both chronic renal failure and nephrotic syndrome are associated with elevation of VLDL levels; in the first there seems to be reduced activity of LPL; in the second, reduced clearance of VLDL has been observed.

Evidence continues to support the strict relation between hypoalphalipoproteinemia (low HDL) and CAD. There are multiple causes for this dyslipidemia, including genetic factors, diabetes mellitus, drugs, hypertriglyceridemia, lack of exercise, malnutrition, obesity, and severe liver disease.

Tangier disease is a form of genetic HDL deficiency. Diabetes mellitus is a frequent cause of low HDL, probably via several mechanisms. Drugs such as progestin, anabolic steroids, and probucol reduce the synthesis of HDL; beta blockers and thiazide diuretics are also associated with low HDL. Hypertriglyceridemia probably increases clearance of HDL. Malnutrition and severe hepatic insufficiency are associated with reduced synthesis of HDL. Factors that increase HDL are cessation of smoking, drugs (estrogen, gemfibrozil, nicotinic acid), and exercise.

## THERAPY OF DYSLIPIDEMIAS

The National Institutes of Health sponsored a conference on cholesterol in 1986. An expert panel recognized the negative effects of hypercholesterolemia on CAD and issued recommendations for the screening and treatment of hypercholesterolemia. The recommendations stem from the analysis of previous studies indicating a decrease in the risk for CAD in patients receiving cholesterol-lowering drugs. An educational program for physicians was also promoted: National Cholesterol Education Program (NCEP). The guidelines for the treatment of hypercholesterolemia have recently been revised and are listed in Tables 4–6 and 4–7. Screening is recommended above age 20 and in children at risk by measuring total cholesterol and HDL cholesterol (HDL-C). The risk factors for CAD are listed in Table 4–8. Patients with total cholesterol levels lower than 200 mg/dl and HDL-C levels of 35 or higher may be given educational material and rechecked in 5 years; those with HDL-C level lower than 35 mg/dl should have a 12-hour fasting lipoprotein analysis. Patients with total cholesterol higher than 200 mg/dl should have it remeasured; those with average total cholesterol between 200 mg/dl and 239 and HDL-C level of 35 mg/dl or higher and fewer than two risk factors for coronary disease should be given educational material and rechecked in 1 or 2 years, while those with HDL-C lower

## TABLE 4–6. TOTAL CHOLESTEROL (TC) AND HDL CHOLESTEROL (HDL-C) SCREENING RECOMMENDATIONS, NATIONAL CHOLESTEROL EDUCATION PROGRAM (ADULT TREATMENT PANEL II)

TC <200 mg/dl: HDL-C ≥ 35 mg/dl: give educational material and remeasure in 5 years
    <35 mg/dl: obtain 12-hr fasting lipoprotein analysis
TC 200–239 mg/dl: HDL-C ≥35 mg/dl and <2 risk factors: give educational material and remeasure in 1 or 2 years
    HDL-C <35 mg/dl or ≥ 2 risk factors: obtain 12-hr fasting lipoprotein analysis
TC ≥ 240: obtain 12-hr fasting lipoprotein analysis

From Summary of the Second Report of the National Cholesterol Education Program (NCEP) Expert Panel on Detection, Evaluation, and Treatment of High Blood Cholesterol in Adults (Adult Treatment Panel II). JAMA 269:3015–23, 1993.

than 35 mg/dl or two or more risk factors should have a 12-hour fasting lipoprotein analysis. Patients with average total cholesterol >240 should have a 12-hour fasting lipoprotein analysis. Therapy is based on LDL cholesterol (LDL-C) level and additional risk factors. In patients with CAD the goal is to reduce LDL-C to less than 100 mg/dl; in patients without coronary artery disease but with two or more risk factors the goal is to reduce LDL-C to less than 130 mg/dl, while in those with fewer than two risk factors to less than 160 mg/dl.

Screening recommendations have been developed also for HDL and triglycerides by the NIH (Table 4–9). Hypertriglyceridemia is defined as moderate when the triglyceride level is between 250 and 500 mg/dl and marked when the triglyceride level is higher than 500 mg/dl. Traditionally, only individuals with marked hypertriglyceridemia have been treated aggressively to prevent pancreatitis. There is less agreement among lipid experts on the treatment of mild and moderate hypertriglyceridemia. Currently there is no definite evidence that decreasing triglyceride levels will reduce the risk for coronary artery disease.

Most endocrinologists would agree that patients with type I or type II diabetes mellitus should have a complete lipid profile. Those individuals with elevated LDL should be treated according to the NCEP recommendations. Obviously the first step is to bring the diabetes under control and to use nonpharmacologic intervention. If these measures are unsuccessful, drug therapy is indicated.

The initial therapy of hyperlipidemias includes achievement of ideal body weight, cessation of smoking, exercise, and diet.

Obesity and smoking are risk factors for CAD. Smoking may also reduce HDL levels by about 6 per cent; the mechanism is unknown.

Exercise may raise HDL levels and reduce triglyceride levels and help patients achieve their ideal body weight. Exercise stimulates the utilization of fatty acids from triglyceride-rich VLDL, which leads to increased activity of LPL and increased clearance of VLDL; it also reduces the hepatic synthesis of VLDL. Patients who plan to enroll in an intense exercise program, especially if older than 40 years, should have an exercise stress test beforehand to rule out existing significant CAD.

The Oslo study was one of the first trials to demonstrate the beneficial effects of diet on cholesterol level. It was a primary prevention

## TABLE 4–7. TREATMENT DECISIONS BASED ON LDL CHOLESTEROL LEVEL*

| PATIENT CATEGORY | INITIATION LEVEL | LDL GOAL |
|---|---|---|
| **Dietary Therapy** | | |
| Without CHD and with fewer than two risk factors | ≥160 mg/dL (4.1 mmol/L) | <160 mg/dL (4.1 mmol/L) |
| Without CHD and with two or more risk factors | ≥130 mg/dL (3.4 mmol/L) | <130 mg/dL (3.4 mmol/L) |
| With CHD | >100 mg/dL (2.6 mmol/L) | ≤100 mg/dL (2.6 mmol/L) |
| **Drug Treatment** | | |
| Without CHD and with fewer than two risk factors | ≥190 mg/dL (4.9 mmol/L) | <160mg/dL (4.1 mmol/L) |
| Without CHD and with two or more risk factors | ≥160 mg/dL (4.1 mmol/L) | <130 mg/dL (3.4 mmol/L) |
| With CHD | ≥130 mg/dL (3.4 mmol/L) | ≤100 mg/dL (2.6 mmol/L) |

*LDL indicates low-density lipoprotein; and CHD, coronary heart disease.
Summary of the Second Report of the National Cholesterol Education Program (NCEP) Expert Panel on Detection, Evaluation, and Treatment of High Blood Cholesterol in Adults (Adult Treatment Panel II). JAMA 269:3015–23, 1993.

## TABLE 4–8.   RISK STATUS BASED ON PRESENCE OF CHD RISK FACTORS OTHER THAN LOW-DENSITY LIPOPROTEIN CHOLESTEROL*

### POSITIVE RISK FACTORS

Age, y
  Male ≥45
  Female ≥55 or premature menopause without
    estrogen replacement therapy
Family history of premature CHD (definite myocardial
  infarction or sudden death before 55 y of age in father
  or other male first-degree relative, or before 55 y of
  age in mother or other female first-degree relative)
Current cigarette smoking
Hypertension (blood pressure ≥140/90 mm Hg,† or
  taking antihypertensive medication)
Low HDL cholesterol (<35 mg/dL† (0.9 mmol/L)
Diabetes mellitus

### NEGATIVE RISK FACTOR‡

High HDL cholesterol (≥60 mg/dL (1.6 mmol/L)

---

*High risk, defined as a net of two or more coronary heart disease (CHD) risk factors, leads to more vigorous intervention. Age (defined differently for men and women) is treated as a risk factor because rates of CHD are higher in the elderly than in the young, and in men than in women of the same age. Obesity is not listed as a risk factor because it operates through other risk factors that are included (hypertension, hyperlipidemia, decreased high-density lipoprotein [HDL] cholesterol, and diabetes mellitus), but it should be considered a target for intervention. Physical inactivity is similarly not listed as a risk factor, but it too should be considered a target for intervention, and physical activity is recommended as desirable for everyone.

†Confirmed by measurements on several occasions.

‡If the HDL cholesterol level is ≥60 mg/dL (1.6 mmol/L), subtract one risk factor (because high HDL cholesterol levels decrease CHD risk).

From Summary of the Second Report of the National Cholesterol Education Program (NCEP) Expert Panel on Detection, Evaluation, and Treatment of High Blood Cholesterol in Adults (Adult Treatment Panel II) JAMA 269:3015–23, 1993.

---

trial enrolling 1232 healthy men age 40 to 49 years with a cholesterol level of 290 to 379 mg/dl, and without clinical evidence of coronary disease. Half of the patients were placed on a relatively high polyunsaturated and low-saturated fat diet; the rest of the patients served as a control group. After five years there was a 13 per cent reduction of the total cholesterol and a statistically significant reduction in the incidence of fatal and non-fatal myocardial infarcts in the intervention group compared to the control group. Diet management is stressed for at least six months before administration of a cholesterol-lowering drug is considered; patients should be observed at two- to three-month intervals by a registered dietitian for reinforcement and to assess compliance. A

lipid profile may be repeated once or twice during this time. In Table 4–10 are typical low cholesterol diets of the American Heart Association, which are also recommended by the American Diabetes Association for diabetic patients. The cholesterol and fat contents of animal products are listed in Table 4–11, and the recommended diet modifications to lower plasma cholesterol are given in Table 4–12.

Presently there is no agreement on what a diabetic diet should be. In a recent article Dr. S. Grundy points out that a universal diet may not be suitable to all diabetic patients; he suggests that the diet should be based on the patient's body weight and the duration and type of diabetes. Obese patients in the early stage of NIDDM may benefit from a caloric reduction of all nutrients (carbohydrate, protein, fat). In nonobese patients with advanced NIDDM a low carbohydrate diet enriched with monounsaturated fatty acids might be preferable. Finally in patients with insulin-dependent diabetes mellitus (IDDM) a high carbohydrate diet might be

## TABLE 4–9.   SCREENING RECOMMENDATIONS FOR HDL AND TRIGLYCERIDES

Measure HDL when total cholesterol is measured to
  determine CHD risk
Measure HDL and triglycerides:
  • to assess risks for progression of disease and
    development of additional cardiovascular
    complications in persons with known CHD
  • to refine CHD risk assessment in those with total
    cholesterol above the desired range, or in those
    with desirable total cholesterol levels who have two
    or more CHD risk factors, or in people with other
    disorders that may be associated with increased
    triglyceride levels and are known to be associated
    with increased CHD risk (diabetes mellitus
    peripheral vascular disease, hypertension, central
    obesity, chronic renal disease)
  • in patients with lactescent serum, lipemia retinalis,
    xanthomas, or pancreatitis, to determine the
    presence of familial hyperlipidemic disorders and/
    or the likelihood for recurrence of pancreatitis and
    to follow triglyceride response to treatment in such
    cases when triglyceride is elevated.
  • to follow results of nonpharmacologic and/or
    pharmacologic therapy directed toward reduction of
    triglyceride levels and/or increases of HDL levels in
    order to assess treatment effect

---

From National Institutes of Health Consensus Development Conference on Triglyceride, High Density Lipoprotein, and Coronary Heart Disease, Bethesda, MD, February 26–28, 1992.

## TABLE 4-10. AMERICAN HEART ASSOCIATION LOW CHOLESTEROL DIETS

| Nutrient | Step 1 | Step 2 |
|---|---|---|
| Total fat | <30% total calories | <30% total calories |
| Saturated fatty acids | <10% | <7% |
| Polyunsaturated fatty acids | <10% | <10% |
| Monounsaturated fatty acids | 10–15% | 10–15% |
| Carbohydrates | 50–60% | <50–60% |
| Protein | 10–20% | 10–20% |
| Cholesterol | <300 mg/day | <200 mg/day |
| Total calories | To achieve and maintain desirable weight | |

From Report of the National Cholesterol Education Program Expert Panel on detection, evaluation, and treatment of high blood cholesterol in adults. Arch. Intern. Med. 148:36–69, 1988.

well tolerated. Two weight-reduction diets compared with a typical American diet are shown in Table 4–13. Dr. Grundy concludes his article by underlying the fact that a simple solution to this problem might not be realistic and that diet recommendations may need to be individualized for each patient.

## DRUG THERAPY

Several classes of drugs are available for the treatment of the various dyslipidemias:

Bile acid–binding resins (BABR)
Vitamins
Hydroxymethylglutaryl-CoA reductase inhibitors
Antioxidants
Fibric acid derivatives

Fish oils and other minor agents will not be discussed because of their limited usefulness.

### Bile Acid–Binding Resins

The resins currently in use are cholestyramine (Questran) and colestipol (Colestid). BABR's bind cholesterol in the gastrointestinal tract and promote its elimination in the stool. They also appear to increase the number of LDL receptors indirectly by lowering the cholesterol level, therefore stimulating LDL clearance indirectly. Cholestyramine was used in the Lipid Research Clinics Coro-

nary Primary Prevention Trial. The characteristics of the study are:

Primary prevention trial
3806 men, age 35 to 59 years
Cholesterol level greater than 265 mg/dl
No CAD
Placebo group on diet
Treatment group received cholestyramine
7- to 10-year follow-up

The results of the study are shown in Table 4–14. Those patients receiving the drug had more pronounced reduction of cholesterol and LDL and a lower incidence of CAD; in addition, patients receiving a full dose of the drug had a much lower incidence of coro-

## TABLE 4-11. CHOLESTEROL AND FAT CONTENT OF ANIMAL PRODUCTS IN THREE-OUNCE PORTIONS (COOKED)

| SOURCE | CHOLESTEROL CONTENT, mg/3 oz | TOTAL FAT CONTENT, gm/3oz |
|---|---|---|
| Red meats (lean) | | |
| Beef | 77 | 8.7 |
| Lamb | 78 | 8.8 |
| Pork | 79 | 11.1 |
| Veal | 128 | 4.7 |
| Organ meats | | |
| Liver | 270 | 4.0 |
| Pancreas | 400 | 2.8 |
| (sweetbreads) | 329 | 2.9 |
| Kidney | 1746 | 10.7 |
| Brains | 164 | 4.8 |
| Poultry | | |
| Chicken (without skin) | | |
| Light | 72 | 3.8 |
| Dark | 79 | 8.2 |
| Turkey (without skin) | | |
| Light | 59 | 1.3 |
| Dark | 72 | 6.1 |
| Fish | | |
| Salmon | 74 | 9.3 |
| Tuna, light, canned in water | 55 | 0.7 |
| Shellfish | | |
| Abalone | 90 | 0.8 |
| Clams | 57 | 1.7 |
| Crab meat | | |
| Alaskan King | 45 | 1.3 |
| Blue crab | 85 | 1.5 |
| Lobster | 61 | 0.5 |
| Oysters | 93 | 4.2 |
| Scallops | 35 | 0.8 |
| Shrimp | 166 | 0.9 |

From Report of the National Cholesterol Education Program Expert Panel on detection, evaluation, and treatment of high blood cholesterol in adults. Arch. Intern. Med. 148:36–69, 1988.

## TABLE 4–12.  RECOMMENDED DIET MODIFICATIONS TO LOWER BLOOD CHOLESTEROL

### THE STEP-ONE DIET

| | Choose | Decrease |
|---|---|---|
| Fish, chicken, turkey, and lean meats | Fish, poultry without skin, lean cuts of beef, lamb, pork or veal, shellfish | Fatty cuts of beef, lamb, pork; spare ribs, organ meats, regular cold cuts, sausage, hot dogs, bacon, sardines, roe |
| Skim and low-fat milk, cheese, yogurt, and dairy substitutes | Skim or 1% fat milk (liquid, powdered, evaporated), buttermilk | Whole milk (4% fat): regular, evaporated, condensed; cream, half and half, 2% milk, imitation milk products, most nondairy creamers, whipped toppings |
| | Nonfat (0% fat) or low-fat yogurt | Whole-milk yogurt |
| | Low-fat cottage cheese (1% or 2% fat) | Whole-milk cottage cheese (4% fat) |
| | Low-fat cheeses, farmer or pot cheeses (all of these should be labeled no more than 2 to 6 gm of fat per ounce) | All natural cheeses (e.g., blue, Roquefort, Camembert, Cheddar, Swiss), low-fat or "light" cream cheese, low-fat or "light" sour cream, cream cheeses, sour cream |
| | Sherbert, sorbet | Ice cream |
| Eggs | Egg whites (2 whites equal 1 whole egg in recipes), cholesterol-free egg substitutes | Egg yolks |
| Fruits and vegetables | Fresh, frozen, canned, or dried fruits and vegetables | Vegetables prepared in butter, cream, or other sauces |
| Breads and cereals | Homemade baked goods: using unsaturated oils sparingly, angel food cake, low-fat crackers, low-fat cookies | Commercial baked goods: pies, cakes, doughnuts, croissants, pastries, muffins, biscuits, high-fat crackers, high-fat cookies |
| | Rice, pasta | Egg noodles |
| | Whole-grain breads and cereals (oatmeal, whole wheat, rye, bran, multigrain, etc) | Breads in which eggs are a major ingredient |
| Fats and oils | Baking cocoa | Chocolate |
| | Unsaturated vegetable oils: corn, olive, rapeseed (canola oil), safflower, sesame, soybean, sunflower | Butter, coconut oil, palm oil, palm kernel oil, lard, bacon fat |
| | Margarine or shortenings made from one of the unsaturated oils listed above, diet margarine | |
| | Mayonnaise, salad dressings made with unsaturated oils listed above, low-fat dressings | Dressings made with egg yolk |
| | Seeds and nuts | Coconut |

From Report of the National Cholesterol Education Program Expert Panel on detection, evaluation, and treatment of high blood cholesterol in adults. Arch. Intern. Med. 148:36–69, 1988.

## TABLE 4–13.  COMPARISON OF TYPICAL AMERICAN DIET WITH TWO WEIGHT-REDUCTION DIETS

| NUTRIENTS | TYPICAL AMERICAN DIET (3000 kcal) | WEIGHT-REDUCTION DIETS | |
|---|---|---|---|
| | | High-Monounsaturated Diet (1800 kcal) | High Carbohydrate Diet (1800 kcal) |
| Fat (gm) | 133 | 80 | 50 |
| Saturated | 47 | 14 | 14 |
| Monounsaturated | 63 | 52 | 22 |
| Polyunsaturated | 23 | 14 | 14 |
| Carbohydrate (gm) | 338 | 203 | 270 |
| Protein (gm) | 113 | 68 | 68 |

From Diet and diabetes. Diabetes Care 14:773–866, 1991.

**TABLE 4–14.  RESULTS OF LIPID RESEARCH CLINICS CORONARY PRIMARY PREVENTION TRIAL**

|  | TREATMENT GROUP (CHOLESTYRAMINE) | |
|---|---|---|
|  | 14 gm | 24 gm |
| Coronary deaths or non fatal myocardial infarct (% reduction) | 19 | 49 |
| LDL cholesterol % reduction | 11 | 35 |

From The Lipid Research Clinics Coronary Primary Prevention Trial. JAMA 251:365–374, 1984.

nary events. The resins are able to reduce LDL and cholesterol by an average of about 20 per cent. The drugs are taken with water or juice. The dosage of cholestyramine is between 4 and 8 gm three times daily; the dosage of colestipol is between 5 and 10 gm three times daily. The most common side effects are epigastric distress, constipation, and hypertriglyceridemia. These drugs interfere with the absorption of medications such as propranolol, thyroxine, and digoxin; to avoid this problem the resins should be taken one hour after or four hours before other medications. Bile acid–binding resins are indicated in hypercholesterolemia of adults and children; they are contraindicated in hypertriglyceridemia. The resins are often used effectively in combination with other lipid-lowering agents.

### Nicotinic Acid

Nicotinic acid (niacin) is a vitamin that becomes an effective lipid-lowering agent when used in high doses. Niacin was used in a secondary drug prevention trial, and it was associated with reduction in the occurrence of coronary events (Table 4–15). Nicotinic acid administration is started in small doses of 100 mg twice daily and gradually increased by 100 mg every two or three days to achieve a dosage of 1 to 1.5 gm three times daily. It is expected to reduce LDL cholesterol and VLDL cholesterol by approximately 20 per cent and 40 per cent, respectively; it also raises HDL cholesterol by about 30 per cent. It exerts its mechanism of action by decreasing hepatic VLDL synthesis. Common side effects include flushing (thought to be prostaglandin-mediated and usually relieved by

one aspirin taken about 30 minutes prior to the first daily dose), pruritus, gastrointestinal distress, activation of peptic ulcer and other bowel diseases, glucose intolerance, hyperuricemia, hypotension, hepatic transaminase increase, acanthosis, hepatic necrosis, and amblyopia. Nicotinic acid is indicated in patients with increased LDL cholesterol or VLDL cholesterol, combined hyperlipidemia, or HDL deficiency. It is contraindicated in patients with hepatic insufficiency, hyperuricemia, gout, peptic ulcer disease, or other bowel diseases. It should be used with caution in diabetic patients because it impairs glucose tolerance.

### Hydroxymethylglutaryl (HMG)-CoA Reductase Inhibitors

Lovastatin (Mevacor) was the first compound of this group to be approved by the FDA. Three other products are now available—pravastatin (Pravachol), simvastatin (Zocor), and fluvastatin (Lescol). Their mechanism of action is by inhibiting HMG-CoA reductase, the rate-limiting enzyme for the synthesis of cholesterol with consequent reduced formation of cholesterol in the liver; this in turn stimulates the synthesis of LDL receptors leading to increased clearance rate of LDL; they are very powerful in reducing LDL cholesterol by 25 to 45 per cent. All of these drugs have a good side effect profile; the most common adverse effects include headaches, allergic reactions, myalgia, myopathy, increase of liver enzymes. The initial fear that lovastatin might cause increased incidence of lens opacities has been disproven by a study carried out in the Boston area. The usual initial dose for lovastatin and pravastatin is 10 to 20 mg at bedtime; it may be in-

**TABLE 4–15.  CORONARY DRUG PROJECT**

|  | NUMBER OF PATIENTS | |
|---|---|---|
| CAUSES OF DEATH | Niacin 1119(%) | Placebo 2789(%) |
| All causes | 582(52) | 1623(58.2) |
| Cardiovascular | 474(42.4) | 1331(47.7) |
| Cancer | 408(36.5) | 1153(41.3) |
| Other noncardiovascular | 33(2.9) | 85(5) |
| Unknown | 30(2.7) | 83(3) |

From Canner, P.L., et al.: Fifteen year mortality in Coronary Drug Project patients: Long term benefit with niacin. J. Am. Coll. Cardiol. 8:1245–1255, 1986.

creased to 40 mg twice daily if necessary; the initial dose of symvastatin is 5 to 10 mg at bedtime, and it may be increased to 20 mg twice daily if needed. Liver function tests, creatine phosphokinase, creatinine, and lipid profile should be rechecked three to four weeks after the beginning of therapy and after any dose change, and every three to six months afterward. Recent studies employing lovastatin in combination with other drugs have demonstrated lack of progression or reduced rate of progression or even regression in patients treated with an aggressive lipid-lowering regimen compared to those receiving conventional therapy (see Familial atherosclerosis Treatment Study and FH Trial studies in discussion of Combination Therapy). The differences among the three drugs are minor; pravastatin is water soluble, it does not seem to cross the blood-brain barrier, and it has a lower incidence of myopathy, possibly because of its limited penetration into the muscular tissue. The indications for this group of drugs include increase of LDL cholesterol, VLDL cholesterol, and combined hyperlipidemias. They are contraindicated in patients with severe liver disease or myopathy and in those taking erythromycin, nicotinic acid, cyclosporin, or gemfibrozil (Lopid) because of the increased incidence of myopathy. Combination with gemfibrozil is tempting, but it is not recommended although I personally have a few patients receiving this combination. They are taking gemfibrozil already and I usually add the smallest available dose of pravastatin. I observe them very closely and give them written instructions; so far none of these patients has had complications.

## Fibric Acid Derivatives

Gemfibrozil and clofibrate are available in the United States; fenofibrate is awaiting approval. Clofibrate is rarely used because of evidence of possible association with an increased incidence of cancer. Gemfibrozil was employed in the Helsinki study (Table 4–16).

The Helsinki Heart Study consisted of:

Primary prevention trial
4081 men, age 40 to 55 years
Non-HDL cholesterol greater than 200
Control group receiving placebo
Treatment group receiving gemfibrozil
Five-year follow-up

### TABLE 4–16.   HELSINKI HEART STUDY

| CORONARY EVENTS | NUMBER OF PATIENTS | |
| --- | --- | --- |
| | Gemfibrozil | Placebo |
| Nonfatal myocardial infarct | 45 | 71 |
| Fatal myocardial infarct | 6 | 8 |
| Sudden cardiac death | 5 | 4 |
| Unwitnessed death | 0 | 1 |
| Total | 56 | 84 |

From Manninen, V., et al.: Lipid alteration and decline in the incidence of coronary heart disease in the Helsinki Heart Study. JAMA 260:641–651, 1988.

The participants receiving gemfibrozil had a reduction of total cholesterol, LDL cholesterol, and triglycerides of 11, 10, and 43 per cent, respectively, as well as an increase of HDL cholesterol of 10 per cent, and a lower incidence of CAD. Its mechanism of action consists of stimulation of LPL and decrease in synthesis of VLDL by the hepatocyte. The recommended dosage is 600 mg twice daily. The expected effects include reduction of triglycerides by as much as 50 per cent, increase in HDL by 20 per cent, and a mild reduction of LDL of 10 per cent. Common side effects include gallstones, myopathy, gastrointestinal distress, blood dyscrasias, and liver enzyme abnormalities. It is contraindicated in patients with liver disease, myopathy, or gallstones; it is not recommended in combination with HMG-CoA reductase inhibitors. Indications include elevation of VLDL cholesterol and mild elevation of LDL cholesterol, with or without low HDL cholesterol. Fenofibrate is well tolerated and more effective in lowering the LDL and also the uric acid levels.

### Antioxidants

Probucol (Lorelco) is a lipophilic antioxidant agent. The interest in this drug stems from the evidence that LDL oxidation is implicated in atherogenesis; its antioxidant properties might play a role in reducing the risk for CAD. Probucol stimulates the clearance of LDL by non-receptor-mediated mechanisms (i.e., pinocytosis); unfortunately it also decreases HDL synthesis. The dosage of probucol is 250 to 500 mg twice daily. After its absorption through the intestine, probucol is stored in the adipose tissue; the drug may remain in the body for more than six months after discontinuation of therapy. Side effects include gastrointestinal distress,

## TABLE 4–17.  DRUGS COMMONLY USED IN THE TREATMENT OF DYSLIPIDEMIAS

| CLASS | DOSE | INDICATIONS | COMMON SIDE EFFECTS |
|---|---|---|---|
| Bile acid–binding resins | | | |
|   Cholestyramine | 4–8 gm tid | High C | Epigastric distress, constipation, elevation |
|   Colestipol | 5–10 gm tid | | of triglycerides |
| Vitamins | | | |
|   Nicotinic acid | 1–3 gm/dl | High C, High T, Low H | Skin flushing, GI distress, hepatic dysfunction, glucose intolerance, hyperuricemia, peptic ulcer activation |
| HMG-CoA reductase inhibitors | | | |
|   Lovastatin | 10–80 mg/dl | High C | Hepatotoxicity, myalgia, myopathy, skin |
|   Pravastatin | 10–80 mg/dl | High T | reactions, GI disturbances |
|   Simvastatin | 5–40 mg/dl | | Potentiated by cyclosporin, fibric acid |
|   Fluvastatin | 20–40 mg/dl | | derivatives, nicotinic acid, erythromycin |
| Antioxidants | | | |
|   Probucol | 0.25–0.5 gm bid | High C | GI distress, ECG: QT prolongation, ventricular arrhythmias |
| Fibric acid derivatives | | | |
|   Gemfibrozil | 0.6 gm bid | High C, High T, Low H | Gallstones, GI disturbances, myopathy, anemia, leukopenia |
|   Atromid | | | |

C = cholesterol; T = triglycerides; H = HDL cholesterol.

prolonged QT interval, and eosinophilia. Indications include hypercholesterolemia. Probucol reduces LDL cholesterol and HDL cholesterol by approximately 15 per cent and 20 per cent, respectively.

A summary of the dosage, indications, and side effects of the drugs commonly used in the treatment of dyslipidemias is presented in Table 4–17.

## Combination Therapy

Combination therapy is very effective in the treatment of dyslipidemias. Recent studies have demonstrated regression of the atherosclerotic lesions with combination therapy.

CHOLESTEROL-LOWERING ATHEROSCLEROSIS STUDY (CLAS) I AND II. One hundred and sixty-two non-smoking men age 40 to 59 years with a history of coronary artery bypass graft (CABG) and with total cholesterol level of 185 to 350 mg/dl were enrolled. The intervention group was treated with low cholesterol diet, colestipol 30 gm daily, and nicotinic acid (up to 12 gm daily). The control group was placed on a low cholesterol diet. Angiography was performed at two years (CLAS I); 103 subjects were observed for two more years (CLAS II); the intervention group experienced a 25, 40, and 18 per cent reduction of total cholesterol, LDL-cholesterol, and triglycerides, respectively, and a 37 per

cent increase in HDL cholesterol (Table 4–18).

FAMILIAL ATHEROSCLEROSIS TREATMENT STUDY (FATS). Enrolled in this study were 146 men with CAD documented by angiography, a family history of vascular disease, and high apo B level; the duration of the study was about 2.5 years. Patients received diet counseling and a placebo (with colestipol subsequently) or colestipol 30 mg with lovastatin 40 mg daily or colestipol 30 mg with nicotinic acid 4 gm daily. The results of the study are presented in Table 4–19.

After $2\frac{1}{2}$ years of therapy the change in the average percentage of stenosis in nine proximal segments was 2.1 per cent in the

## TABLE 4–18.  CHOLESTEROL-LOWERING ATHEROSCLEROSIS STUDIES (CLAS) I AND II

| | TREATMENT GROUPS | |
|---|---|---|
| | Placebo (%) | Drugs (%) |
| Angiogram at two years (CLAS I) | | |
|   New lesions | 22 | 10 |
|   Progression | 61 | 39 |
|   Regression | 2.4 | 16.2 |
| Angiogram at four years (CLAS II) | | |
|   Nonprogression | 15 | 52 |
|   Regression | 6 | 18 |

From Blackenhorn, D. H., et al.: Beneficial effects of combined colestipol-niacin therapy on coronary atherosclerosis and coronary venous bypass grafts (CLAS I and II). JAMA 257:3233–3240, 1987.

### TABLE 4–19.  FAMILIAL ATHEROSCLEROSIS TREATMENT STUDY (FATS)

| | TREATMENT GROUPS | | |
| | Placebo with Colestipol | Colestipol with Nicotinic Acid | Colestipol with Lovastatin |
|---|---|---|---|
| Cardiac events | 10 | 2 | 3 |
| LDL reduction % | 7 | 32 | 46 |
| HDL increase % | 6 | 43 | 15 |
| Average % stenosis in 9 proximal segments | 2.1 | −0.9 | −0.7 |

From Brown, G., et al.: Regression of coronary artery disease as a result of intensive lipid lowering therapy in men with high levels of apolipoprotein B. N. Engl. J. Med. 323:1289–1298, 1990.

placebo-colestipol group, −0.9 per cent in the niacin-colestipol group, and −0.7 per cent in the lovastatin-colestipol group; digital angiography was used to quantitate the lesions.

Another recent trial conducted at the University of California at San Francisco demonstrated regression of coronary artery stenotic lesions (detected by digital angiography) in men and women with familial hypercholesterolemia treated with combination therapy (colestipol, nicotinic acid, and lovastatin).

These are some examples of drug combinations and their indications:

Elevation of LDL cholesterol
  BABR + nicotinic acid
  BABR + fibric acid derivative
  BABR + probucol

BABR + HMG-CoA reductase inhibitors
Combined hyperlipidemia
  BABR + nicotinic acid
  BABR + fibric acid derivative
  Nicotinic acid + fibric acid derivative
  HMG-CoA reductase inhibitor + fibric acid derivative (cautiously)

Combination therapy is indicated in all forms of hyperlipidemias that cannot be corrected with one drug alone, and in those patients who cannot tolerate maximal doses of one drug but are able to tolerate lower doses of two different drugs.

### Estrogens

Currently, estrogens are widely used for replacement therapy in perimenopausal and

### TABLE 4–20.  EFFECTS OF ESTROGEN REPLACEMENT ON PLASMA TRIGLYCERIDE, TOTAL CHOLESTEROL, AND LIPOPROTEIN CHOLESTEROL CONCENTRATIONS IN POSTMENOPAUSAL DYSLIPIDEMIC WOMEN

| PLASMA PARAMETER (n = 20) | ESTROGEN REPLACEMENT (MEAN ± SD) | | % CHANGE | P VALUE |
| | Before | During* | | |
|---|---|---|---|---|
| Triglyceride | | | | |
| mg/dl | 187 ± 100 | 244 ± 156 | +30 | .003 |
| mmol/L | 2.11 ± 1.12 | 2.75 ± 1.77 | | |
| Total cholesterol | | | | |
| mg/dl | 288 ± 50 | 252 ± 43 | −13 | .0001 |
| mmol/L | 7.45 ± 1.28 | 6.52 ± 1.11 | | |
| VLDL cholesterol | | | | |
| mg/dl | 42 ± 27 | 47 ± 35 | +12 | .4 |
| mmol/L | 1.09 ± 0.70 | 1.22 ± 0.90 | | |
| LDL cholesterol | | | | |
| mg/dl | 197 ± 49 | 143 ± 40 | −27 | .0001 |
| mmol/L | 5.09 ± 1.27 | 3.70 ± 1.03 | | |
| HDL cholesterol | | | | |
| mg/dl | 49 ± 13 | 61 ± 14 | +24 | .001 |
| mmol/L | 1.27 ± 0.33 | 1.58 ± 0.36 | | |

From Granfone, A., et al.: Effects of estrogen replacement on plasma lipoproteins and apolipoproteins in postmenopausal, dyslipidemic women. Metabolism 11:1193–1198, 1992.
*During estrogen replacement for a period of 13 ± 4 weeks.

TABLE 4-21.   EFFECTS OF ESTROGEN REPLACEMENT ON PLASMA APO A-1 AND APO B CONCENTRATIONS AND LDL PARTICLE SCORE IN POSTMENOPAUSAL, DYSLIPIDEMIC WOMEN

| PLASMA PARAMETER | ESTROGEN REPLACEMENT (MEAN ± SD) | | % CHANGE | P VALUE |
|---|---|---|---|---|
| | Before | During | | |
| Apo A-I (mg/dl; n = 17) | 163 ± 39 | 254 ± 61 | +56 | .001 |
| Apo B (mg/dl; n = 17) | 170 ± 47 | 148 ± 48 | −13 | .03 |
| LDL particle score (n = 12) | 4.09 ± 1.27 | 4.52 ± 1.26 | +11 | .01 |

From Granfone, A., et al.: Effects of estrogen replacement on plasma lipoproteins and apolipoproteins in postmenopausal, dyslipidemic women. Metabolism 11:1193–1198, 1992.

postmenopausal syndromes and for the treatment of osteoporosis. Although estrogens are not approved for the treatment of dyslipidemias, they have a profound effect on lipid metabolism (Table 4–20). This was well described by Tikkanen et al. in 1978; more recent studies have confirmed their findings and have demonstrated an effect on apolipoprotein metabolism (Table 4–21). Studies in animals and humans have revealed that estrogen administration is associated with increased clearance of LDL through an increased number of hepatic LDL receptors; increased synthesis and decreased clearance of VLDL; and increased synthesis of HDL and apo A-I. Therefore, it is important to monitor the lipid profile a few weeks after the beginning of estrogen therapy and every few months afterward; patients with combined hyperlipidemia and hypertriglyderidemia are at risk for developing massive hypertriglyceridemia and pancreatitis.

## CONCLUSIONS

Atherogenesis is a complex process that now is being studied at cellular and molecular levels. Most of this chapter was devoted to lipoprotein metabolism and treatment of dyslipidemias in normal and diabetic patients. As the pathogenetic mechanisms of atherosclerosis become more precisely defined, therapeutic intervention will eventually become more specifically tailored to the detected abnormalities. Diabetes mellitus is an important risk factor for cardiovascular disease. It is hoped that additional and more specific markers for atherosclerosis will enable us to better identify those individuals who are at increased risk for atherosclerotic cardiovascular disease and treat them more aggressively.

## SUGGESTED READING LIST

Blackenhorn, D.H., et al.: Beneficial effects of combined colestipol-niacin therapy on coronary atherosclerosis and coronary venous bypass grafts (CLAS I and II). JAMA 257:3233–3240, 1987.

Brown, G., et al: Regression of coronary artery disease as a result of intensive lipid lowering therapy in men with high levels of apolipoprotein B. N. Engl. J. Med. 323:1289–1298, 1990.

Canner, P.L., et al: Fifteen year mortality in Coronary Drug Project patients: Long term benefit with niacin. J. Am. Coll. Cardiol. 8:1245–1255, 1986.

Castelli W.P., et al: Incidence of coronary heart disease and lipoprotein cholesterol levels. The Framingham Study. JAMA 256:2835–2838, 1986.

Ginsberg, H.N.: Lipoprotein physiology in non diabetic and diabetic states: Relationship to atherogenesis. Diabetes Care 14:839–855, 1991.

Granfone, A., et al: Effects of estrogen replacement on plasma lipoproteins and apolipoproteins in postmenopausal, dyslipidemic women. Metabolism 11:1193–1198, 1992.

Grundy, S.M.: Dietary therapy in diabetes mellitus: Is there a single best diet? Diabetes Care 14:796–801, 1991.

Hjermann, I., et al: Effect of diet and smoking intervention on the incidence of coronary heart disease (Oslo Diet Study). Lancet 2:1303–1310, 1981.

LaRosa, J.C. (ed.): Lipid Disorders. Endocrinol. Metab. Clin. North Am. 19:211–467, 1990.

Lipid Research Clinics Coronary Primary Prevention Trial. JAMA 251:365–374, 1984.

Manninen, V., et al: Lipid alteration and decline in the incidence of coronary heart disease in the Helsinki Heart Study. JAMA 260:641–651, 1988.

Multiple Risk Factor Intervention Trial Research Group: Mortality Rates after 10.5 years for participants in the Multiple Risk Factor Intervention Trial. JAMA 263:1795–1801, 1990.

National Institutes of Health Consensus Development Conference on Triglyceride, High Density Lipoprotein, and Coronary Heart Disease. Bethesda, Md., February 26–28, 1992.

Report of the National Cholesterol Education Program Expert Panel on detection, evaluation, and treatment of high blood cholesterol in adults. Arch. Intern. Med. 148:36–69, 1988.

Schaefer, E.J., et al: Pathogenesis and management of lipoprotein disorders. N. Engl. J. Med. 312:1300–1310, 1985.

Schwartz, C.J., et al: Pathogenesis of the atherosclerotic lesion. Implications for diabetes mellitus. Diabetes Care 15:1156–1167, 1992.

Stout, R.W.: Insulin and atheroma: 20 year perspective. Diabetes Care 13:631–654, 1990.

Summary of the Second Report of the National Cholesterol Education Program (NCEP) Expert Panel on Detection, Evaluation, and Treatment of High Blood Cholesterol in Adults (Adult Treatment Panel II). JAMA 269:3015–3023, 1993.

Tikkanen M.J., et al.: Natural estrogen as an effective treatment for the type II hyperlipoproteinemia in postmenopausal women. Lancet 2:490–491, 1978.

# Chapter 5

# PATHOLOGY OF THE DIABETIC FOOT

## URMILA KHETTRY, M.D.

The pathological hallmark of the diabetic foot is premature senescence. Certain lesions not uncommonly seen in the general population, but with their particular complications in this setting, make the diabetic foot a clinical challenge. The classic pathological triad of the diabetic foot is vascular disease, neuropathy, and infection. Each of these may be present alone or in combination with others, making the clinical picture rather complex. Intelligent and worthwhile therapeutic approach demands understanding the pathology and interrelationships of these three problems. While neuropathy may be partly blamed for the problems that plague a diabetic's foot, by far the most important and devastating lesions appear secondary to disease of the blood vessels (see Plates 4 and 5).

## CHARACTERISTICS OF GANGRENE

Gangrene resulting from extreme vascular compromise is one of the most feared complications of diabetes. Warren et al. in their study involving 1854 autopsies on diabetic patients found 543 cases of gangrene. One hundred and thirty patients in this group had diabetes for over 15 years. The lower extremities are by far the most common site of involvement. Often these patients at autopsy are seen to have evidence of previous amputation and, when amputated leg specimens are received in the pathology laboratory, it is not uncommon to find all or some of the toes missing.

Gangrene or ischemic necrosis can result in a variety of ways. The most common is arteriosclerosis of major vessels. This is also the underlying cause of gangrene in almost all cases in diabetes. In this setting, i.e. in a diabetic, the word *gangrene* also seems to include, probably incorrectly, an element of infection along with the ischemic injury. The incidence of an embolic type of gangrene is the same for diabetics as for nondiabetics. Gas gangrene is rarely seen in the modern era.

It is rather difficult if not impossible to distinguish between the vascular disease of a diabetic and a nondiabetic on morphological grounds alone. However, the extent and severity of the disease tend to be more marked in diabetic patients. Also, the distribution of vascular involvement is somewhat different in the two groups. Smaller arteries below the knee are most likely to be involved in diabetics as compared with the aortic and iliac involvement seen in nondiabetics. This situation is noted clinically as well, when good popliteal and pedal pulses may be felt in the presence of small areas of gangrene involving the toes.

Arteriosclerotic gangrene that is usually seen is almost always of the dry type and histologically shows changes of coagulative necrosis, whereas the gangrene seen in diabetics is commonly the moist, or wet, type. Histologically, it is characterized by liquefactive necrosis of tissues, but this distinction is not absolute. We have seen instances of both in our surgical specimens; however, the moist type is more common. Infections probably play a major role in the second type of necrosis.

Arterial occlusion in typical diabetic gangrene is a gradual process. Usually a delicate balance is attained to meet the vascular demands of a limb, but any unusual and untimely stress such as infection can result in compromised circulation. Moist gangrene can result.

Bell's classic study of atherosclerotic gangrene of legs involved a phenomenal number of cases. He reviewed the autopsy records of 2130 diabetics and 59,733 nondiabetics and found the incidence of gangrene to increase with age. He found gangrene of the lower extremity to be 156 times more common in diabetics than in nondiabetics in the fifth decade, 85 times more common in the sixth decade and 53 times more common in the seventh decade.

Histologically, the gangrenous area shows changes of necrosis and as has been mentioned before it is usually of the liquefactive type. The skin surface may or may not be ulcerated. Cellular outlines and details are lost and so is the basic architecture. Collections of inflammatory cells consisting of predominantly polymorphonuclear leukocytes are scattered through the tissues. Infrequently the coagulative type of necrosis is seen; in this the basic architecture is preserved but cells are converted into "tombstones," with loss of nucleus and other cytologic details.

## ARTERIAL CHANGES IN DIABETICS

Since gangrene is largely related to diseases of arteries, we will discuss the arterial changes seen in diabetics. It must be noted at the outset that all these changes can be seen in nondiabetics as well, but these changes usually have a characteristic distribution and are more extensive in diabetics. The changes also tend to appear early in younger individuals. Calcified vessels in a young patient should raise the suspicion of diabetes.

There are two types of arteries, the elastic arteries, with a heavy inlay of elastic tissue in their walls, and the muscular arteries, in which smooth muscle is the most prominent component of the wall, with elastic tissue arranged in two layers. The aorta, the carotids, and iliacs are elastic arteries, while the peripheral vasculature is almost entirely muscular. Vascular problems in the diabetic can be divided into two major categories: large vessel disease (macroangiopathy) and small vessel disease (microangiopathy). Large vessel disease, or macroangiopathy, is most often seen in popliteal and tibial arteries. Small muscular arteries are more severely affected with the arteriosclerotic process. Strandness et al. in their study of the vessels of the lower extremity found that 81 per cent of diabetic persons have stenosis or occlusion of the three major vessels below the knee as compared with 57 per cent involvement of the same vessels in nondiabetics. According to Cecile et al., 40 per cent of diabetics have characteristic lesions in small arteries of the foot.

There are no distinctive histopathological lesions of diabetic macroangiopathy. The question of whether or not there is any qualitative difference in the atherosclerotic process in diabetics and nondiabetics has troubled many investigators. Atherosclerotic plaques in diabetics have been shown to contain more mucopolysaccharides: Coronary artery lipid composition has been reported to be different and also the total content of ash, calcium, and cholesterol has been reported to be increased in diabetics. Regardless of these qualitative differences, it must be emphasized that quantitatively the macrovascular process is much more extensive in diabetics.

Macrovascular disease in a diabetic consists of *arteriosclerosis*. The term arteriosclerosis encompasses a group of lesions that results in thickening and loss of elasticity of the arterial wall. Histopathologically, three distinct changes are included within the term arteriosclerosis. *Atherosclerosis,* a word that has unfortunately gained popularity as a synonym for arteriosclerosis, is characterized by formation of atheromas. It is the most important and common change that is encountered in the large arteries. The other two changes are *Mönckeberg's sclerosis,* or *medial calcific sclerosis,* and *diffuse intimal fibrosis.* Mönckeberg's sclerosis is characterized by calcification of the media of muscular arteries, whereas the intimal fibrosis is a normal aging process. Some authors consider arteriolosclerosis as a form of arteriosclerosis, but we shall discuss the changes in arterioles and capillaries under the term *diabetic microangiopathy.*

Each of the three aforementioned types of arterial thickening has a distinct morphological appearance. However, more than one change can be present in the same individual and even in the same artery. Atherosclerosis and medial calcific sclerosis are often seen together in the vessels of the lower extremity of the elderly. A similar situation may exist in diabetics.

## ATHEROMA

Atherosclerosis in diabetics appears within a few years of the clinical manifestations of the disease. The lesions tend to be more extensive and florid. Morphologically, the lesions are heterogeneous. Fatty streaks may be seen early in the disease, but the important histological lesion we are concerned with in this context is the atheroma, which is the basic lesion of atherosclerosis.

An atheroma or atheromatous plaque may be fibrous or fibrous and fatty. Sometimes it may almost exclusively consist of lipid and is then referred to as a *fatty* or *lipid plaque*. Depending upon the lipid or fibrous tissue content, it may be yellow, tan, or white. A plaque, as opposed to a flat fatty streak, protrudes into the vessel lumen. Large plaques are formed by coalescence of smaller ones. An uncomplicated plaque generally has a smooth surface formed by a fibrous cap, underneath which lies a mass of soft, pasty, grumous material. In advanced disease, a variable amount of fibrosis and calcification can convert this soft mass into firm to hard nodules with a concrete-like consistency. An extreme state of calcification can turn the artery into "pipestem" with total loss of elasticity of the wall. A soft to firm atheroma can ulcerate when the abundant grumous material can no longer be contained within the arterial wall and the fibrous cap, or when there is hemorrhage into the plaque. The ulcerated surface allows the atheromatous material to enter the bloodstream. Frequently, portions of atheroma are swept away into distant sites by the bloodstream. Superimposed thrombosis is the most feared complication. In a small artery it may cause a sudden occlusion, whereas in a larger vessel such as the aorta, more often than not it becomes incorporated into the plaque. The plaque then turns brown or reddish-brown.

Histologically, plaques are composed of smooth muscle cells, fibrous tissue, and lipid in variable amounts, thus giving a spectrum of changes under the microscope. The fibrous cap contains essentially fibrous tissue and collagen. Occasional smooth muscle cells may be found as well. The central part of the grumous material is essentially a disorganized mass of lipid, cellular debris, fibrin, and amorphous proteinaceous material. Needle-shaped cholesterol clefts are present in abundance. Inflammatory cells are difficult to find; however, lipid-laden macrophages are not infrequent. We have occasionally seen aggregates of lymphocytes in the adjacent arterial wall. Fibrous or fibrous and fatty plaques are composed predominantly of fibrous tissue enmeshed in collagen, giving it a scar-like appearance. A calcified plaque contains irregular masses of "calcium" that histologically is highly basophilic and has no structural details.

## MEDIAL CALCIFIC SCLEROSIS

Medial calcific sclerosis, or Mönckeberg's sclerosis, is morphologically a distinctive form of arteriosclerosis. It involves the muscular arteries and, unlike atherosclerosis, spares the elastic arteries. Anatomically, Mönckeberg's sclerosis is easily distinguished from atherosclerosis. However, the two disorders may be present in the same vessel, thus complicating the picture. In a diabetic, this is more often than not the case.

As the name implies, in medial calcific sclerosis, the brunt of injury is borne by the media of the arterial wall. Calcification occurs in and around the smooth muscle cells. Initially calcium is deposited in fine granules, but as the process advances small particles fuse to form a large homogeneous structureless basophilic mass. These deposits tend to form imperfect rings or plates around the vessel; this gives the characteristic "goose trachea" nodularity on palpation. In far-advanced cases, the vessel may be one long rigid tube made of calcium. At this stage, the radiographic picture has the classic "pipestem" or "trolley track" appearance. The calcification here is continuous and irregular and in the atheromatous type it is discontinuous and regular. Within the large masses of dystrophic calcification, osseous metaplasia may occur. Bony trabeculae contain normal-appearing osteocytes. In between the trabeculae, marrow may be found.

Uncomplicated medial calcific sclerosis does not compromise the vascular lumen. Intimal injury in most cases is insignificant. Atherosclerosis with or without superimposed thrombosis can complicate the histological picture. Inflammatory cells are usually absent.

Electron microscopy has been performed on the tibial arteries from diabetics. The most prominent ultrastructural feature was the presence of calcium in appreciable amounts. The calcium deposits were found in three successive morphological states from granules to pools. In the granular state it tends to occur along the intimal elastic membrane; this gives it a "speckled" appearance. With the larger deposits, this relationship is lost. Calcium is also present close to the collagenous fibrous bundles.

Calcification is probably related to the age of the patient and the duration of diabetes. Its relationship to neuropathy has been suggested.

## DIABETIC MICROANGIOPATHY

Microangiopathy, or small vessel disease, consists of changes seen in small arteries, arterioles, and capillaries. These vessels show rather severe and extensive involvement. The arteries included in this group are smaller than 115 mμ in diameter. The pathological lesions in these vessels lead to narrowing and occlusion of the vascular lumen with resultant small and patchy areas of gangrene—for example, in a toe.

The severity and extent of small vessel involvement distinguish the vascular disease of diabetics from that of nondiabetics. It is also generally believed that macroangiopathy and microangiopathy are not present at the same time. Usually microangiopathy precedes the large vessel disease.

Arteriolosclerosis, or thickening of arterioles, forms part of the microangiopathic process in a diabetic. Similar changes are also frequently encountered in elderly patients, particularly in those who have a history of hypertension. A given arteriole from a diabetic with hyaline sclerosis is morphologically indistinguishable from a given arteriole of a nondiabetic, in whom the vessel disease may be related to the age or hypertensive state.

The arteriolar lesion consists of thickening of the vessel wall with deposition of positive periodic acid–Schiff (PAS) material. There is hypertrophy and proliferation of intima and endothelium. The PAS-positive material imparts a homogeneity and hyalinization to the wall with loss of structural details.

The vessel lumen at this stage is markedly narrowed. The mural thickening is an end result of many pathological processes taking place simultaneously. Besides endothelial proliferation, there is also pericytic proliferation. Irregular thickening of the basement membrane has been found by electron microscopy. Mural collagen deposition adds to the hyaline change of the wall. Immunofluorescent studies have shown plasma proteins entrapped in this material; this probably reflects leakage of plasma proteins across the injured endothelium.

Hyaline arteriolosclerosis has been found in intraneural arterioles in diabetics. This prompted one investigator to suggest angiopathy as the basic lesion of neuropathy and to suggest that the latter should be grouped with other manifestations of diabetic angiopathy.

The capillaries are a frequent site of diabetic microangiopathy. Homogeneous, PAS-positive thickening of the capillary wall is considered a hallmark of diabetic microangiopathy. These patients are almost always insulin dependent. This change results because of basement membrane thickening, which also envelops the pericyte and is present in all parts of the body. However, the most advanced degree of this capillary wall thickening occurs in the most dependent areas of the body. Therefore, it is not surprising to find the greatest degree in the lower extremity vessels.

Banson and Lacy in their study involving 18 diabetics and 17 nondiabetics found capillary basement membrane thickening in 88 per cent of the diabetics and only 23 per cent of the nondiabetics. Of interest also is the difference in the average basement membrane thickness in the two groups, 5900 Å for nondiabetics and 13,000 Å for the diabetics.

More recently, Tilton et al. have studied the ultrastructure of skeletal muscle capillaries in diabetics and nondiabetics. Capillary circumference was essentially the same for the two groups. However, the capillary basement membrane thickness was consistently greater in the diabetics, and this difference was greatest in the lower extremity muscles. Pericyte debris was found much more frequently in diabetics, suggesting that pericyte degeneration and turnover are somewhat enhanced in diabetics. These investigators also found a strong correlation between the presence of pericyte debris and the capillary basement membrane thickening.

## PERIPHERAL NEUROPATHY

Peripheral neuropathy involving the lower extremity in a diabetic imparts its own unique set of problems to the clinical presentation. There is degeneration of nonmyelinated nerve fibers and foci of demyelination and degeneration of myelinated nerve fibers. Loss of sensory perception results in formation of Charcot joints and neuropathic ulcers, which are discussed in detail elsewhere. Charcot joint is a chronic degenerative arthropathy that is microscopically characterized by atrophy and loss of bone. The articular surface is usually eroded and destroyed with proliferation of synovium. Joint effusion may be present. Osteoclastic activity is rather prominent. Gross evidence of cartilage and bone material embedded within the synovium is considered pathognomonic for this entity.

A neuropathic ulcer often occurs concomitantly with neuropathic joints. The most common location for a neuropathic ulcer is on the medial side of the ball of the foot. There may be a localized area of hyperkeratosis. Occlusive angiopathy may be present simultaneously, thus complicating the picture.

Diabetic mononeuropathies are probably vascular in origin, representing ischemic damage secondary to angiopathic involvement of the intraneural arterioles. Amyotrophic syndrome related to diabetes has been shown to have a characteristic histopathological lesion. The single fiber atrophy distinctively seen with the clinical presentation has been described.

## INFECTION

Infection can complicate the pathological picture of a diabetic foot. Its probable role in the development of moist gangrene has already been mentioned. When the infectious process dissects deep into the soft tissue and breaches the periosteum, osteomyelitis results. In acute stages of osteomyelitis, the process is a suppurative one. There is necrosis of both cortical and cancellous bone with formation of sequestrum. Later, as the reparative processes set in, the histological picture changes to that of chronic osteomyelitis with fibrosis of marrow spaces and variable osteoblastic activity.

## SUGGESTED READING LIST

Arenson, D. J., Sherwood, C. F., and Wilson, R. C.: Neuropathy, angiopathy, and sepsis in the diabetic foot. J. Am. Podiatr. Assoc. 71:618, 1981.

Arenson, D. J., Sherwood, C. F., and Wilson, R. C.: Neuropathy, angiopathy, and sepsis in the diabetic foot. J. Am. Podiatr. Assoc. 71:661, 1981.

Banson, B. B. and Lacy, P. E.: Diabetic microangiopathy in human toes. Am. J. Pathol. 45:41, 1964.

Bell, E. T.: Atherosclerotic gangrene of the lower extremities in diabetic and nondiabetic persons. Am. J. Clin. Pathol., 28:27, 1957.

Cecile, J. P., Descamps, C. L., Guaquiere, A., and Faille, J. C.: Diabetic foot arteriography. J. Cardiovasc. Surg., 15:12, 1974.

Clouse, M. E., Gramm, H. F., Legg, M. A., and Flood, T.: Diabetic osteoarthropathy: Clinical and roentgenographic observations in 90 cases. Am. J. Roentgenol. Rad. Therap. Nucl. Med., 121:22, 1974.

Edmonds, M. E., Morris, N., Laws, J. W., and Watkins, P. J.: Medial arterial calcification and diabetic neuropathy. Br. Med. J., 284:928, 1982.

Fagerberg, S. E.: Diabetic neuropathy, clinical and histological study on the significance of vascular affection. Acta Med. Scand. 345 Suppl. 1959.

Gendre, P. and Tinguard, R.: Ultrastructure of the human arterial wall in diabetic patients. J. Cardiovasc. Surg., 15:21, 1974.

Giabbani, V., Agrifoglio, G., Sironi, G., and Benedetti, G.: Nosological, clinical, topographic and histological elements of diabetic arteriopathy. J. Cardiovasc. Surg., 15:33, 1974.

Lithner, F. and Tornblom, N.: Gangrene localized to the lower limbs in diabetics. Acta Med. Scand., 208:315, 1980.

Locke, S., Lawrence, D. G., and Legg, M. A.: Diabetic amyotrophy. Am. J. Med., 34:775, 1963.

Rice, J. S.: Diabetic infection, ulceration and gangrene. J. Am. Podiatr. Assoc., 64:774, 1974.

Robbins, S. L. and Cotran, R. S.: Pathologic Basis of Disease, 2nd ed. Philadelphia, W.B. Saunders Company, 1979.

Shagan, B. P.: Is diabetes a model for aging? Med. Clin. North Am., 60:1209, 1976.

Sinha, S., Munichoodappa, C. S., and Kozak, G. P.: Neuroarthropathy (Charcot joints) in diabetes mellitus. Medicine, 51:91, 1972.

Strandness, D. E., Jr., Priest, R. E., and Gibbons, G. E.: Combined clinical and pathologic study of diabetic and nondiabetic peripheral arterial disease. Diabetes, 13:366, 1964.

Tilton, R. G., Hoffmann, P. L., Kilo, C., and Williamson, J. R.: Pericyte degeneration and basement membrane thickening in skeletal muscle capillaries of human diabetics. Diabetes, 30:326, 1981.

Warren, S., LeCompte, P. M., and Legg, M. A.: The Pathology of Diabetes Mellitus, 4th ed. Philadelphia, Lea & Febiger, 1966.

# Chapter 6

# DIABETIC NEUROPATHIES: LOWER EXTREMITIES

GEORGE P. KOZAK, M.D., and JOHN M. GIURINI, D.P.M.

The nervous system is so frequently involved in diabetes mellitus that neuropathy has been included in that triad of pathological conditions ("triopathy") characteristic of this disease—retinopathy, nephropathy, and neuropathy. Diabetic neuropathies comprise a polymorphous group of disorders ranging from those characterized by acute onset and reversibility to those characterized by insidious onset, continuous progression, and complete irreversibility. The etiology, pathogenesis, pathology, and diagnosis of these neurological disorders are quite diverse and contradictory. From a morbidity standpoint, the various neuropathies are certainly the most common among the major complications of diabetes. Although no definite figures are available, at least 50 per cent of patients with long-standing diabetes develop neurological complications. Diabetic neuropathy is rarely diagnosed before the fifth year of juvenile-onset (insulin-dependent) diabetes. In non-insulin-dependent diabetics, prior undetected hyperglycemia may have played a role in neuropathy noted at time of diagnosis. A referral-based cohort study consisting mainly of older non-insulin-dependent diabetic patients reported an 8 per cent overall incidence of neuropathy at time of diagnosis of diabetes. This increased with time to 40 per cent after 20 years of diabetes.

Despite this frequent occurrence, neuropathies are perhaps the most inadequately studied of the complications of diabetes, and little is known about them. Nevertheless, despite our ignorance, symptomatic treatment is possible. The development of clinical symptoms is usually related to duration of diabetes and periods of poor control. There are certainly many interesting inconsistencies related to various neuropathies and diabetic control. On occasion the neuropathic disorder can be the presenting feature of the newly diagnosed diabetes. The neuropathic disorders may certainly occur with presumed good control. The most frustrating is the paradoxical precipitation of neuropathy, particularly distal polyneuropathy, following institution of attempts at good control of the diabetic state by diet and oral agents or insulin. The onset of neuropathic symptoms with institution of treatment, particularly insulin, can be quite disconcerting to the patient. The patient should be forewarned of such a possibility.

## PATHOGENESIS

Pathogenesis of diabetic neuropathies is not yet fully understood. Possible explanations of the mode of development of different forms of this complication of diabetes mellitus are based on theories of changes in blood vessels or abnormalities of metabolism, or both (Table 6–1). No one as yet has attempted to correlate both vascular and metabolic theories. The vascular theory attributes diabetic neuropathy to the development of microangiopathy with thickening of the nutrient vessels (vasa nervorum), which may progress to complete occlusion of these vessels. Supporting this vascular theory of pathogenesis is the recovery seen in some forms of diabetic neuropathy after recanalization of blood vessels.

Currently the most popular theory for pathogenesis of diabetic neuropathy is the increased activity of the polyol (sorbitol—sugar alcohol of glucose) pathway in diabetic

## TABLE 6–1. THEORETICAL PATHOGENETIC MECHANISMS IN DIABETIC NEUROPATHY

Sorbitol (polyol) pathway: Schwann cell hyperosmolality due to sorbitol excess, swelling, and destruction
Occlusion of vasa nervorum
Decreased nerve *myo*inositol
Decreased nerve conduction
Altered myelin synthesis and deficient repair
Motor and sensory neuropathy
Autonomic disorders
Neurotropic factors: Nerve growth factors

Modified from Kozak, G.P.: Clinical Diabetes Mellitus. Philadelphia, W.B. Saunders Company, 1982.

neural tissue (Fig. 6–1). For excessive activity of the polyol (sorbitol) pathway to be present, the uncontrolled diabetic state associated with the following conditions is required: (1) hyperglycemia (insulin deficiency) and (2) tissues that contain the enzyme aldose reductase and tissues (nerve tissue, lens, aorta, red blood cell) in which intracellular glucose entry is not regulated by insulin.

In a normal individual, approximately 1 per cent of glucose is shunted through the polyol pathway, producing sorbitol and fructose. In the late 1950s, it was realized that sorbitol and fructose could be synthesized from glucose in mammalian tissues. To have healthy and motile sperm, fructose is required as a substrate for glycolysis. Plasma fructose is less than 2 mg/dl, whereas seminal fluid fructose is approximately 200 mg/dl. This crucial role in reproduction has to be taken into account if one considers the possibility of using enzyme inhibitors for future treatment. Besides nerve tissue, sorbitol and fructose accumulate in diabetic lenses

and play a definite role in production of "sugar cataracts." Accumulation of sorbitol has also been demonstrated in aortic intima and media of rabbits and humans. In animals, studies have shown localization of aldose reductase in Schwann cells and sorbitol dehydrogenase in axons. It is interesting to speculate that in diabetic patients, excessive sorbitol may accumulate in Schwann cells. Since the sorbitol lacks cell membrane permeability, the excess sorbitol may produce a toxic effect, resulting in segmental demyelination and impaired velocity of peripheral nerve conduction.

Pathological findings of segmental demyelination have been seen in human diabetic neuropathy. This possible toxic effect of sorbitol accumulation is an attractive biochemical hypothesis, and it would encourage the best metabolic control possible for diabetic patients. The polyol pathway offers one explanation of how hyperglycemia could contribute to development of peripheral neuropathy.

Recent studies suggest that a decrease in neurotrophic factors may play a role in the pathogenesis of diabetic neuropathy. Neurotrophic factors are proteins that promote the morphological differentiation, survival, and maturation of specific neuronal populations. A number of investigative studies are going on in regard to this possible etiology of neuropathy. The best characterized neurotrophic factor is called nerve growth factor. Future investigations might prove its clinical usefulness. Other neurotrophic factors include brain-derived neurotrophic factor, neurotrophin 3, neurotrophin 5, and ciliary neurotrophic factor. Insulin and the insulin-like growth factors are also being studied in re-

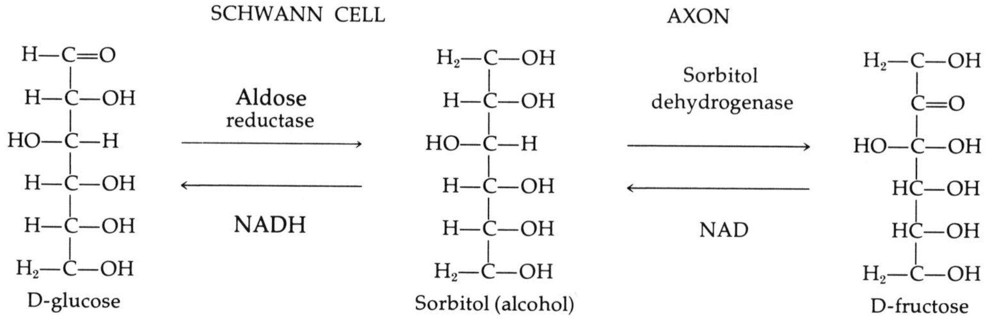

**Figure 6–1.** Polyol (sorbitol) pathway in nerve tissue. NADH = nicotinamide adenine dinucleotide (reduced form) and NAD = nicotinamide adenine dinucleotide. (From Kozak, G.P.: Clinical Diabetes Mellitus. Philadelphia, W.B. Saunders Company, 1982.)

## TABLE 6–2. CLASSIFICATION OF DIABETIC NEUROPATHIES ACCORDING TO THE STRUCTURE AFFECTED

| DIABETIC NEUROPATHY | AFFECTED STRUCTURE | PROBABLE ETIOLOGY | SIGNS AND SYMPTOMS |
| --- | --- | --- | --- |
| Radiculopathy | Nerve root | Vascular | Pain and sensory loss in distribution of a dermatome |
| Mononeuropathy | Mixed spinal or cranial nerve | Vascular | Pain, weakness, reflex change, sensory loss in distribution of mixed spinal or cranial nerve |
| Polyneuropathy | Nerve terminals | Metabolic (sorbitol) | Glove-and-stocking sensory loss, mild peripheral weakness, absence of reflexes |
| Diabetic amyotrophy | Nerve terminal? Muscle? | Unknown | Anterior thigh pain, weakness of pelvic girdle muscles, muscle atrophy, cachexia |
| Autonomic neuropathy | Sympathetic ganglion | Unknown | Postural hypotension, anhidrosis, impotence, gastropathy, diarrhea, vesical atony, gustatory sweating, cardiorespiratory arrest |

gard to possible pathogenesis and treatment of neurological problems.

Altered *myo*inositol metabolism may also play a role in the pathogenesis of peripheral neuropathy. *Myo*inositol (cyclic hexitol) is a normal constituent of plasma and cells. Approximately 0.5 gm of dietary *myo*inositol is ingested daily by humans. In uncontrolled diabetes, urinary excretion of *myo*inositol is greatly increased. This increase is attributed to the effects of high glucose concentrations on renal tubule absorption of *myo*inositol. Decreased nerve *myo*inositol concentrations have been shown to impair conduction nerve velocity in experimental animals. The decreased *myo*inositol is another biochemical upset that could explain how uncontrolled diabetes and hyperglycemia might contribute to development of peripheral neuropathy.

## CLASSIFICATION

Classification of diabetic neuropathies can be based on the anatomical locations of structures affected (Table 6–2 and Fig. 6–2). From a clinical standpoint, this has proved a useful tool. The lesions affecting the peripheral nervous system may be classified under five major headings: radiculopathy, mononeuropathy, polyneuropathy, amyotrophy, and autonomic neuropathy. There is most likely a vascular basis for the etiology of radiculopathy and mononeuropathy. The hypothesis of sorbitol accumulation is perhaps most likely in the most common form of diabetic neuropathy—distal symmetrical polyneuropathy. One can only speculate about the probable etiology of diabetic amyotrophy and the

number of disorders related to autonomic dysfunction.

## CLINICAL NEUROPATHIC DISORDERS

The major emphasis will be the discussion of the most common distal polyneuropathy and the rare diabetic amyotrophy. Limited discussion will be given to radiculopathy, mononeuropathy, postural hypotension, sweating disorder, and cardiorespiratory arrests. These are conditions that cause problems in management of diabetic foot and leg problems.

## RADICULOPATHY

Pain and sensory loss in the distribution of dermatomes overlying the thorax or abdomen are infrequently due to diabetic radiculopathy. Prior to considering a diabetic etiology, one needs to rule out other possible intrathoracic or intra-abdominal pathology as the cause of the pain. Radicular pain can be noted quite frequently as a prelude to herpes zoster lesions.

## MONONEUROPATHY

Mononeuropathy is a disorder of a single peripheral nerve, either mixed spinal or cranial. The most common peripheral nerve involvements include the ulnar, median, radial, axillary, femoral, peroneal, and the lateral cutaneous nerve of the thigh (meralgia par-

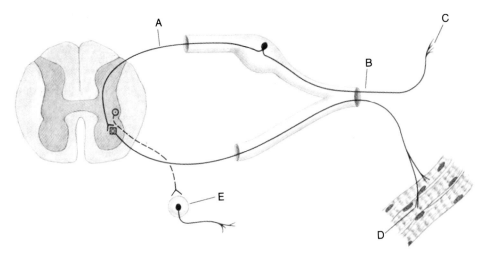

**Figure 6-2.** Spinal segment—anatomical localization. (From Kozak, G.P.: Clinical Diabetes Mellitus. Philadelphia, W.B. Saunders Company, 1982.)

| *Structure* | *Disorder* |
|---|---|
| A. Nerve root | Radiculopathy |
| B. Mixed spinal or cranial nerve | Mononeuropathy |
| C. Nerve terminals | Polyneuropathy |
| D Nerve terminal? Muscle? | Diabetic amyotrophy |
| E. Sympathetic ganglion | Autonomic neuropathy |

esthetica). Severe involvement of the femoral nerve will be discussed under Diabetic Amyotrophy. Involvement of all cranial nerves has been reported, but the most common disorders are oculomotor and abducens palsy. On rare occasions, phrenic, long thoracic, or obturator nerves are involved. The less frequent mononeuropathy multiplex is characterized by simultaneous or successive dysfunction of several peripheral nerves remote from one another. The onset is more rapid, and motor involvement usually outweighs the sensory. Recovery is the rule in the asymmetrical diabetic neuropathies, including mononeuropathies, mononeuropathy multiplex, and cranial nerve palsy. These differ from the most common polyneuropathy, which is a more diffuse and symmetrical disorder of the nerves. This will be discussed in the next section of disorders. A vascular etiology has long been suspected in the asymmetrical neuropathies. Multiple small infarcts in peripheral nerves and brain stem nuclei have been noted. Postmortem study of neuropathic disorders has, however, been extremely limited.

## POLYNEUROPATHY

### Clinical Features

The most common form of peripheral neuropathy is the slowly progressive symmet-
rical distal polyneuropathy involving both the lower and upper extremities. Subjective neuropathy symptoms may precede objective neurological findings. Two outstanding symptoms are pain and paresthesias. The nocturnal intensification of the pains is quite characteristic. Although the pain and paresthesias can be quite mild, the pains can be severely disabling in many patients. The discomfort can be unremitting, with characteristic cutaneous hypersensitivity leading to acute discomfort on contact with shoes and clothing. Constant burning symptoms tend to be especially severe at night, leading to insomnia and depression. Emotional upset, loss of appetite, and severe weight loss can be noted with severe pains. The polyneuropathy syndrome is more common in men than in women and occurs mainly with diabetes of long duration.

The severe forms of polyneuropathy do not occur solely in insulin-dependent patients. The condition may also be found in those with relatively mild diabetes not requiring insulin and sometimes without other complications. On rare occasions the polyneuropathy can be the presenting sign of diabetes. The lower extremity involvement usually occurs initially with sensory symptoms and signs, and reflex loss also can be noted. The ankle reflex loss precedes the loss of deep tendon reflexes of the knee. Diminished sensation to such stimuli as vibration, pinprick, or temperature can also be noted. Upper extremity involvement is also quite common in diabetes of long duration. Disabling pain in the hands is not common, but atrophy of intrinsic muscles can be noted in addition to sensory impairment. Severe hand pain should raise the possibility of carpal tunnel entrapment syndrome, which appears to be more common in diabetic patients. Entrapment syndrome should also be considered at other sites along nerve pathways, such as compression of the posterior tibial nerve behind the medial malleolus (tarsal tunnel syndrome). Symptoms of distal polyneuropathy can obscure the diagnosis of carpal or tarsal tunnel syndrome. Motor nerve conduction studies can be helpful in confirming the diagnosis in both carpal and tarsal tunnel syndromes.

## Prognosis

In diabetic polyneuropathy one can be optimistic that clearing of sensory disturbance (pain) should usually occur within six months to two years. Return of the patient's appetite and the ability to sleep undisturbed throughout the night are encouraging signs. Rapid improvement can then be expected. On occasion, recurrence of distal polyneuropathy has been noted at a later stage of the patient's diabetes.

## Treatment

Currently it appears that most important in prevention of neuropathic pains even after symptoms have appeared is tight diabetes management. This can be accomplished by using diet and oral agents or insulin as required. During the painful phase, symptomatic and supportive measures are indicated. The most popular drug therapy at the present time for pain control consists of the tricyclic antidepressants. Other medications used have included anticonvulsants (carbamazepine, phenytoin, and valproic acid) and topical agents (capsaicin). Amitriptyline is most commonly used, starting with a low dose of 10 to 25 mg/day; usually at least 100 mg is required for relief; maximal dose range would be 150 to 200 mg. Nortriptyline is used similarly with a maximal dose of 100 mg/day.

The anticonvulsant most commonly tried is carbamazepine (Tegretol). In view of possible toxicity and hazards, use of this medication should be followed with serial blood counts to check for possible bone marrow suppression or liver function abnormalities.

Capsaicin, a drug that presumably depletes substance P from nerve endings, can be applied topically as a cream to the burning extremities. Easing of the dysesthetic neuropathic pains may be noted perhaps on a counterirritant basis.

In our experience, simple analgesics, either singly or in combination, have been helpful. The use of single-agent aspirin, acetaminophen, or propoxyphene (Darvon) every four hours has been helpful in mild cases. The combination of propoxyphene hydrochloride with aspirin or acetaminophen every four hours and promazine hydrochloride (Sparine), 50 mg at bedtime, has been helpful in moderately painful cases. For severe pains, 25 mg promazine can be given every four hours during the day in addition to the 50 mg at bedtime.

Freedom from discomfort at night is the major desire of the patient. Instead of promazine, other drugs such as diazepam (Valium), 5 to 10 mg, or hydroxyzine (Vistaril), 25 mg, can be used. Some physicians have advocated stronger phenothiazines such as fluphenazine (Prolixin) or trifluoperazine (Stelazine), either singly or in combination with amitriptyline (Elavil, Etrafon), as being helpful. In our experience, amitriptyline has been occasionally helpful when depression is a major problem. With grossly uncontrolled diabetes, the patient may improve rapidly after starting treatment with insulin. Paradoxically, some patients temporarily become worse with onset of insulin therapy. This is certainly difficult for the patient to comprehend and accept.

Although there is no evidence of effectiveness, one might add a B complex with a C vitamin. Our experience with diphenylhydantoin (phenytoin, Dilantin) has been disappointing. The same applies to vitamin $B_{12}$ injections. Vitamin $B_{12}$ had the benefit of giving something over a temporal period during which spontaneous subsidence of symptoms is frequently noted. During the severe painful phase, sometimes a period of bed rest is helpful. On rare occasions, patients can become addicted to opiate-type medications. Such drugs are not usually required, and if at all possible, should be avoided. In view of the hematological and hepatic toxicity, one should have reservation about prescribing carbamazepine. Carbamazepine should be perhaps considered if one thinks about the use of opiate-type medication. This drug has been helpful in treating the severe neuralgia related to tic douloureux and glossopharyngeal neuralgia. In our limited experience, pain relief with the newer nonsteroidal analgesics has been inconsistent and variable. From a clinical investigational standpoint, one might consider the use of a high *myo*-inositol diet or an enzyme inhibitor for aldose reductase. In view of the effect upon fructose production, one might have some reservation about using the enzyme inhibitors for fear of interfering with normal sperm production.

## DIABETIC AMYOTROPHY

A rather striking, but infrequent, neuromuscular disorder is the syndrome of diabetic amyotrophy. In the early 1950s, when the clinical picture was described and popularized by Garland and Taverner, this disorder was named diabetic myelopathy, since extensor plantar responses were thought to signify disease of the spinal cord. Inability to demonstrate pathological defects in the central nervous system caused the name to be changed to diabetic amyotrophy. In 1890, the German pathologist Ludwig Bruns incriminated diabetes mellitus as a cause of wasting and weakness of the pelvic girdle muscles without sensory impairment. In addition, Bruns first described the distinct muscle pathological change of single-fiber atrophy. Whether diabetic amyotrophy is an appropriate name or whether it exists as a distinct clinical entity is under dispute. Some neurologists prefer the term *femoral motor neuropathy*. When one deals with a large number of diabetic patients, a rather striking clinical picture of diabetic amyotrophy is seen occasionally.

### Clinical Features

Diabetic amyotrophy was thought to occur only in elderly men in whom the abnormality of glucose metabolism was mild. In our experience, it occurs in females as well. The process is somewhat insidious and usually appreciated only when features are full blown. It is indeed a most striking abnormality. Extreme catabolism produces marked weight loss. Weakness and wasting of pelvic girdle muscles (iliopsoas, quadriceps, gluteal) and hamstring muscles are typical. In the initial stages, pain or other sensory disturbances can be noted in the muscles. On occasion, motor features can be predominant without any detectable sensory impairment. Severe myalgia and dysesthesia of the anterior thigh are noted quite frequently. These symptoms can be associated with an ill-defined sensory loss to pinprick. Although the disorder may begin unilaterally, it ultimately becomes bilateral. On occasion, muscle fasciculations and extensor plantar toe responses are present. The spinal fluid protein level in amyotrophy tends to be higher than that seen in distal polyneuropathy. Diabetic amyotrophy was aptly called neuropathia cachexia by Ellenberg.

Diabetic amyotrophy is usually a self-limited disease with a protracted course of approximately two years. In view of the extreme cachexia resulting from the catabolic state and muscle wasting, the major disease to be differentiated is polymyositis associated with occult carcinoma or with collagen disease. Other clinical features might be suggestive of hyperthyroid myopathy, amyotrophic lateral sclerosis, subacute necrotic myelitis, and other myopathies. As in other diabetic neurological disorders, diabetic amyotrophy is suggested by the clinical picture, but is indeed a diagnosis of exclusion.

### Diagnosis

Electromyography is not specific for diabetic amyotrophy. Electromyographic findings are suggestive of primary muscle disease as well as of a neurogenic lesion. Muscle biopsy can be helpful in confirming the clinical impression if diagnostic studies exclude the differential diagnostic possibilities mentioned earlier. Muscle biopsy reveals a characteristic pattern of single-fiber atrophy that does not conform to the pattern seen in atrophy of a motor unit or to that involving ischemic changes in muscle. Single-fiber atrophy and diabetic amyotrophy contrast with the usual picture of muscle atrophy due to nerve damage in which the smallest group of atrophic muscle fibers is that of a motor unit. In diabetic amyotrophy isolated muscle fibers become markedly narrow without losing cross-striations and myofibril pattern. No granular degeneration or necrosis is noted. The sarcolemmal cells condense around the atrophic muscle fiber, giving a false appearance of proliferation of these cells. Similar muscle biopsy findings can be seen in alcoholic myopathy.

## Prognosis

Symptoms associated with diabetic amyotrophy usually clear within 18 to 24 months, although microscopic changes on biopsy may persist after clinical recovery. Once the painful phase is over, a program of physical rehabilitation and muscle-strengthening exercises is beneficial. It is indeed quite gratifying to see someone who has been bedridden walk again after a period of two years. The same symptomatic and supportive measures used in diabetic polyneuropathy are applicable to diabetic amyotrophy during the painful phase.

## AUTONOMIC NEUROPATHY

### Postural Hypotension

#### Clinical Features

Postural hypotension is a common manifestation of autonomic neuropathy, usually occurring after 15 or more years of diabetes. The most common symptoms are lightheadedness or unsteadiness when standing or walking. Some patients experience associated nausea and vomiting. Sometimes these symptoms occur as soon as the patient arises in the morning. Symptoms often disappear after the patient is upright for a variable period. Postural hypotension should be distinguished from the unsteadiness of the diabetic with severe retinopathy and neuropathy whose visual failure prevents compensation for proprioceptive loss. Differentiation from hypoglycemic episodes can be difficult. Symptoms are usually transient, lasting only a few minutes, but sometimes they are sustained and cause falls during which frank loss of consciousness and skeletal fractures may occur.

Symptoms of postural hypotension may be markedly aggravated by various medications, particularly antihypertensive diuretics, phenothiazines, or tranquilizers. They are also often aggravated by dehydration, which is commonly associated with uncontrolled diabetes. A lack of compensatory tachycardia in association with a drop in blood pressure in the upright position may differentiate the neuropathy of postural hypotension from that of volume contraction.

A surprising number of patients will remain asymptomatic despite significant falls of systolic pressure—greater than 40 to 50 mm Hg. Postural hypotension must be recognized before it can be treated. This emphasizes the need to always check the standing blood pressure in diabetic patients. This is especially important prior to embarking on antihypertensive therapy, since some diabetic patients paradoxically may have hypertension with associated postural hypotension.

Symptoms may be ameliorated by cautious salt loading and use of 9 alpha-fludrocortisone acetate (Florinef). Florinef causes an increase in volume by sodium and water retention, but a direct effect on arterial tone has also been proposed. The dose required is usually 0.1 to 0.2 mg/day; on occasion, some patients have required 0.4 mg/day. A reasonable starting dose is 0.1 mg daily with close follow-up of weight gain, edema formation, and blood pressure changes. Since limited cardiac reserve with congestive failure and deteriorating renal function are quite common in those with long-term diabetes, these measures must be used cautiously and judiciously in such patients. Slight ankle edema toward the end of the day is often compatible with satisfactory control. Support garments such as elastic stockings and abdominal binders are probably of limited value.

Further clinical investigation and use will be required to determine the clinical benefits of ergot drugs and pindolol. Dihydroergotamine has direct and sustained vasoconstrictor actions, particularly affecting the venous circulation. Caution is definitely warranted in diabetic patients with generalized arteriosclerosis. Pindolol acts as a beta-adrenoreceptor agonist in orthostatic hypotension.

### Sweating Disorders

Sweating disorders are frequent in diabetic patients. Hyperhidrosis has been recorded at the time of initial diagnosis. Some patients with long-term diabetes complain of severe nocturnal sweating unrelated to hypoglycemia. Loss of sweating (self-sympathectomy) is common in the lower limbs, and hyperhidrosis tends to occur in unaffected areas. Many patients complain of discomfort in warm weather or at night, associated with drenching sweats of the face, neck, and upper chest. Damage to sudomotor fibers produces dry skin. Gustatory sweating is a less common symptom, but can be a sign of diabetic autonomic neuropathy. Within a few seconds of eating certain foods, the diabetic experiences profuse sweating of the face, neck, and upper chest. Cheese is the most powerful stimulus, but pickles, alcohol, and vinegar may also contribute. Relief from excessive sweating may be obtained by use of an anticholinergic such as propantheline (Pro-Banthine). Anticholinergics unfortunately give rise to their own unpleasant side effects and are not always well tolerated. The area affected is sharply demarcated and confined to the anatomical regions supplied by the superior cervical sympathetic ganglion (face, scalp, neck) and sometimes the shoulders and upper chest.

## Cardiorespiratory Arrest

In view of the wide anatomical distribution of diabetic neuropathy, it is not surprising that the cardiorespiratory system should also be involved. Although diabetic patients with advanced autonomic neuropathy are subject to unexpected cardiorespiratory arrest, anesthesia and surgery are usually tolerated. As a consequence of control of cardiac autonomic neuropathy, imbalance between the sympathetic and parasympathetic nervous system can be noted. Apnea is generally the primary event. Standard cardiac tests of autonomic regulation (amyl nitrite–provoked hypotension, carotid sinus pressure, Valsalva maneuver, and administration of phenylephrine) have had minimal, at times paradoxical, or no significant effect on heart rate in patients with diabetes of long duration. This is similar to the denervated heart following cardiac transplantation. Such patients have a tendency for unexplained tachycardia and development of arrhythmias. Infrequently, unexpected cardiac arrest has been noted. In such patients, physicians should be cautious in use of respiratory depressants and anesthetics. Pulmonary infections should be treated vigorously to avoid stressing the autonomous heart with limited responses due to autonomic neuropathy.

## Role of Neuropathy in Foot Ulcerations

While all three forms of diabetic neuropathy (i.e. sensory, motor, autonomic) play a role in the etiology of ulcerations, the major predisposing factor for plantar ulcerations is peripheral sensory neuropathy. The inability to detect painful stimuli or injury to the lower extremity results in the loss of an important protective mechanism. The ability is lost to detect the presence of a pebble in the shoe or the wrinkling of a sock, either of which can lead to skin irritation. Sharp objects such as an insulin needle can penetrate the sole of the foot without detection. Loss of this early warning signal allows relatively simple and minor problems to quickly progress to limb-threatening situations.

In 1959, Kosiak demonstrated that ulcerations can develop in neuropathic limbs even at low pressures if applied continuously over long periods. Kosiak and Brand both outlined mechanisms of injury that typically lead to ulcerations:

1. Low pressure, continuous stress: When relatively low pressures are applied for long periods, the classic signs of early ulceration were seen to develop, i.e. redness, warmth, swelling, and blistering. Pressures as low as 2 to 3 psi when applied continuously for eight hours were sufficient to cause ulcerations. The classic example of this type of stress is heel decubitus ulceration.

2. High pressure, short duration stress: Certain pressures are significantly high enough to cause primary ulceration of the neuropathic foot. When those pressures are applied over a very small area of the foot, they need to be applied only for a very short time to cause injury to the foot. The pressures are typically in the range of 700 to 1000 psi. The prime example of this principle is the puncture wound, i.e. insulin needle or sharp tack.

3. Moderate pressure, repetitive stress: This is the most common mechanism for the development of neuropathic ulcerations.

While the pressures involved are not especially high (20 to 60 psi), the repetitive nature of these injuries has a cumulative effect on the diabetic neuropathic foot. This does not take into account any structural or biomechanical deformities that may further increase local pressure on the foot. While pressure plays an important role in ulcer formation, areas with bony prominences are especially vulnerable. Deformities such as plantar flexed metatarsals, bunion deformities, or hammer toe deformities result in areas of increased focal pressure and increased susceptibility to ulceration. These deformities often lead to excessive callus formation that subsequently develops subepidermal blistering. With continued ambulation, the blister becomes a penetrating ulcer.

Motor neuropathy, while less common than sensory neuropathy, may also play a significant role in the etiology of ulcerations. Specifically, motor neuropathy contributes to ulceration in two ways: (1) With increasing levels of motor neuropathy there is loss of intrinsic muscle function. These muscles, the interossei and the lumbricales, are important in maintaining digital stability at the metatarsophalangeal joint level. With the loss of intrinsic muscle function, the larger and stronger long extensors of the foot begin to overpower the long flexors, thus causing progressive musculoskeletal deformities such as claw toes, hammer toes, and plantar flexed metatarsals to develop. This results in potential shoe irritation over the dorsum of the toes and excessive pressures and callus formation on the plantar surface of the foot, thus increasing the risk of ulceration. (2) Motor neuropathy may selectively affect the larger muscles of the leg, specifically the anterior tibial and extensor hallucis longus muscles, which are supinators and dorsiflexors of the ankle. Loss of function of these large leg muscles adversely affects the foot during gait so that instability and drop-foot deformities develop. Additionally, the normal phasic activity of agonist-antagonist muscles is altered so that the foot is pronated and plantar flexed and consequently spends more time in contact with the ground. This allows moderate pressures to build up over a small area and to act over a longer time.

Autonomic neuropathy has received a great deal of interest in the past five years. Its role in gastroparesis, impotence, and cardiovascular abnormalities is well known and well documented. However, its role in ulcer formation is only now beginning to be investigated. It has been widely known that autonomic neuropathy is responsible for diminution or absence of sweating in the lower extremity. This lack of sweat production, or anhidrosis, leads to dry skin with cracking and fissuring. Interestingly, while anhidrosis is commonly seen in the lower extremity, patients with autonomic neuropathy suffer from hyperhidrosis in the upper half of the body, as seen in gustatory sweating—profuse sweating following meals.

Recently, however, there has been increased interest in the vasomotor disturbances produced by autonomic neuropathy. These disturbances can lead to abnormal vasodilatation and vasoconstriction resulting in distention of dorsal veins. It has been well documented that this leads to arteriovenous (AV) shunting in the foot. Several investigators believe that the AV shunting is a major cause of neuropathic ulcerations based on the fact that microvascular changes occurring in the skin result in decreased oxygenation. Along this same line of thought, Edmonds et al. have postulated that AV shunting plays a significant role in the pathogenesis of Charcot joint disease in diabetic patients. The increased blood flow to bones of the feet leads to increased demineralization and osteopenia in neuropathic feet. This results in weakening of the bony structure and increased susceptibility to fractures.

While this theory has been difficult to prove conclusively, it is a well-described observation that Charcot joint disease is rarely seen in diabetic patients with documented peripheral vascular disease. However, much controversy still exists on the effect of autonomic neuropathy on the foot. Young et al. investigated 106 diabetic patients: 33 with no symptoms of neuropathy, 28 with newly painful neuropathy, 24 with chronic painful neuropathy, and 21 with painless neuropathy and recurrent foot ulcers. In the three symptomatic groups, both electrophysiology and autonomic function were more abnormal than in the asymptomatic group. When each group was evaluated individually, autonomic function was abnormal to an equal degree in the three symptomatic groups while electrophysiologic function was significantly more abnormal in the foot ulcer group.

In a similar study performed by Seshiah et al., 96 diabetic patients were studied. Clinical evaluation showed 32 patients had sexual dysfunction, 25 patients had peripheral neuropathy, and 10 patients had foot ulcerations. Of the 96 patients, 76 (79.16 per cent) had abnormal responses to autonomic function testing. The authors further noted that all 10 patients with foot ulcerations tested abnormally, as did 21 of the 32 and 16 of the 25 in the other two groups. Based on these data, the authors conclude that autonomic neuropathy leads to the initiation and propagation of diabetic foot ulcers. What the authors fail to explain is the fact that 66 of the 76 (86.8 per cent) abnormal respondents on autonomic function testing had no history of foot ulceration. One can conclude that autonomic neuropathy is a common feature of diabetic neuropathy, but its contribution to the etiology of diabetic ulcerations is not fully understood.

Finally, mention should be made about the patient's perception of his own neuropathy, i.e., the psychology of sensation. Several years ago, Brand wrote a marvelous monograph that described the psychology of sensation in these neuropathic patients. In it he states that a normal person's body image is based on the sensory input that person receives from his body. Because the neuropathic patient loses this input, that limb is removed from the person's consciousness. Consequently, patients will neglect wounded hands and feet to the point of gross sepsis and destruction. They will describe walking as though their feet were blocks of wood and not attached to their legs. They will continue to walk normally and avoid any shoes or assistive devices that may label them as disabled. We as physicians must temper our disgust or impatience, as this often reinforces a patient's already low self-image. This attitude may lead to a feeling of inevitability on the part of patients that their limbs are not worth saving.

## SUGGESTED READING LIST

Albert, I.W., and Greene, D.A.: Diabetic polyneuropathy: The importance of insulin deficiency, hyperglycemia and alterations in myoinositol metabolism in its pathogenesis. N. Engl. J. Med. 295:1416, 1976.

Apfel, S.C., and Kessler, J.A.: Diabetic neuropathy: Current management and future treatments. Drug Therapy May:17–30, 1993.

Asbury, A.K.: Focal and multifocal neuropathies of diabetes. In Dyck, P.J., Thomas, P.K., Winegrad, A.L., Porte, D., (eds.): Diabetic Neuropathy. Philadelphia, W.B. Saunders, 1987, pp. 45–55.

Boulton, A.J.M., Scarpello, J.H.B., and Ward, J.D.: Venous oxygenation in the diabetic neuropathic foot: Evidence of arteriovenous shunting. Diabetologia 72:6–8, 1981.

Brand, P.W.: Pathomechanics of diabetic (neuropathic) ulcers and its conservative management. In Bergan and Yao: Gangrene and Severe Ischemia of the Lower Extremities. Grune & Stratton, New York, 1978, pp. 117–130.

Brand, P.W.: Pathomechanics of pressure ulcerations. In Symposium on the Neurologic Aspects of Plastic Surgery. C.V. Mosby, St. Louis, 1978, pp. 185–189.

Edmonds, M.E., Roberts, V.C., and Watkins, P.J.: Blood flow in the diabetic neuropathic foot. Diabetologia, 22:9–15, 1982.

Gabbay, K.H.: The sorbitol pathway and the complications of diabetes. N. Engl. J. Med. 15:831–836, 1973.

Garland, H.T.: Diabetic amyotrophy. Br. J. Clin. Pract. 15:9, 1961.

Garland, H., and Taverner, D.: Diabetic myelopathy. Dr. Med. J. 1:1405–1408, 1953.

Greene, D.A., Sima, A.A.F., Stevens, M.J., et al.: Complications: Neuropathy, Pathogenic Considerations. Diabetes Care 15:1902–1915, 1992.

Kosiak, M.: Etiology and pathology of ischemic ulcers. Arch. Phys. Med. Rehabilitation 40:62–69, 1959.

Kozak, G.P.: Diabetic Neuropathies. In Kozak, G.P. (ed.): Clinical Diabetes Mellitus. Philadelphia, W.B. Saunders, 1982, pp. 228–301.

Leedman, P.J., Davis, S., and Harrison, L.C.: Diabetic amyotrophy. Aust. NZ J. Med. 18:768–773, 1988.

Locke, S., Lawrence, S.G., and Legg, M.A.: Diabetic amyotrophy. Am. J. Med. 34:775, 1963.

Seshiah V., Venkataraman S., Madhavan R., et al.: Autonomic neuropathy and sexual dysfunction, peripheral neuropathy and foot syndrome in diabetes mellitus. In Ward and Goto, eds. Diabetic Neuropathy. New York, John Wiley & Sons, 1990, pp. 425–428.

Vinik A.I., Holland M.T., Le Beau J.M., et al.: Diabetic neuropathies. Diabetes Care 15:1926–1975, 1992.

Vinik, A.I.: Management of painful syndromes in diabetes mellitus. Clinical Diabetes July/August 57–62, 1991, 1992.

Watkins, P.J.: Natural history of the diabetic neuropathies. Q. J. Med. 77:1209–1218, 1990.

Young R.J., Zhou Y.Q., Rodriguez E. et al.: Variable relationship between peripheral somatic and autonomic neuropathy in patients with different syndromes of diabetic polyneuropathy. Diabetes 35:192–197, 1986.

# Chapter 7

# BIOMECHANICAL CONSIDERATIONS OF THE DIABETIC FOOT

GEOFFREY HABERSHAW, D.P.M.,
and JAMES CHZRAN, D.P.M.

## THE PROBLEM

The highest priority in managing foot problems in the diabetic is prevention, and there is more to prevention than the simple cautioning of patients to never go barefoot. The concern from the physician's point of view is to identify those factors that have already caused or have the potential to cause damage to the foot. To make this more than an admonition, let us consider how damage to the foot can occur.

## FORCES AFFECTING THE FOOT

*Friction* is the resistance that any body meets in moving over another body. The more irregular the surfaces in contact, the greater the friction. The smoother the surfaces in contact, the less the friction. Thus the more irregular the shape of the foot, the greater the chance of friction-induced tissue breakdown over its irregularities. Constant and rapid friction against the skin forms blisters, such as a heel blister from a new shoe. Intermittent and slow friction causes calluses and corns, such as the hard corn on the little toe from tight shoes and the even-thickness callus across the ball of the foot in those who are obese or wear high-heeled shoes.

*Pressure* is the force exerted by one body on another by its weight. For a given weight, the pressure is inversely proportional to the area the body rests on. As the area increases, the pressure goes down; as it decreases, the pressure goes up (Fig. 7–1). Unremitting direct pressure against tissue causes ischemia and necrosis. The skin over a bunion in a tight shoe will die when subjected to such pressure. Decubitus ulcer on a heel is another example. Intermittent direct pressure against tissue above the normal limits of tolerance causes localized hyperemia, edema, and eventual tissue breakdown if the pressure is not relieved. Periodic relief allows for tissue recovery and eventual toughening or keratin-

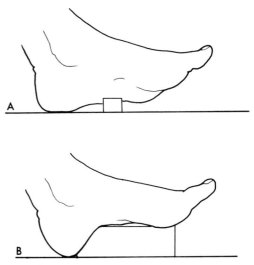

**Figure 7–1.** As the surface area of the object increases, the pressure decreases. The pressure beneath the foot about to step on a small object will be much greater than that beneath the foot about to step on a large object. Soft tissue damage can be expected in *A,* but only minor irritation in *B.*

**53**

on hard modern surfaces has not been compensated for genetically. Natural selection may eventually correct this, but for now accommodation becomes necessary. Shoes provide support for the musculoskeletal elements and cushioning for shock absorption and alteration of forces, especially shear. This "shoe environment" allows for potential situations in which skin and tissue breakdown may occur rapidly with concurrent insensitivity and/or ischemia.

A cross section of the foot within a shoe through the metatarsophalangeal joints is illustrated in the upper portion of Figure 7–6. Forces acting on the foot may be represented by three circles, designated A, B, and C in the lower portion of Figure 7–6. The pressure generated by the dynamic action of the foot, transmitted through the skin to the leather of the shoe, is a direct function of the radius of each circle, while the frictional forces generated are inversely proportional to the radius of the circle. This illustration is indicative of forces generated in a single plane. A wide foot with a hallux valgus bunion deformity in a narrow shoe will have frictional forces acting in the frontal, sagittal, and transverse planes, and it is not uncommon to see medial tissue breakdown over a first metatarsal head in a patient with hallux valgus.

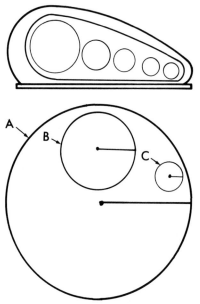

**Figure 7–6.** Relative pressures on different parts of the foot are proportional to the sizes of the circles. A, The dorsum of the foot; B, The first metatarsal head; and C, The fifth metatarsal head.

This simple principle is true for many other situations that may cause tissue breakdown in the insensitive, ischemic foot. Stiff, rigid leather against hammer toes, the rough liner of a shoe chafing a toe or a bunion, the back portion or counter of a shoe rubbing against the heel or chafing the lower surface of the lateral malleolus or ankle bone, a nail protruding through a worn heel, creasing of the shoe upper against a tight, contracted tendon on the top of the foot—these are just some shoe problems that must be taken into consideration when dealing with insensitive feet.

Shoe selection for a particular foot must be dictated by the shoe's mechanical structure, the observed or purported dynamic action of the foot, and the degree to which insensitivity or ischemia has affected the lower extremity. Shoe selection must be influenced if not determined by the health care team.

## THE DIABETIC FOOT

The term "diabetic foot" indicates that there are specific qualities about the feet of people with diabetes that sets this disease apart from other conditions that affect the lower extremity. This is true because of the concurrent neurological and circulatory involvement. Taken separately, anything that can affect the feet of the patient with diabetes can also affect the nondiabetic. The dynamic function and static structure of the diabetic foot are indirectly affected by changes in the neurological and circulatory systems of the lower extremity. The most significant changes occur in the presence of neurological deficit (Fig. 7–7). Examination of these feet rapidly demonstrates the alteration of sensory impulses transmitted proximally as evidenced by decreased vibratory, pinprick, and light touch sensation. It also becomes apparent that sensory deficit is accompanied by motor involvement, that of muscular atrophy attended by weakness. Most apparent are the cocked-up toes, plantarly prominent metatarsal heads, intrinsic muscular wasting, equinus deformity of the ankle, and varus position of the hindfoot. These deformities are commonly observed in rigid cavovarus foot types, which are characterized by stiffness, lack of motion, low tolerance to shock, an inability to compensate for irregularities

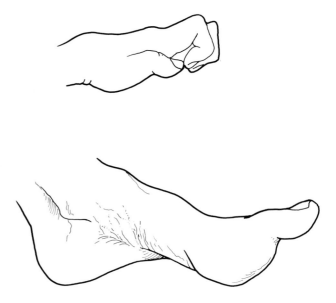

**Figure 7–7.** The "intrinsic minus foot" is characterized by atrophy of the small muscles that are responsible for metatarsophalangeal stabilization. Claw toes, prominent metatarsal heads, and pes cavus attitude are some of the developments. Comparison of the intrinsic minus foot with the intrinsic minus hand shows many similarities. Proximal phalangeal extension becomes prominent because of intrinsic failure, placing the powerful long flexors at a mechanical advantage. This accentuates the claw finger or claw toe phenomenon.

in terrain, and proximal malalignment (Fig. 7–8).

The intrinsic muscles of the foot are mid-stance phase muscles that function as stabilizers of the metatarsophalangeal joints. They stabilize the phalanges against the metatarsal heads, immediately before the powerful push-off motions of the foot. Although the functions of the intrinsic musculature of the hand and foot are different, atrophy produces very similar-appearing deformities. The result is the loss of fine motor control in the hand, and loss of stability at the metatarsophalangeal joints in the foot. There is flexion of the hand at the wrist and of the foot at the ankle, extension of the proximal phalanges at the metacarpophalangeal and metatarsophalangeal joints, and flexion of the proximal interphalangeal joints of both the hand and the foot.

Deformities arising from neuropathies are attributable not only to the intrinsic musculature; depending upon the severity and level of the neuropathy, the proximal musculature will also be affected. The extensor hallucis longus muscle is affected early. Weakness of this muscle allows hammering of the hallux by the overriding pull of the long flexor (Fig. 7–9). Bony prominences develop as shown in the drawing, with possible tissue breakdown in the neuropathic foot. Some feel that the effect is displacement of the protective subcutaneous fat from the metatarsal heads, which are then unprotected during stance and ambulation, leading to added soft tissue trauma and eventual ulceration.

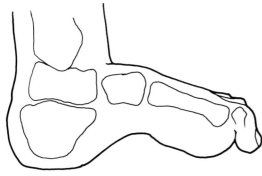

**Figure 7–8.** The pes cavus is a poor functional machine characterized by rigidity and lack of ability to accommodate to irregular terrain—it is a poor shock absorber. This type of foot is in constant peril if sensory neuropathy begins to emerge.

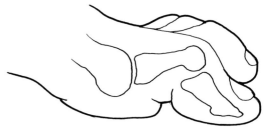

**Figure 7–9.** Hammered hallux deformity is depicted in this drawing. With weakness of the extensor hallucis longus muscle, affected early in diabetic neuropathy, the long flexor overpowers it, extending the proximal phalanx and flexing the distal phalanx. With concomitant sensory deficit, ulceration could occur at the distal aspect or over the dorsum of the toe.

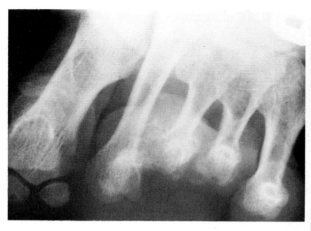
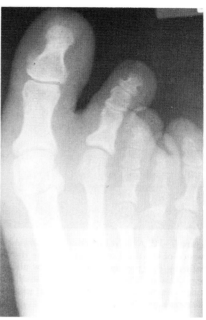

**Figure 7–16.** Brachymetatarsia or congenitally short metatarsals disturb the metatarsal parabola in that adjacent normal-length metatarsals will encounter undue stress and compromise soft tissue.

essarily changed. Removal of one of the lesser toes usually has little effect on the posture and function of the foot, whereas ablation of the hallux or a lesser toe and a metatarsal head can have a dramatic effect on pressure points and function of the foot in gait. As was stated earlier, as the weight-bearing surface area beneath the foot decreases, the pressure on the remaining weight-bearing surface area increases. Identical pressure on less surface area can cause rapid soft tissue breakdown.

The course of weight distribution along the plantar surface of the foot during gait is depicted in Figure 7–17. At toe-off the force of the body weight exits through the hallux.

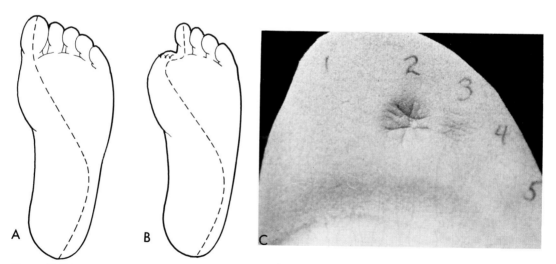

**Figure 7–17.** *A,* The course of weight distribution along the plantar surface of the normally functioning foot during the gait cycle. At toe-off, the main force exits through the hallux. *B,* When the hallux has been amputated the force exits through the next toe, the second. This is why it is not uncommon to see an ulceration develop at the tip of the second toe after hallux amputation. *C,* An insole was removed from the shoe of a diabetic patient who had prior hallux amputation. The imprint of the second toe clearly shows the excessive pressure through this toe.

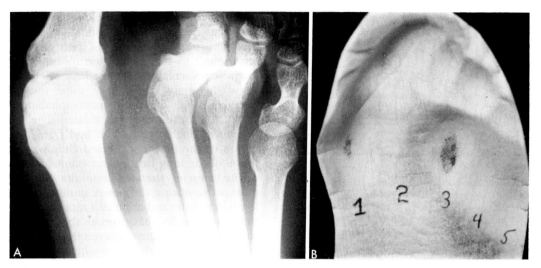

**Figure 7–18.** *A,* Radiograph after second toe and metatarsal head amputation. The removal of a metatarsal head lessens the effective weight-bearing surface in the forefoot. Excess pressure is distributed to the remaining metatarsal heads with possible tissue compromise. *B,* The same patient. Excessive pressure is demonstrated beneath the third metatarsal head. Tissue breakdown is prevented by the use of appropriate shoes and accommodative orthotics.

After hallux amputation, the forces and weight are the same during gait, but the hallux is no longer there to dissipate the force at push-off. Instead, the force is transmitted laterally to the lesser digits through the long flexor tendons, causing hammering of the toes. The greatest force lies beneath the second toe and to a lesser degree laterally. Neglect of this phenomenon may result in rapid ulceration of the distal tips of the lesser toes with the possibility of further amputation. Treatment is directed toward maintaining the foot on a molded total contact device to provide functional hindfoot control and cushioning for the forefoot. Flexor tenotomy is sometimes necessary when recurrent ulceration persists in a flexible toe. Arthroplasty is necessary when the toe is no longer flexible. Amputation of a second toe and metatarsal head similarly shifts push-off force laterally (Fig. 7–18).

The forefoot may be divided into three columns in the sagittal plane (Fig. 7–19). The medial column consists of the hallux, first metatarsal, and medial cuneiform. The central column comprises the second, third, and fourth toes, their metatarsals, and the connecting cuneiforms. The lateral column consists of the fifth toe, fifth metatarsal, and proximally located cuboid. The medial and lateral columns have independent ranges of motion that go through full excursion during gait and are as a result more flexible than the central column. The central column functions as a unit during gait and is typically rigid, having firm proximal interosseous ligamentous attachments. Amputation of parts of the central column is more likely to result in ulceration beneath the metatarsal head directly adjacent to the site of previous ulceration (so-called transfer ulceration), whereas loss of the distal medial or distal lateral columns (first toe and metatarsal head or fifth toe and metatarsal head) is tolerated more readily by the foot. We always recommend protective shoe gear and accommodative orthotic devices after any type of partial foot amputation. The possibility of transfer ulceration depends on age, body morphology, and activity level resumed after surgery.

The transmetatarsal amputation as performed at the New England Deaconess Hospital is the most radical amputation confined solely to the foot. Chopart's and Syme's amputations are not commonly performed because of the need for cumbersome prostheses and because of functional problems that may occur after surgery. The unique combination of the transmetatarsal amputation and vascular surgical techniques has saved hundreds of legs, as has the transmetatarsal amputation alone.

The transmetatarsal amputation is performed as a salvage procedure in order that

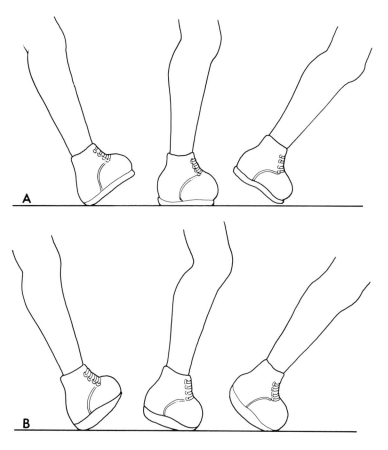

**Figure 7-23.** Three positions of the foot during gait: heel contact, midstance, and toe-off, after transmetatarsal amputation. *A,* in a short shoe without a rocker sole, the foot remains on the ground longer at midstance. *B,* with a rocker sole the knee rapidly flexes at midstance when the short shoe *touches* the ground. This allows a rapid forward motion of the leg with early heel-off, causing pressure to traverse the plantar surface of the foot more rapidly. The disadvantage is the need for rapid motion, which may require some external support such as a cane or walker, until the patient is accustomed to the alteration of gait.

commodative devices like the one pictured in Figure 7–24 can be used.

Achilles tenotomy has sometimes been performed to dramatically diminish the force across the distal aspect of a transmetatarsal amputation that is chronically ulcerated, despite exhaustive conservative measures. This procedure is done only when the clinical sit-

uation is ideal as to medical condition, mechanical considerations, and proposed activity levels after surgery. When this tendon is severed the patient is able to ambulate quite effectively at low velocities. High-speed ambulation is not comfortable because of the effective loss of the gastrocnemius-soleus muscle group. A noticeable limp will occur

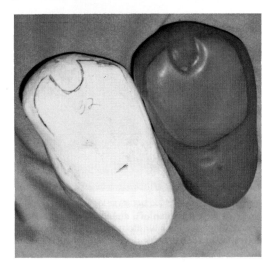

**Figure 7-24.** Chronic ulceration at the distal plantar aspect of a transmetatarsal amputation stump is sometimes controllable with a device such as this latex sock. It allows for pressure to be directed away from the site of the chronic problem.

with high velocity that will subside when velocity is diminished. Some power in plantar-flexion will remain with the tibialis posterior, peroneus longus, and peroneus brevis muscles.

## ABOVE THE FOOT

The mechanics of the foot are complicated, fascinating, and certainly not completely understood. It must be remembered, however, that all motion in the foot, diabetic or nondiabetic, is complicated further by the structure and function of the musculoskeletal units above the foot. The proximal structures must be scrutinized in great detail to fully appreciate what forces may be jeopardizing insensitive tissue. Anything that compromises the ideal parallel and perpendicular arrangement of the hip, thigh, and leg to the foot is potentially a problem. Congenital anomalies, the arthritides, and progressive vascular occlusion are obvious in their contribution to foot pathology. More subtle are the neurological changes, sensory and motor, that can occur with the neuropathy of diabetes mellitus. Examples are weakening or paralysis of the anterior leg muscles causing a drop foot and paralysis or weakness of proximal thigh and pelvic muscles. All of these entities must be fully understood and their relationship to foot function evaluated before effective therapy for an insensitive diabetic extremity can be achieved.

## SUGGESTED READING LIST

Asbury, A.K.: Understanding diabetic neuropathy. N. Engl. J. Med. 319:577–578, 1988.

Boulton, A.J.M.: The importance of abnormal foot pressures and gait in the causation of foot ulcers. *In* Connor H., Boulton A.J.M., and Ward J.D. (eds.): The Foot in Diabetes. Chichester, U.K., John Wiley & Sons, 1987, pp. 11–21.

Brand, P.W.: Insensitive Foot Seminar. Rehabilitation Branch, United States Public Health Service Hospital, Carville, LA, 1982.

Brink, S.J.: Limited joint mobility as a risk factor for diabetes complications. Clin. Diabetes 5:123–127, 1987.

Brownlee, M., Cerami, A., and Vlassara, H.: Advanced glycosylation endproducts in tissue and the biochemical basis of diabetic complications. N. Engl. J. Med. 318:1315–1321, 1988.

Buell, T., Green, D.R., and Risser, J.: Measurement of the first metatarsophalangeal joint range of motion. J. Am. Podiatr. Med. Assoc. 78:439–448, 1988.

Cavanagh, P.R., Hennig, E.M., Rodgers, M.M., and Sanderson, D.J.: The measurement of plantar pressure on the plantar surface of diabetic feet. *In* Whittle, M., and Harris, D. (eds.): Biochemical measurement in orthopedic practice. Oxford; Clavendon Press, 1985, pp. 234–243.

Cavanagh, P.R., and Rodgers, M.M.: The arch index: A useful measure from foot prints. J. Biomechanics 20:547–551, 1987.

Coleman, W.C., Brand, P.W., and Birke, J.A.: The total contact cast: A therapy for plantar ulceration on insensitive feet. J. Am. Podiatry Assoc. 74:548–552, 1984.

Diabetes Control and Complications Trial Research Group: Factors in development of diabetic neuropathy. Diabetes 37:476–481, 1988.

Delbridge, L., et al.: The aetiology of diabetic neuropathic ulceration of the foot. Br. J. Surg. 72:1–6, 1985.

Duckworth, T., Boulton, A.J.M., Betts, R.P., et al.: Plantar pressure measurements and the prevention of ulceration in the diabetic foot. J. Bone Joint Surg. 67B:79–85, 1985.

Edmonds, M.E.: The diabetic foot: Pathophysiology and treatment. Clin. Endocrinolog. Metab. 15:889–915, 1986.

Hall, C.O., and Brand, P.W.: The etiology of neuropathic plantar ulceration. J. Am. Podiatry Assoc. 69:173–177, 1979.

Lawrence, A. M. and Abraira, C.: Diabetic neuropathy. A review of the clinical manifestations. Ann. Clin. Lab. Sci., 6:78–83, 1976.

Locke, S.: The peripheral nervous system in diabetes mellitus. Diabetes 13:307–311, 1964.

LoGerfo, F.W.: Vascular disease, matrix abnormalities, and neuropathy: Implications for limb salvage in diabetes mellitus. J. Vasc. Surgery 5:793–796, 1987.

LoGerfo, F.W., and Coffman, J.D.: Vascular and microvascular disease of the foot in diabetes. N. Engl. J. Med. 311:1615–1619, 1984.

Root, M. L., William, P., and Weed, J. H.: Normal and Abnormal Function of the Foot. Clinical Biomechanics Corporation, 1977.

Thompson, D.E.: The effects of mechanical stress on soft tissue. *In* Levin, M.E., and O'Neal, L.W. (eds.): The Diabetic Foot, 4th ed. St. Louis, CV Mosby Co., 1988, pp. 91–103.

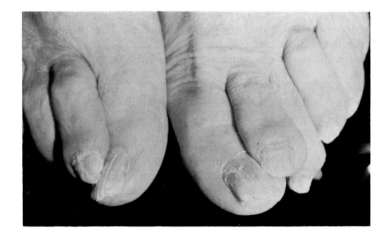

**Figure 8-1** Onychomycosis. Note the opaque white appearance of the thickened nails.

be idiopathic, iatrogenic, or secondary to injured or displaced matrix tissue, hypertrophic skin folds, and subungual exostoses (Fig. 8–2). Tight shoes and injudicious nail care often lead to an inflamed nail fold due to an offending nail border or spicule. Patients in the habit of "digging out" the corners often leave a deep portion of the nail intact in the distal nail groove. This spicule acts as a lance that eventually grows into the distal skin, becoming extremely painful (Fig. 8–3). A paronychia develops when the ungualabia (nail fold) becomes inflamed and/or infected (Fig. 8–4). A chronic paronychia will incite the "proudflesh," or granuloma, formation.

The primary goal of treatment is to remove the portion of nail that is irritating the skin. Only after this is accomplished will the paro-

nychia subside. A simple debridement of the distal corner may very well suffice. In the more advanced cases avulsion of the involved nail border under local anesthesia may be necessary. Additionally, wet compresses or soaks and topical applications of hexylresorcinol (S.T. 37) or povidone-iodine (Betadine) are used until the inflammation has resolved. Rarely are systemic antibiotics required for a simple paronychia. However, in the presence of cellulitis, peripheral vascular disease, or significant neuropathy, antibiotics should always be included in the therapy.

Chronic recurring onychocryptosis is best treated by excision of the nail border and matrix (matrixectomy). This will permanently eradicate the offending nail border, as opposed to the temporary relief offered by simple avulsion. If the entire nail plate is

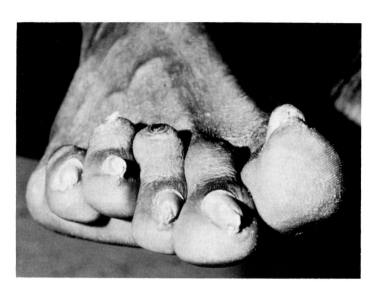

**Figure 8-2** Onychocryptosis. All nails are severely incurvated and painful. They are difficult to cut.

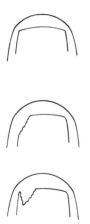

**Figure 8–3** *Top,* Properly trimmed nail. *Center* and *bottom,* Improperly trimmed nail results in a spicule that grows forward and incites development of a paronychia.

troublesome, a total matrixectomy should be performed. In the diabetic it is wiser to have the matrix removed surgically rather than with phenol or sodium hydroxide solutions (chemocautery). The latter techniques result in a prolonged period of drainage and susceptibility to infection. Of course in the ischemic "high-risk" foot, periodic podiatric care should be the only method of treatment.

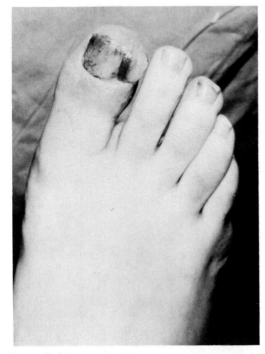

**Figure 8–4** Paronychia. The entire toe has become inflamed. Note the granuloma formation from chronic irritation to the lateral nail border.

*Tinea pedis* is especially common in the diabetic foot. Once again, host resistance is an associated factor. Very commonly the patient with a chronic dermatophytosis will be found to have mycotic toenails as the source of the infection. The infecting organisms for onychomycosis and tinea pedis are the same. *Trichophyton mentagrophytes, T. rubrum,* and *Epidermophyton floccosum* are the most frequent offenders. Less commonly, *Candida albicans* will be found.

The patient will usually have a slightly pruritic, desquamating, erythematous rash on the soles of both feet. One foot may show more involvement than the other. Looked at closely, there may be evidence of small superficial vesicles, especially at the periphery of the rash. This is the typical "moccasin" distribution associated with a chronic *T. rubrum* infection. In the more acute cases caused by *T. mentagrophytes* the rash will be more localized and severe. Larger weeping vesicles may predominate, with surrounding crusted lesions and secondary bacterial infection. The interdigital spaces will often have a white macerated appearance with fissuring at the skin creases. Diagnosis is confirmed by KOH examination or culture of skin scrapings from active peripheral lesions. Dermatophytosis must be distinguished from candidiasis, dyshidrotic eczema, contact dermatitis, atopic dermatitis, erythrasma, and psoriasis, to name but a few differential diagnoses. The reader is referred to appropriate dermatology texts for specific characteristics of each.

Treatment consists of drying the moist lesions and applying topical antifungal agents. Burow's solution, soaks, or wet compresses will have a drying and soothing effect on the macerated areas. This should be followed by twice daily applications of antifungal cream or solutions. Clotrimazole (Lotrimin) and miconazole nitrate (Micatin) have been found to be very effective, owing to their broader spectrum, which is also active against *Candida albicans.* Solutions are more efficacious for interdigital lesions because of their drying properties. Since the fungi thrive in moist environments, efforts must be made to keep the feet dry. This includes drying between the toes after bathing, dusting lightly with talcum powder, and wearing absorbent nonsynthetic stockings. Sneakers and vinyl shoes should be avoided in favor of leather shoes, which can breathe and allow evaporation of moisture.

*Hyperkeratotic lesions* (corns, calluses, and so forth) are no more frequent in the diabetic than in the nondiabetic. However, such lesions in the neuropathic or ischemic foot are potential sources of trouble. Hyperkeratosis is a normal protective response of the skin to intermittent pressure and friction. Therefore, each corn or callus has an underlying etiology, whether it be shoe pressure, bony prominence, faulty biomechanics, or inclusion cyst. On the plantar aspect of the foot, intractable plantar keratoses are the result of excessive pressure being borne by prominent metatarsal heads. Familiar to all are corns on the dorsal aspect of the contracted hammer toes, which are due to shoe pressure on the toe. Histologically, there is no difference between a hard corn, soft corn, and callus. Each shows areas of hyperkeratosis and acanthosis to varying degrees. Clinically a corn will have a central keratotic plug that extends deeper than the surrounding callus. This is the same appearance as a cyst or plugged sweat duct lesion, which is very common on the sole of the foot. Verruca, on the other hand, is of viral origin. It has a typical speckled appearance with multiple pinpoint bleeding sites upon debridement and should not be confused with other hyperkeratotic lesions.

Focal keratoses are often quite painful when they thicken. If left untreated, the pressure creates painful subkeratotic ulcerations, hematomas, and sinus tracts. In the neuropathic foot these lesions often go unnoticed. As the pressure increases, the microcirculation becomes impeded and frank ulceration eventually occurs. This then sets the stage for infections, necrosis, and gangrene.

Treatment is initially directed toward relieving the pressure to underlying tissues by mechanical debridement of the hyperkeratosis. Salicylic acid is always avoided because of its caustic effect on surrounding healthy skin. The lesions are reduced to the level of adjacent normal healthy skin. Frequently subkeratotic sinuses or hematomas will be encountered during debridement. Prompt relief is usually noticed after evacuation of the accumulated fluid. Next the etiology of the lesion must be determined. Often digital keratoses are a direct result of tightly fitting shoes, which must be stretched or discarded before permanent resolution can occur. Structural deformities such as hammer toes or plantar-flexed metatarsals very frequently underlie the lesions. Once again, proper-fitting shoes with generous toe room should be recom-

mended. For the intractable plantar keratosis of any nature, treatment with custom-fabricated orthoses ("arch supports") should be initiated. Such orthoses can redistribute weight-bearing forces across the sole of the foot and thus alleviate excessive pressure on the callus. If conservative measures fail, minor surgical procedures can be performed to correct the deformity in the suitable patient. Hammer toe correction, metatarsal osteotomies, bunionectomies, and other procedures are frequently done under local anesthesia with little risk to the patient's general health. Such measures are taken in the patient with severe recurring lesions, near ulcerations, and recurrent noninfected ulcerations. In these instances, surgery is undertaken at the optimum time to prevent otherwise inevitable complications from occurring.

## NEUROPATHIC ULCERS

Neuropathic ulcerations (mal perforans) are often the result of neglected callosities, infections, or other traumatic lesions (Figs. 8–5 and 8–6). In the presence of neuropathy

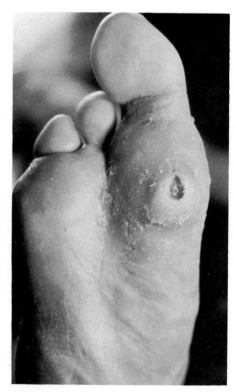

**Figure 8–5** Neuropathic ulcer developed under a prominent first metatarsal head after second and third rays had been amputated for the same reason.

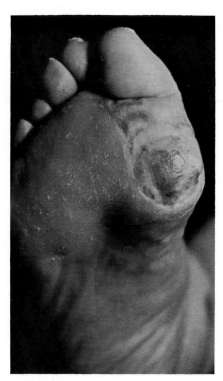

**Figure 8–6** Superficial ulcer secondary to neglect of a blister.

such lesions either go unnoticed or are undertreated because of the lack of symptoms. Failure to adequately treat these primary lesions allows their progression to ulceration, necrosis, and gangrene. The neuropathic foot is often found to have rather good arterial circulation, as demonstrated by palpable dorsalis pedis and posterior tibial pulses. The development of ulceration in these feet is perhaps most influenced by microvascular disease in the presence of neuropathy. Ischemic diabetic ulcerations are occasionally quite painful in the absence of significant neuropathy. They too result from excessive pressure, injury, or infection in a compromised foot. In this instance, however, there is occlusion of one or more of the large vessels with little or no collateral circulation.

Treatment of any type of ulceration must begin with rest and avoidance of pressure. In most instances this necessitates bed rest. Appropriate cultures and sensitivity studies, blood tests, and x-ray studies should be done initially. Anaerobic foot infections are quite prevalent in the diabetic, although these are rare in the nondiabetic patient. Foul-smelling exudate and subcutaneous crepitus (gas formation) therefore warrant an anaerobic culture. Mechanical debridement of the ulcer and surrounding callus tissue is extremely important. All pus must be evacuated and all necrotic tissue must be removed before healing can begin. Probe the ulcer under sterile conditions for depth and any hidden sinus tracts. If the bone or joint is exposed, there will most likely be a need for surgical intervention.

The more fulminant diabetic foot lesions require hospitalization and absolute bed rest in conjunction with aggressive therapy. Appropriate intravenous antibiotics and surgical debridement and drainage are of course essential. Vascular studies are indicated for ischemic lesions to assess their prognosis and necessity for arterial reconstruction. Levels of amputation or bone resection are determined after the infection has subsided or stabilized.

In the noninfected superficial neuropathic ulcer, topical therapy and rest will often heal the ulcer. Twice daily applications of Betadine or S.T. 37 and sterile dressings keep the area clean and promote healing. Topical enzymes and xenografts (pigskin) are of questionable value and infrequently used. Do not allow the patient to soak or bathe the foot. Weight bearing may be permitted, although this should be restricted as much as possible. The ulcer should be protected from excessive pressure by a "donut" or "horseshoe" accommodative pad around the lesion, which will disperse the weight to surrounding tissues (Fig. 8–7). Then apply a sterile gauze pad over this, which can be changed daily by the patient after topical care to the ulcer. For dorsal digital lesions, the shoe should be cut out over the involved area. Plantar lesions may require that the shoe be discarded and replaced with a "healing sandal" or extra-depth shoe that will allow generous room for the forefoot and toes (Figs. 8–8 and 8–9). Eventually, a pair of protective insoles or orthoses should be fabricated to prevent future recurrence of plantar ulcerations (Fig. 8–10). For the more resistant or recurring lesions, additional shoe therapy with molded shoes, metatarsal bars, or rocker soles may be of value in redistribution of weight-bearing forces. Selective bone resections and osteotomies are often quite successful and should be considered when conservative measures fail.

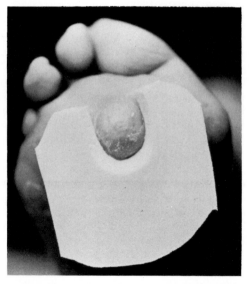

**Figure 8–7** Accommodative pad around the ulcer disperses weight to surrounding areas, enabling the superficial lesion to heal while the patient is ambulatory. Paper tape or gauze holds the pad in place. A sterile gauze pad is then applied over the ulcer.

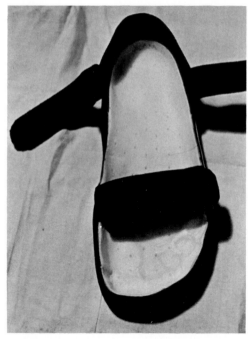

**Figure 8–8** "Healing sandal" is custom fabricated from Plastazote cushions and protects the sole of the foot.

## PODIATRIC ORTHOPEDIC DISORDERS

Musculoskeletal foot disorders primarily involve the forefoot. Although flatfoot and cavus foot conditions often have their origin in the rear foot, it is the metatarsal and digital areas that are most affected. Hammer toes, bunions, and "metatarsalgia" are by far the most frequent musculoskeletal findings in any patient population regardless of foot type.

A *hammer toe* refers to a condition whereby the toe is contracted at one or more joints, thus becoming prominent dorsally. Strictly speaking, a hammer toe is a flexion contracture at the proximal interphalangeal joint and an extension contracture at the metatarsophalangeal joint. A *claw toe* refers to a hammer toe that is also contracted at the distal interphalangeal joint. A *mallet toe* is similar to a mallet or "trigger" finger in that only the distal joint is contracted. Although the differences are subtle, the results are the same. A contracted toe does not bear weight alone on

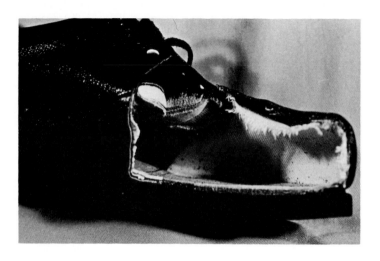

**Figure 8–9** Cross section of an extra-depth shoe. Note the abundant space for the toes.

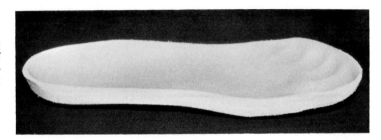

**Figure 8-10** Plastazote insole made from a direct impression of the patient's foot. This can be further trimmed and placed inside an extra-depth shoe.

the plantar pad but also, and sometimes only, on its distal tip. Just as significant, the dorsal prominences created constantly abut against the top of the shoe. The results are abnormal friction and the development of hyperkeratotic lesions at these sites. The hammer toe may be caused by intrinsic muscle atrophy, neuropathy, cavus foot, flatfoot, or trauma. In any case the normal stability of the toe is lost, resulting in its contracted state.

*Bunion* is the common term referring to a hallux valgus deformity whereby the great toe drifts laterally and the medial aspect of its metatarsal becomes prominent. This medial exostosis of the first metatarsal head is actually the bunion. A painful adventitious bursa develops over the bunion secondary to shoe pressure. As the great toe drifts toward and crowds the lesser toes, they become hammered. Frequently the second toe will overlap the hallux, thus becoming a dorsally subluxed hammer toe (Fig. 8–11). Hallux valgus is more of a syndrome than a simple deformity because of its progressive nature. It can cause havoc to the lesser toes and forefoot in general, especially when jammed into a toe. Excessive pressure is exerted in all directions,

owing to the widening of the foot and hammer toes. Therefore, adventitious bursae and dorsal and plantar hyperkeratoses are commonly associated with the digital deformities. Hallux valgus may be caused by hereditary factors, tight shoes, the pronated flatfoot, and degenerative, rheumatoid, and, occasionally, gouty arthritis.

The initial goal of treatment of hammer toes and bunions centers on the avoidance of excessive shoe pressure and prevention of hyperkeratosis. This is especially important in the neuropathic patient. Therefore, shoes with adequate depth and width are required to accommodate the forefoot. Such extra-depth shoes are available commercially. Periodic podiatric care is usually necessary to reduce the almost inevitable soft interdigital corns and plantar calluses. In those symptomatic patients with adequate neurovascular status, surgery is often advisable. The primary objective of such elective surgery is to correct structural deformities with the potential for progression, thereby preventing the development of secondary skin lesions and associated complications.

*Metatarsalagia* is a frequently used term de-

**Figure 8-11** Hallux valgus deformities with overlapping hammer toes and associated digital keratoses. Adventitious bursae overlie the bunions.

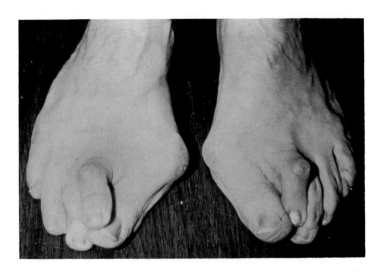

noting pain or discomfort in and around the ball of the foot. The pain (burning, aching, cramping) may stem from a great variety of causes. Most obvious would be that associated with intractable plantar keratoses, bunions, and flat and high arched feet as well as vascular disorders. A frequent finding, especially in women, is a Morton neuroma between the third and fourth toes. This is a painful lesion caused by irritation to plantar digital nerves from tight shoes. In the diabetic foot an additional etiology for metatarsal and forefoot discomfort may be peripheral neuropathy. However, it seems all too easy to assign forefoot pain in the diabetic to neuropathy. Therefore, other likely causes must be ruled out prior to the establishment of this particular diagnosis. Generally metatarsalgia responds well to treatment with orthotic devices designed to improve foot function and stability (Fig. 8–12). Such orthoses are usually fabricated from a plaster impression cast of the foot to ensure proper fit. Over-the-counter products that are commercially available are for the most part ineffective. Occasionally the placement of cushioned insoles into the shoe will alleviate symptoms related to friction and shearing forces. External shoe modifications such as Jones' bars and rocker soles may also aid in the relief of these symptoms.

## NEUROPATHIC JOINT DISEASE (CHARCOT JOINT)

Neuropathic arthropathy is a relatively painless, progressive, and destructive process that occurs in single or multiple joints and is due to underlying neurological deficits and trauma. The reader is referred to Chapter 9 for an in-depth discussion of the pathophysiology and clinical and radiographic findings of the diabetic Charcot foot.

Treatment of the acute Charcot foot consists primarily of cessation of weight bearing and elevation. The simple act of walking or standing on the compromised neuropathic joint is traumatic and will exacerbate the condition. Therefore rest and elevation are required to convert the active and destructive process to the quiescent healing stage. A minimum of three to four weeks is necessary for the condition to stabilize. Once radiographic signs of healing (absorption of debris, bone callus formation, and so forth) become evident, the patient may be weaned from bed rest to limited ambulation. It is of utmost importance to protect and support the foot, thereby preventing additional trauma and deformity. This is accomplished by the fabrication of temporary Plastazote healing sandals, which are worn whenever weight is borne on the foot (Fig. 8–13). The Plastazote is molded directly to the foot, thereby capturing its shape. The impression is then incorporated into a wooden-soled postoperative shoe. This temporary healing sandal allows the patient to ambulate with a cushioned support under the affected foot. It is wise to have the patient also use crutches or a walker, since partial weight bearing is preferred to full weight bearing initially. Ace wraps applied to the foot (or feet) will minimize edema formation and offer some support at

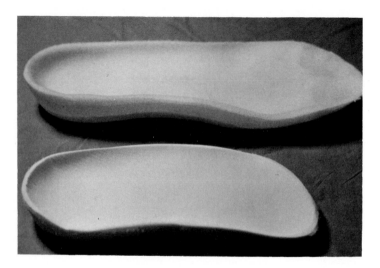

**Figure 8–12** Functional orthoses support and balance the feet to improve function. *Top,* Full length orthosis also provides cushioning under the toes and metatarsal heads. *Bottom,* Conventional orthosis ends just proximal to the metatarsal heads.

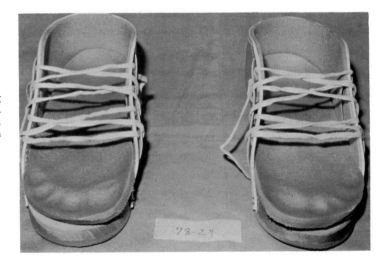

**Figure 8–13** Temporary healing sandals used for initial ambulation. Eventually the Plastazote insoles can be transferred to an extra-depth shoe.

this time. Some physicians may prefer to apply a plaster short leg cast to these patients in lieu of the Plastazote healing sandal. If so, great care must be taken to ensure that adequate padding protects the neuropathic skin from abrasion and pressure points.

Long-term therapy must be based on the degree of deformity in the foot. In those patients receiving early diagnosis and treatment the foot should show little deformity. These feet may be managed by placing the Plastazote orthosis into an extra-depth shoe. This therapy accomplishes the two primary goals: support and protection. Patients should always be cautioned against wearing conventional shoes with a "built-in" arch support. Such supports do not allow for variation in foot shape and often cause ulceration to the neuropathic foot (Fig. 8–14). Rocker-bottom Charcot feet (Fig. 8–15) must be protected and supported by custom-molded shoes, since they cannot be fitted with conventional footwear (see Figs. 9–10 and 9–12). This requires taking plaster impression casts of the feet from which the custom shoes can be fabricated. The inner sole of this shoe should be constructed of a relatively soft and cushioning material such as Plastazote. The patient should then be checked periodically for any progression of the disease that might require adjustments in footwear and cessation of weight bearing.

## PODIATRIC SURGERY

Podiatric surgery in the diabetic foot is frequently undertaken for preventive as well as corrective measures. Diabetes itself is not a contraindication to elective foot surgery. On the contrary, such surgery may be an important facet in the long-term management of the diabetic patient's foot health. Prior to contemplating such procedures, however, two important criteria must be considered. The patient's diabetes must be in good control and good vascular perfusion to the foot must be present. If these criteria are satisfied

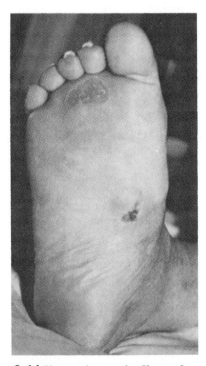

**Figure 8–14** Plantar ulcer on the Charcot foot caused by conventional footwear.

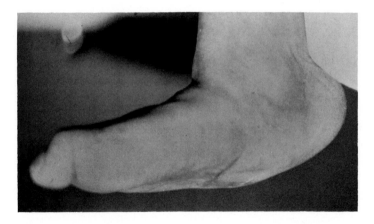

**Figure 8–15** Rocker-bottom Charcot foot.

and proper postoperative management is employed, the diabetic patient will have as satisfactory an outcome as would the nondiabetic patient.

Elective foot surgery is amenable to use of local anesthesia and easily performed on an ambulatory basis. Accordingly, there are potentially fewer operative risks and postoperative complications. Also, this method is more cost-efficient in an age of soaring health care costs. This section will concentrate on the more common and easily performed podiatric procedures that the podiatrist and physician might employ in treating specific foot disorders. The more complicated procedures have been purposely omitted because these should be performed only by the more experienced podiatrist or surgeon. The reader is referred to the appropriate podiatric or orthopedic text for in-depth coverage of these procedures.

## Preoperative Considerations

When ambulatory (outpatient) surgery is planned, the preoperative work-up should be done within a week of the surgery date. The laboratory studies should include a complete blood count, fasting blood sugar, and urinalysis at a minimum. Coagulation studies (PT and PTT) and a chemistry profile including electrolytes are often desirable as well. Medical consultation from the patient's primary physician will serve to elucidate any contraindications to surgery (uncontrolled diabetes, renal failure, and so on) and also to simply inform him of the anticipated surgery. On the morning of surgery, the patient is permitted a light breakfast and should take his usual

medications, including insulin or oral hypoglycemic agents. When circumstances dictate that the patient be hospitalized, the work-up is done on the day of admission and the surgery is performed on the following morning. When general anesthesia is desired, the patient is given nothing by mouth, and half the usual dose of insulin is administered preoperatively (see Chapters 17 and 18).

On the night preceding or the morning of surgery, the foot is initially cleansed by the patient or nurse with Betadine or pHISoHEX scrub. In the operating room the foot receives another Betadine scrub by the OR nurse followed by a "painting" with Betadine solution by the gowned doctor. A sterile stockinette is then applied and the sterile drapes are then put in place. Local or general anesthesia is usually administered prior to the sterile prep and drape.

## Local Anesthesia

Basically, the purpose of the local anesthetic is to produce anesthesia of a given site through blockade of neural transmission in the sensory nerves supplying this area. Certain conditions may require either local infiltration, digital blocks, specific nerve blocks, or regional blocks. Which type to use depends upon the nature of the problem and its location. When dealing with paronychia, it is far better (and less painful) to perform a digital block than to attempt local infiltration at the end of the toe. Conversely, when removing a wart, it is simpler to locally infiltrate around the lesion than to perform a nerve block. The various types and characteristics of the more common local anesthetics are

## TABLE 8-1.    COMMON LOCAL ANESTHETICS

| AGENT | TYPE* | SUGGESTED CONCENTRATIONS | MAX DOSE (MG) | ONSET | DURATION |
|---|---|---|---|---|---|
| Procaine hydrochloride (Novocaine) | Ester | Infiltration 0.5% Peripheral nerves 1–2% | 1000 mg | 1–3 min | ¾–1 hr |
| Lidocaine hydrochloride (Xylocaine) | Amide | Infiltration 0.5% Peripheral nerves 1–2% | 500 mg | 1–2 min | 2 hrs |
| Bupivacaine hydrochloride (Marcaine) | Amide | Infiltration 0.025–0.75% Peripheral nerves " " | 200 mg | 5–7 min | 6+ hrs |
| Mepivacaine hydrochloride (Carbocaine) | Amide | Infiltration 0.5–1.0% Peripheral nerves 1–2% | 500 mg | 3–5 min | 2–2½ hrs |
| Prilocaine hydrochloride (Citanest) | Amide | Infiltration 0.5% | 600 mg | 3 min | 2½–3 hrs |

*Esters are detoxified by plasma esterases (pseudo-cholinesterases). Amides are detoxified by liver enzymes.

listed in Table 8–1. The most frequently used agents are lidocaine hydrochloride and bupivacaine hydrochloride (Marcaine). They are often used in combination with each other, either with or without epinephrine. Such a mixture combines the rapid action of lidocaine with the long duration of anesthesia provided by bupivacaine (6 to 12 hours). The use of epinephrine in the anesthetic creates local vasoconstriction. This prolongs anesthesia by retarding absorption of the agent as well as providing a degree of hemostasis when infiltrated near the operative site. The use of epinephrine in digits is controversial, although it has been used in thousands of digital blocks without sequelae. It can be a valuable aid during digital procedures when discretion and proper patient selection are employed.

### Digital Blocks

Most digital operations are best performed utilizing a toe block at the base of the toe. Here the skin is more supple and allows for expansion of the tissues as the anesthetic is injected. Since the four nerves in each toe are quite small, concentrations of 0.5 per cent lidocaine and/or Marcaine are very adequate. A total of 3 cc is usually sufficient for the great toe and 2 cc for the lesser toes. If there is any doubt, another cubic centimeter or two can be added.

The preferred injection technique for the great toe is illustrated in Figure 8–16. Using a 25 gauge, 1½ inch needle on a 3 cc syringe, make a wheal on the dorsal-lateral aspect of

the toe adjacent to the web space. Inject slowly. Aspiration is not necessary owing to the minute size of the vessels. Proceed plantarly with the needle while palpating the plantar surface of the toe. When the plantar aspect is reached, start injecting slowly while

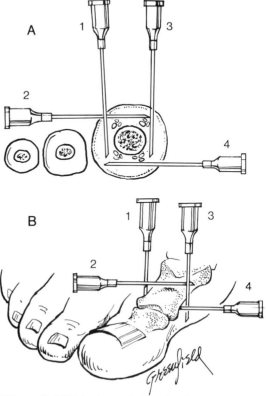

**Figure 8–16** Injection technique for the great toe. *A*, Cross-sectional view. *B*, Dorsal view. See text for details.

made. The second incision is carried obliquely from the proximal end of the first incision proximally and plantarly about 0.8 cm. This "hockeystick" incision will create a proximal flap for excellent exposure of the underlying matrix. The third incision is semi-elliptical and is carried from the distal end of the first incision into the hypertrophic nail fold, and reconnects with the first incision at a point 2.0 mm proximal to the eponychium. This incision is also carried deeply, angling centrally toward the bone. The proximal flap is then developed, gently dissecting the skin and subcutaneous fat from the underlying matrix on the surface of the bone. Be sure to expose the condyle of the distal phalanx for complete visualization of the glistening white matrix. The ellipse of nail matrix and skin is then sharply dissected off the surface of the bone and removed in toto as a wedge. Any remaining matrix tissue is then sharply excised. The bone and periosteum visible are then rasped to ensure removal of any remaining cells. The wound is then flushed with a povidone-iodine and saline solution. The proximal flap is then sutured in place with 4–0 nylon. The elliptical incision can then be closed with either Steri-Strips or a suture placed from the nail fold to under and through the nail plate itself.

The tourniquet is then released and a large dressing is applied, because these tend to bleed postoperatively. The dressing is first changed within one week and sutures removed at two weeks.

The *Zadik* total matrixectomy is used to completely eradicate a deformed nail (Fig. 8–21). Under tourniquet hemostasis the entire nail plate is avulsed. At each corner of the eponychium an oblique 1 cm incision is made extending posteriorly and plantarly. A posterior flap is then developed, gently dissecting the skin and subcutaneous tissue off the matrix, which in this area actually forms an envelope. A third incision is made transversely across the nail bed just distal to the lunula and carried to both medial and lateral nail folds and down to the bone. In each corner, the nail fold should be incised to further expose the medial and lateral portions of the matrix. Following adequate exposure, the matrix is sharply dissected off the bone from distal to proximal. It is sometimes easier to longitudinally incise the matrix in half, then remove each half separately. Be sure to adequately remove the matrix over the con-

dyle, then each side. Once again, rasp the bone surface and flush. A simple suture is placed on each side of the posterior flap and the central portion is partially coapted with a Steri-Strip and left to granulate. The tourniquet is removed and a dressing is applied. Postoperative care is the same as for a partial matrixectomy.

### Subungual Exostosis

Occasionally the tuft of the distal phalanx becomes enlarged to form an exostosis under the nail plate. In some cases it can actually deform the nail and become quite painful from overlying shoe pressure. Removal of the exostosis is simple and can be done independently or in conjunction with surgery on the nail itself (Fig. 8–22).

A transverse stab incision is made on the tip of the toe about 2 mm below the plane of the nail bed. A Freer elevator or periosteal elevator is then tunneled proximally to the dorsal surface of the distal phalanx. Soft tissues are bluntly dissected off the surface and the exostosis is defined. A small rasp or rotary bur is inserted into the tunnel and the exostosis is removed. Care must be taken to adequately remove all bone fragments and debris from the wound. This is accomplished by inserting a rasp upside down (teeth dorsally) and rasping the soft tissues. The toe is then squeezed from proximal to distal to expel any remaining bone paste when using a rotary bur. Bleeding is beneficial in this case, because it helps in flushing out the debris. Finally, the wound is flushed with sterile saline and Betadine in a syringe. Closure is done with one stitch of 4–0 nylon and the dressing is applied. The suture can be removed at 7 to 10 days.

## Verruca Plantaris Removal

The common plantar wart can sometimes be exceedingly difficult to eradicate. It is of viral origin and not directly related to an underlying osseous etiology. There are many treatments for warts, indicating the recalcitrance of these lesions. Such therapies include salicylic acid, vesiculants, vitamin A, fulguration, cryotherapy, excision, curettage, and even carbon dioxide laser vaporization.

*Blunt dissection* or curettage is generally very effective for a single wart. The area sur-

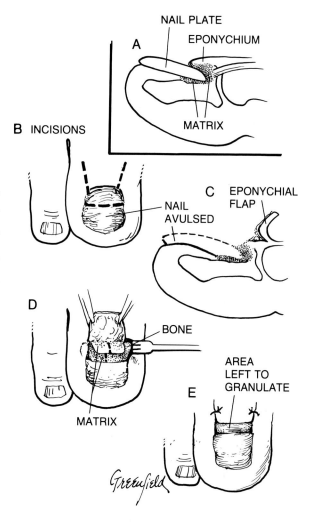

**Figure 8-21** Zadik matrixectomy. *A*, Anatomy of the nail and matrix. *B*, Three incisions performed after avulsion of the nail. *C*, Longitudinal section showing proximal eponychial flap retracted. *D*, Dorsal view: flap retracted, showing matrix at the base of the wound lying on the distal phalanx. Dotted line represents the incision bisecting the matrix. *E*, Sutures in place. Note the gaping, open area, which is left to granulate.

rounding and under the lesion is infiltrated with a local anesthetic containing epinephrine for hemostasis. The perimeter of the wart is visualized as a whitish ring encompass-ing the entire lesion. This is the capsule that should not be broken during the dissection. With a No. 15 blade, score the skin just outside the capsular border completely around

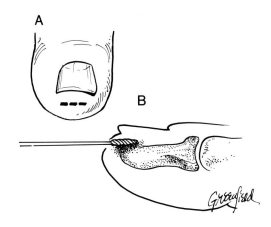

**Figure 8-22** Subungual exostectomy. *A*, Horizontal incision carried to bone. *B*, Rasp or bur tunneled subcutaneously to the exostosis, which is then removed.

the lesion. This incision should go down to but not penetrate the dermis. With a thumb forceps, grasp the wart and apply tension on it. With the other hand, using a thin blunt instrument such as a Freer elevator or curette, the wart is bluntly dissected from the surrounding normal tissue. If the capsule is not penetrated, the wart will shell out nicely when dissection is done from side to side. Once it is removed, there will be a crater-like defect in its place. Since the wart is located at the dermal-epidermal junction, there should be no fat protruding into the wound. The edges of the crater are saucerized (beveled) and a dry sterile dressing is applied. Some prefer to touch the base with phenol to kill any remaining viral cells. Healing should be complete within a few weeks, without any scarring.

## Metatarsal Osteotomy

Disabling intractable plantar keratoses and recurrent plantar ulcerations can often be remedied by an appropriate metatarsal osteotomy. Despite the widespread belief that there is a normal anterior metatarsal arch, this is not so. All five metatarsal heads should be on the same plane. When one metatarsal head comes to lie lower than the adjacent one (plantarflexed), it consequently bears a greater load than normal. The excessive friction and pressure lead to the formation of a plantar keratosis. In the neuropathic foot these keratoses often progress to the point of ulceration. The purpose of the metatarsal osteotomy is simply to elevate the metatarsal head and thereby alleviate the excessive pressure on the underlying skin.

The longitudinal incision is placed dorsally and centered over the affected metatarsal head and shaft, staying medial to the extensor tendon (Fig. 8–23). If two adjacent metatarsal osteotomies are to be done, one incision is made in the corresponding metatarsal interspace. Skin edges are retracted and a sharp dissection is carried to the metatarsal neck, which is fully exposed. It is not always necessary to enter the capsule, but if this is desired for a more distal osteotomy, the proximal capsule is incised and the surgical neck exposed. The osteotomy can be performed with bone-cutting forceps or power equipment. A complete transverse osteotomy is performed at the anatomical neck with bone

forceps. If a power saw is used, a V-shaped osteotomy can be performed with the apex distally placed (Fig. 8–24). Care is taken to stay proximal to the level of the condyles on the plantar aspect of the metatarsal head. From the plantar surface of the foot, the head is pushed dorsally until its plantar surface is at the same level as the adjacent metatarsals. This usually requires a 1- to 2-mm elevation. The cut surfaces of bone are then impacted together with digital pressure. Although not usually required, a K wire may be used to fix the osteotomy for three weeks. The wound is flushed and then closed in layers. It is very important to use vertical mattress skin sutures in this area to prevent inverted skin edges. The patient can ambulate almost immediately for short periods when wearing a wooden-sole postoperative shoe. Clinical union of the osteotomy occurs in about four weeks, at which time regular shoes can be worn.

## Metatarsal Head Resection

For severe metatarsal deformities, metatarsophalangeal joint arthritis, subluxated hammer toes, and deep ulcerations, a metatarsal head resection may be indicated. If a chronic ulceration is present, the metatarsal head can be resected from a plantar approach by extending the incision through the ulcer. The ulcer can also be thoroughly debrided at this time. Otherwise, the traditional dorsal approach is utilized as in the metatarsal osteotomy. Transfer lesions to adjacent metatarsals must be anticipated because of the shift of weight bearing. However, these can be minimized through the use of postoperative orthoses.

The dorsal incision should be carried more distally than that used for an osteotomy because the entire head must be exposed. When crossing over the metatarsophalangeal joint it is advisable to make a "lazy S" incision to avoid skin contractures. The capsule is then exposed and a longitudinal capsulotomy is performed. The metatarsal head is then freed of the collateral ligaments and capsular attachments. The bone is then transected at the anatomical neck, well behind the plantar condyles. The cut should be beveled so that more is taken off plantarly and dorsally. Grasping the metatarsal head with a towel clip at this point will facilitate its re-

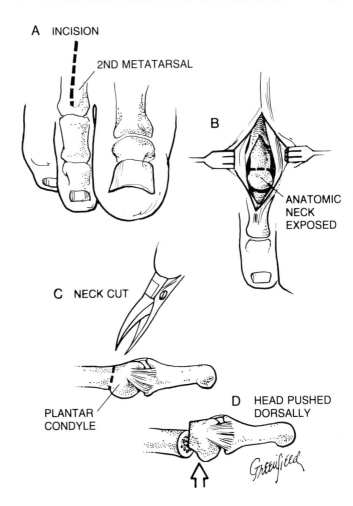

**Figure 8–23** Second metatarsal osteotomy. *A*, Dorsal incision placed over the head and neck of the metatarsal. *B*, Longitudinal capsulotomy exposes the anatomical neck. Dotted line represents the location of the transverse osteotomy. *C*, Osteotomy must be performed proximal to the plantar condyles. *D*, The head is pushed dorsally to reduce the plantarflexed position.

moval. While it is pulled distally and upward, any remaining attachments can be easily released. Note that the entire resection is done within the capsule; therefore, all tendons should be left untouched. The capsule should be stitched in "hourglass" fashion to close off the dead space. Once again, vertical mattress skin sutures should be used.

## Postoperative Care

In most cases the patient may ambulate on the foot that was operated on for limited periods almost immediately. Individual consideration must always be given with regard to the reliability of the patient and the extent of surgery performed. The standard postoperative shoe accommodates even the bulkiest of dressings and allows walking with the necessary degree of immobilization for the first few weeks.

Dressings should be changed at weekly intervals by the surgeon or his staff. It is wise to remember that the dressing provides protection to the wound, splinting of the operated area and, very importantly, a sterile environ-

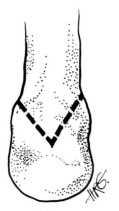

**Figure 8–24** V osteotomy.

ment. The initial dressing can be left in place for about one week, unless there is a reason to remove it sooner (excessive bleeding, hematoma, infection). Bleeding into the dressing is normal and should be expected. It is usually dry by the morning after surgery. To limit the extent of the staining, the foot should be kept elevated and mild compression should be applied. In fact, all patients are routinely instructed to sit with the foot elevated and perhaps apply an ice bag to the dorsum of the ankle. This will also prevent excessive swelling and discomfort while reinforcing the need for resting the foot. Walking to the bathroom and dinner table is permitted.

Sutures are removed around day 14. Minor gapping of the incision can be treated with Steri-Strips for another week or so. At this time the patient may begin bathing his foot. The wearing of normal footwear can be resumed when swelling has subsided and clinical evidence of osseous union is apparent. A jogging or recreational shoe is an excellent choice of footwear for the initial period of unrestricted ambulation. They are fairly wide, cushioned, and allow room for swelling. Most patients find this approach much more acceptable than the traditional "orthopedic" shoe regimen.

## FOOT CARE GUIDELINES

The recommended approach to foot care is based primarily on common sense and discretion. The patient must be made aware that until a problem is recognized it cannot be treated—hence the great importance of daily foot inspection. Since most serious diabetic lesions can be prevented or arrested by proper attention, it is the physician's duty to emphasize the need for conscientious diabetic foot care. Neuropathy and vascular disease are of course the two factors that most directly influence the following guidelines:

Daily bathing and inspection of the feet should be stressed. It is not necessary (and sometimes inadvisable) to soak the feet, as many patients have the habit of doing. (As a rule, soaking should be avoided in the presence of open lesions.) Rather, a gentle washing with warm water, mild soap, and a wash cloth is to be preferred. The water should be hand- or wrist-tested for temperature to prevent scalding. Afterward it is especially important to dry well between the toes. The feet

should then be carefully inspected for any new or suspicious lesions of the heels, soles, interdigital, and/or dorsal aspects. If none are found, a moisturizing cream should be massaged into the skin everywhere except the interdigital areas. Recommended moisturizers are Eucerin, Carmol, Nivea, Vaseline Intensive Care, and LacHydrin. Almost any product will be beneficial if used regularly. Finally, a light dusting of nonmedicated talcum or foot powder should be used, especially between the toes. Caking of the powder should be avoided. Any open lesions should be treated with a mild antiseptic such as diluted Betadine and dry sterile dressing followed by a consultation with a podiatrist or physician.

Toenails should be trimmed straight across with nail clippers or nail scissors. The corners and rough edges can then be filed with an emery board. Do not allow any cutting or digging into the corners to remove ingrown nails. Of course, if the patient has poor eyesight or the nails are thick and difficult to cut, he should not attempt to do so himself. Occasionally a family member may be able to assist the patient, but most often regular podiatric care should be sought.

Thick calluses may sometimes be reduced by gentle filing with a pumice stone or callus file after bathing. Under no circumstances should "bathroom surgery" with razor blades, knives, or scissors be permitted. Just as harmful are over-the-counter preparations of corn and callus removers that remove healthy as well as hyperkeratotic skin. Generally, lesions that are symptomatic enough to warrant such types of self-care should always be treated professionally.

Footwear is a major cause of neuropathic lesions and accordingly should be of concern to both the patient and the doctor. Although shoes and stockings are necessary and extremely important in preventing problems, such ill-fitting footwear can be limb- or life-threatening. The high-risk ischemic or neuropathic foot deserves extra-special attention to footwear. Generally, stockings should be made of natural fibers (cotton or wool) that are absorbent. Many synthetics can cause undue perspiration and its associated problems. Socks should not be constrictive and should fit properly without irritating folds, wrinkles, and seams. Of utmost importance regarding shoe fitting is comfort. Expensive "orthopedic" shoes are often quite heavy and cumbersome in their attempt to support the feet.

Rarely are these beneficial. Instead, a lightweight tie shoe (oxford) with adequate room for the toes and proper heel fit is recommended. Rockport, S. A. S., Easy Spirit, and various types of recreational shoes frequently satisfy these conditions. The shoe should slip on fairly easily (without being too large) and should be comfortable at the time of fitting. It should not have to stretch before proper fit is achieved. A natural leather or suede upper will provide breathability and a small amount of stretchability to conform to the shape of the foot. If support is needed, an orthotic device most often is indicated rather than a stiff-soled or steel-shanked shoe. Cushioning can be provided by crepe soles, Plastazote, or Spenco insoles. However, be aware that increasing the bulk of the inner sole diminishes the available toe space. If the toes are cramped by the shoes, as in those feet with hammer toes, an extra-depth shoe will provide the necessary toe room. Feet that are extremely difficult to fit because of significant deformity may benefit from a custom-molded shoe.

## SUGGESTED READING LIST

Coleman, W.: Footwear Considerations. In Frykberg, R. G. (ed.): The High Risk Foot in Diabetes Mellitus. New York, Churchill Livingstone, Inc., 1991.

Donovan, J. C., et al.: New England Deaconess Hospital Podiatry Service, Sport Orthotic Device. J. Am. Podiatry Assoc. 69:571, 1979.

Frykberg, R. G.: Diabetic Foot Ulcerations. In Frykberg, R. G. (ed.): The High Risk Foot in Diabetes Mellitus. New York, Churchill Livingstone, Inc., 1991.

Frykberg, R. G.: The diabetic Charcot foot. Arch. Podiatric Med. Foot Surg. 5:4:15, 1978.

Frykberg, R. G.: Podiatric problems in diabetes. In Kozak, G. (ed.): Clinical Diabetes Mellitus. Philadelphia, W. B. Saunders Co., 1982, pp. 426–438.

Frykberg, R. G., and Kozak, G. P.: Neuropathic arthropathy in the diabetic foot. Am. Fam. Physician 17:105, 1978.

Harkless, L. B., and Higgins, K. R.: Evaluation of the diabetic foot and leg. In Frykberg, R. G. (ed.): The High Risk Foot in Diabetes Mellitus. New York, Churchill Livingstone, Inc., 1991.

Johng-Nicklaus, B.: Prophylactic Foot Surgery. In Frykberg, R. G. (ed.): The High Risk Foot in Diabetes Mellitus. New York, Churchill Livingstone, Inc., 1991.

Levin, M. E., O'Neal, L. W., and Bowker, J. (eds.): The Diabetic Foot. 5th ed. St. Louis, Mosby–Year Book Co., 1993.

McGlamey, E. D. (ed.): Comprehensive Textbook of Foot Surgery. Baltimore, Williams & Wilkins, 1987.

Pardo-Castello, V., and Pardo, O. A.: Diseases of the Nails, 3rd ed. Springfield, Ill., Charles C Thomas, 1960.

Root, M. L., Orien, W. P., and Weed, J. H.: Normal and Abnormal Function of the Foot. Los Angeles, Clinical Biomechanics Corporation, 1977.

Samitz, M. H., and Dana, A. S.: Cutaneous Lesions of the Lower Extremities. Philadelphia, J. B. Lippincott Co., 1971.

Sanders, L. J., and Frykberg, R. G.: Diabetic Neuropathic Osteoarthropathy. In Frykberg, R. G. (ed.): The High Risk Foot in Diabetes Mellitus. New York, Churchill Livingstone, Inc., 1991.

# Chapter 9

# THE DIABETIC CHARCOT FOOT

ROBERT G. FRYKBERG, D.P.M.,
and GEORGE P. KOZAK, M.D.

In 1868 Jean-Martin Charcot first described neuropathic joint changes associated with tabes dorsalis. More importantly, he believed these changes to be a secondary effect of the neurological deficit related to tertiary syphilis. Since that time, there have been scattered reports and studies in the literature concerning the entity that bears his name. Yet it is surprising how often physicians misdiagnose this condition as arthritis or fallen arch because they are unaware of this diabetic complication.

For many years neuroarthropathy was primarily considered to be a lesion of tertiary lues (syphilis), as Charcot had first described. However, with the gradual decline in cases of tabes dorsalis and the concomitant increased life span of the diabetic population, there has been a shift toward diabetes as the most common cause of Charcot joints. The first such description of neuropathic arthropathy in diabetes was by Jordan in 1936. The first published series of cases of diabetic neuroarthropathy came from the Joslin Clinic in 1947 and placed the incidence of diabetic Charcot joints at approximately one in 1100 patients. In 1972, a more extensive study involving 68,000 Joslin Clinic admissions revealed 101 patients having Charcot joint of the feet, thus raising the incidence to 1 in 680. Even then, it was believed that the incidence is actually greater because of the number of patients with the condition that remain undiagnosed.

## GENERAL CONSIDERATIONS

Neuropathic arthropathy may be defined as a relatively painless, progressive, and degenerative arthropathy of single or multiple joints caused by underlying neurological deficits. Peripheral joints are most commonly affected. The location of the joint involved is dependent upon the nature of the disease causing the underlying neuropathy. There are a host of these diseases, the most notable being diabetes mellitus, tertiary syphilis, syringomyelia, and leprosy (Table 9–1). Certain diseases also have a predilection for sites of involvement (Table 9–2). Tabes dorsalis usually presents as monoarticular involvement of large joints of the lower extremity such as the hip or knee. Conversely, syringomyelia involves the joints of the upper extremities, i.e. shoulder, elbow, and cervical vertebrae. In diabetes mellitus, the areas primarily affected are the foot and ankle, al-

### TABLE 9–1. DISEASES WITH POTENTIAL FOR CAUSING NEUROPATHIC ARTHROPATHY

| | |
|---|---|
| Diabetes mellitus | Congenital insensitivity to pain |
| Tertiary syphilis | Hysterical insensitivity to pain |
| Leprosy | Paraplegia |
| Syringomyelia | Riley-Day syndrome (familial dysautonomia) |
| Myelodysplasia | Peripheral nerve lesions |
| Pernicious anemia | Spinal cord injuries |
| Multiple sclerosis | Intra-articular injection of corticosteroids |
| Poliomyelitis | |

From Frykberg, R. G., and Kozak, G. P.: Neuropathic arthropathy in the diabetic foot. Am. Fam. Physician, 105–113, May, 1978.

**TABLE 9–2.  JOINT PREDILECTION OF CERTAIN DISEASES**

| | |
|---|---|
| Diabetes mellitus | Ankle, tarsus, metatarsophalangeal (knee, spine) |
| Tabes dorsalis | Knee, hip, ankle, spine |
| Syringomyelia | Cervical spine, shoulder, elbow |

though some authors note the neuroarthropathy that occurs infrequently in the knees and the spine. The largest study to date places the most frequent sites of involvement at the tarsal-metatarsal joints (60 per cent), followed by the metatarsal-phalangeal joints (61 per cent), and the ankle joint (9 per cent).

## PATHOPHYSIOLOGY

The two primary components involved in the development of a Charcot joint are neuropathy and trauma (Table 9–3). Although some investigators have postulated an intrinsic osseous defect in the neuropathic extremity, researchers have demonstrated no definite predisposing weakness of the bone. The neuropathy consists primarily of a loss or diminution of pain perception, proprioception, and sympathetic activity. With such sensory losses, joints are subjected to their extreme ranges of motion without the benefits of normal protective mechanisms. This re-

sults in capsular and ligamentous stretching, joint laxity, distention, and subluxation—all of which will remain unheralded in the neuropathic foot. As weight bearing continues, the instability increases and dislocated articular surfaces grind on adjacent bone. This results in cartilage fibrillation, osteochondral fragmentation, and joint fractures. This period of joint destruction brings about a natural hyperemic response to injury. The increased blood supply promotes resorption of debris with a concomitant softening and resorption of normal bone. Further trauma to these osteoporotic areas will create more destruction of the compromised joint, the process will be enhanced, and a vicious cycle ensues.

Often it is a fracture, either intra-articular or extra-articular, that initiates the destructive process (Fig. 9–1). Additionally, amputation of the great toe, often a consequence of osteomyelitis or gangrene in the diabetic, may lead to neuropathic joint changes in the lesser metatarsophalangeal joints (Fig. 9–2).

**TABLE 9–3.  PATHOGENESIS OF THE DIABETIC CHARCOT JOINT**

Long-standing, poorly controlled diabetes
↓
Neuropathic diseases → Neuropathy ← Nerve injury
↓
Ambulation on insensitive joint
↓
Joint instability
↓
Trauma ⟶ Joint degeneration ⟵ Infection
and subluxation
↑                              ↓
Continued
weight bearing        Charcot Joint

From Frykberg, R. G., and Kozak, G. P.: Neuropathic arthropathy in the diabetic foot. Am. Fam. Physician, 105–113 May, 1978.

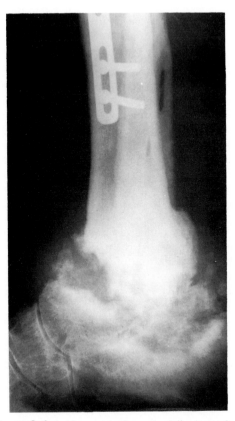

**Figure 9–1** Ankle neuroarthropathy following a fracture of the tibia.

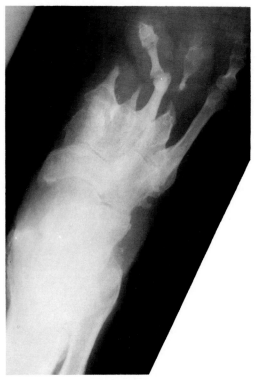

**Figure 9-2** Metatarsophalangeal and interphalangeal arthropathy following amputation of the first and second toes.

Presumably this is a stress-related factor secondary to an acquired biomechanical deficiency. Septic arthritis, with its severe joint destruction, can easily progress to a neuropathic arthropathy. In that case, it is often difficult to distinguish one disease process from the other because of rather similar joint changes. Essentially, any type of destructive or inflammatory process introduced to a neuropathic joint has the potential for creating a Charcot joint.

The disease process can be divided into three stages based on pathological findings. The first stage, that of *development,* is the initial destructive phase, characterized by joint laxity, subluxation, osteochondral fragmentation, and debris formation (Fig. 9–3). At this stage, a synovial biopsy showing osseous debris embedded in a thickened synovium is considered pathognomonic of the disease. The *stage of coalescence* is marked by absorption of much of the fine debris and fusion of the larger fragments to adjacent bone (Fig. 9–3). The *stage of reconstruction* is an attempt to restore joint architecture by revascularization and remodeling of bone and fragments.

The fate of any Charcot joint is greatly dependent upon the amount of destruction taking place during the initial stage of development. This is directly a function of the amount of trauma or weight bearing sustained by the joint during the active process of the disease. If such stress is continually introduced to the neuropathic joint, the destructive cycle is perpetuated, healing is greatly prolonged, and there is a poor prognosis for the foot. In these cases the final result is often pseudoarthrosis, severe deformity, instability, abnormal weight-bearing surfaces, ulcerations, and infections. If, however, the disease is diagnosed early and nonweight bearing is instituted, there will be less destruction and morbidity, and there is a greater likelihood of stable fusion or reconstruction or both taking place.

## CLINICAL FEATURES

Various studies of diabetic Charcot feet indicate a high incidence in those patients with an average duration of diabetes of 12 to 18 years, ranging from 8 months to 43 years. There is apparently no definite predilection for either sex. In the majority of patients only one foot is affected; however, there is an 18 per cent incidence of bilateral involvement (Fig. 9–4). Although most are in their fifth or sixth decades, their ages range from mid twenties to late seventies, once again depending upon the duration of diabetes.

In most patients, the diabetes is poorly controlled, regardless of treatment with diet and oral hypoglycemic agents or insulin. Neuropathy of some degree is always present, whether of recent onset or of long duration. Neuropathic manifestations may include absence of knee and ankle jerks, diminished vibratory, pain, and position sensations, and various paresthesias consistent with diabetic neuropathy (Table 9–4). Autonomic neuropathy is manifested by anhidrosis, neuropathic stomach or nocturnal diarrhea, and neurogenic bladder.

The patient seeks medical help for a markedly swollen foot, often associated with recent trauma. *The foot may or may not be painless.* When there is some pain or discomfort, it is usually much less than expected for such pathology. On examination, the foot may appear to be grossly deformed with a typical *rocker bottom* subluxation of the mid tarsal re-

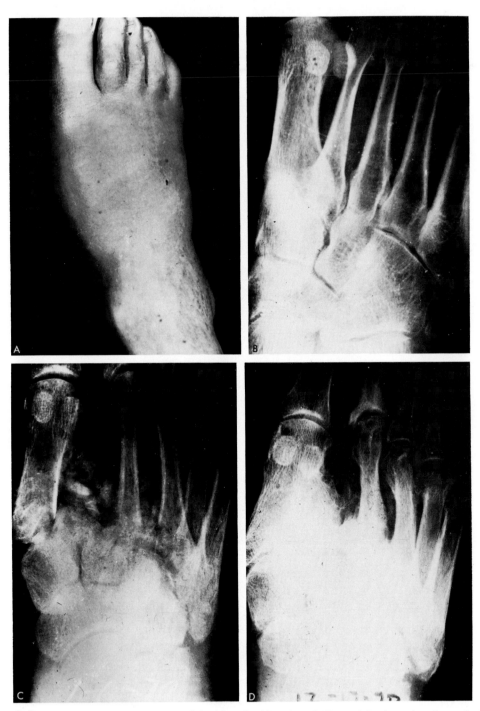

**Figure 9–3** *A,* Acute Charcot foot. Note medial midtarsal subluxation. *B,* X-ray of the foot taken 5 months before onset of neuroarthropathy. There are no significant joint abnormalities. *C,* X-ray showing marked joint destruction. *D,* X-ray taken 11 months later, showing coalescence of the fragments in destroyed joints.

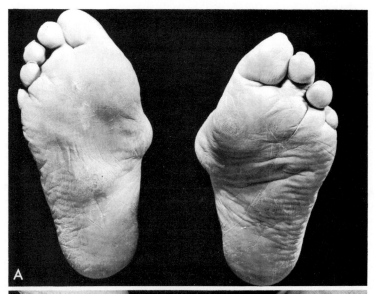

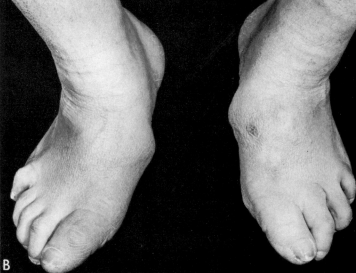

**Figure 9–4** *A* and *B,* Bilateral tarsal neuroarthropathy. Twenty per cent of patients have bilateral disease.

## TABLE 9–4.    CLINICAL FEATURES OF THE ACUTE CHARCOT JOINT

| VASCULAR | NEUROPATHIC | SKELETAL | CUTANEOUS |
|---|---|---|---|
| Bounding pulse | Absent or diminished | Rocker bottom deformity | Neuropathic ulcer |
| Erythema | Pain | Medial tarsal subluxation | Hyperkeratoses |
| Swelling | Proprioception | Digital subluxation | Infection |
| Warmth | Vibration | Crepitus | |
| | Deep tendon reflexes | Hypermobility | |
| | Hyperhidrosis | | |

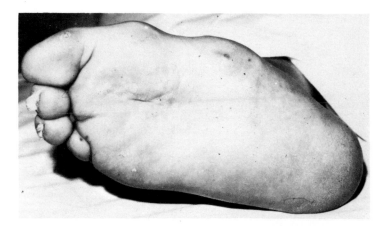

**Figure 9–5** A typical presentation of tarsometatarsal neuroarthropathy involves a bony deformity causing medial convexity of the affected foot.

gion or subluxations of the metatarsophalangeal joints (Fig. 9–5). The foot will be very erythematous, quite warm to the touch, and show signs of anhidrosis. Almost invariably the *pulses will be bounding*. This finding in association with that of relatively mild pain to absence of pain is the cornerstone of the diagnosis. Neurological examination should reveal the impaired sensory status of the extremity as already described.

Infection often plays a role in the pathogenesis of the disease, and accordingly the examiner may find an infected neuropathic ulcer overlying or adjacent to the affected joint (Figs. 9–6 and 9–7). If the joint is palpated, some degree of hypermobility and crepitus will be revealed, caused by the effusions and destructive process taking place within it.

Adequate circulation is needed for the neuroarthropathy process to occur. This principle is exemplified by three Joslin patients. All had ischemic foot ulcers and absence of pulses below the femoral area. With revascularization by femoral-popliteal bypass, foot ulcers healed and Charcot deformity subsequently developed. In one patient who had bilateral arterial bypasses, bilateral Charcot foot deformities developed. With closure of bypass graft in two patients, nonhealing ischemic ulcers were again noted in a Charcot deformed foot.

## X-RAY FINDINGS

Radiologically, the osteoarthropathy takes on the appearance of a severely destructive form of degenerative arthritis (Table 9–5). If serial x-rays are taken, it is possible to follow the events taking place in the process. Early changes (stage I) consist of joint effusion, subluxations, and bone alteration. The bone changes seem to be an exaggeration of those found in osteoarthritis—cartilage fibrillation,

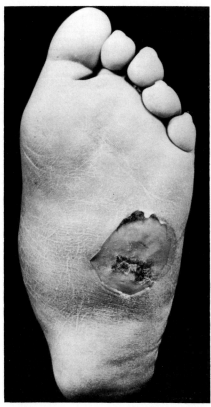

**Figure 9–6** Neuropathic ulcer overlying Charcot joint on the plantar surface of the foot. Rocker-bottom deformity.

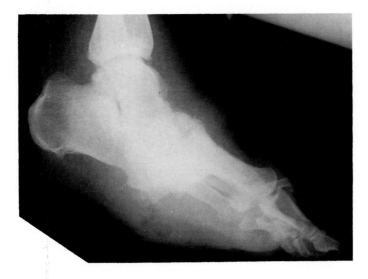

**Figure 9–7** X-ray of rocker-bottom Charcot foot with neuropathic plantar ulcer.

loose body formation, subchondral sclerosis, and marginal osteophytes. These hypertrophic changes are primarily found in the solid bones of the tarsal regions of the foot (Fig. 9–8).

As the disease process continues, there is complete destruction of the involved joints. The tubular bones of the metatarsus and toes show atrophic bone changes consisting of reabsorption of metatarsal heads and shafts (penciling) and "hourglass" resorption of phalangeal diaphyses (Fig. 9–9). These peri-articular findings often seem to mimic those seen in osteomyelitis. Hence, the terms *diabetic osteoarthropathy* and *diabetic osteolysis* have been introduced to identify such lesions. Although sometimes classified as distinct entities, the atrophic changes of the tubular bones of the foot are herein considered to be consistent with osteoarthropathy.

The types of bone reaction found in neuroarthropathy include sclerosis, fragmentation, periosteal new bone formation, resorption, and subchondral osteoporosis. These

## TABLE 9–5.  X-RAY FINDINGS IN DIABETIC OSTEOARTHROPATHY

| STAGE | ATROPHIC* | HYPERTROPHIC | MISCELLANEOUS |
|---|---|---|---|
| 1. Development | Phalangeal "hourglassing" | Osteochondral fragmentation | Joint effusion |
|  | "Pencil pointing" metatarsal resorption | Intra-articular debris and joint mice | Subluxation |
|  |  |  | Soft tissue swelling Arterial calcification Fracture |
| 2. Coalescence |  | Marginal osteophytes Periosteal new bone formation Subchondral sclerosis (avascular necrosis) | Resorption of debris |
| 3. Reconstruction |  | Ankylosis                    OR | Rounded bone ends Decreased sclerosis Diminished swelling |

From Frykberg, R. G., and Kozak, G. P.: Neuropathic arthropathy in the diabetic foot. Am. Fam. Physician, 105–113, May, 1978.
*Some classify these changes as a distinct entity called diabetic osteopathy or osteolysis. Since they are frequent findings in diabetic Charcot foot, they have been included with the classic x-ray findings of neuroarthropathy.

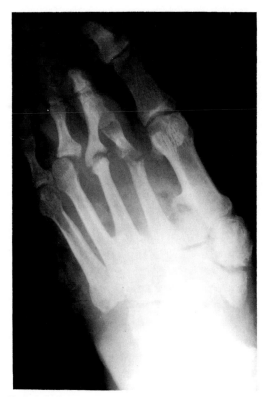

**Figure 9-8** Hypertrophic neuropathic bone changes in the tarsus.

reactions require an abundant blood supply, thereby invalidating hypotheses relating them to an ischemic etiology. While generalized osteoporosis is probably a function of inflammatory hyperemia, areas of subchondral osteoporosis with adjacent sclerosis may actually represent subchondral fractures with subsequent healing. Furthermore, there may possibly be episodes of avascular necrosis occurring in some of the sclerotic zones that

eventually revascularize and heal with normal bone.

The progression of the Charcot joint is dependent upon the therapy instituted and the time at which it was started. Serial x-rays will provide radiographic evidence of this progression and, hence, the efficacy of treatment. The end stage or cessation of destruction is noted by decreased soft tissue swelling, diminished sclerosis, and greater definition of bony contours. The most satisfactory end point is either reconstruction or complete ankylosis of the joint. Poor results are indicated by continued destruction, repetition of the processes, intercurrent infections, fractures, pseudoarthrosis, and instability.

## DIFFERENTIAL DIAGNOSES

The diagnosis of diabetic neuropathic arthropathy is primarily dependent upon the physician's clinical suspicion for the disease. Consideration of the patient's medical history in combination with the characteristic appearance of the foot is often enough for a tentative diagnosis. Of course, a detailed examination and bilateral x-rays are mandatory to confirm changes consistent with the disease. One may even find indications of early changes or quiescent deformity in the contralateral foot.

It is important to realize that all problems arising in the diabetic are not necessarily caused by the diabetes. This patient is still subject to the same multitudinous illnesses from which the nondiabetic population suffers. Therefore, the possibility of intercurrent disease as a cause of the disorder must always be ruled out through appropriate serological

**Figure 9-9** "Diabetic osteopathy" (osteolysis). Note the distal tapering of the metatarsal shafts in this example of Charcot foot.

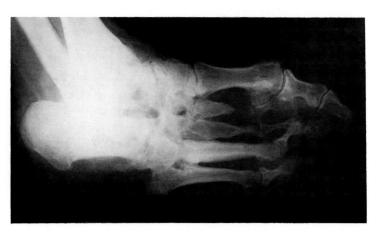

**TABLE 9-6. CONDITIONS CAUSING JOINT CHANGES SIMILAR TO CHARCOT JOINTS**

| | |
|---|---|
| Gout | Osteoarthritis |
| Acute septic arthritis | Tuberculous arthritis |
| Rheumatoid arthritis | Paraplegia |
| Psoriatic arthritis | Neoplasms |

and laboratory tests. In this same regard, a knowledge of joint involvement characteristic of each pertinent disease is helpful in narrowing the differential diagnoses. A useful clinical guide to follow is that the luetic arthropathy primarily affects the larger joints of the lower extremity, syringomyelia involves the larger joints of the upper extremity, and diabetic neuroarthropathy affects the joints of the foot.

Various arthritides may often mimic Charcot joint changes but to a much lesser extent. They will usually not show the progression or staging characteristics of osteoarthropathy, nor will they demonstrate a notable halt in progression upon cessation of weight bearing. Such arthritides include the systemic varieties (osteoarthritis, rheumatoid arthritis, and so on) and the pyogenic processes (Table 9–6). Serological and laboratory tests are indicated to detect histocompatibility antigens and certain immunoglobulins, while blood, sputum, and joint cultures may be necessary to exclude the presence of a pyogenic process.

## TREATMENT

Prevention of further trauma is the goal of treatment. Cessation of weight bearing will stop the progressive destruction and thereby promote eventual healing of the joint. Weight bearing must be completely avoided, with the affected leg elevated. Hospitalization is usually necessary to accomplish this and to provide proper treatment of infected neuropathic ulcers. The edema will subside in a matter of days to weeks, depending upon the duration and extent of joint destruction. Serial x-rays should be taken to note the efficacy of treatment.

Cast immobilization is indicated for severe joint destruction and fractures. Casts should not be applied until the edema has subsided and the condition has stabilized (one to two weeks). *Additional care must be taken to ensure that the neuropathic foot is adequately protected beneath the cast.* More often than not, an Unna boot, Jones dressing, or simple elastic bandage wrap will offer sufficient stabilization. Only after adequate immobilization may the patient walk on crutches, without bearing weight on the affected foot. As clinical and radiological improvement continues, a walking cast is applied. Immobilization is maintained until osseous repair is complete, or for a minimum of 8 to 12 weeks.

Essential to long-term management is the use of accommodative footwear. Molded or contour shoes will support the misshapened foot as well as help to prevent ulcerations over prominent bony surfaces (Fig. 9–10). Many hospital admissions of these patients are the result of ulcerations caused by ill-fitting shoes. These infected ulcers may reactivate the whole process of destruction.

Impression casting and fabrication of the therapeutic shoes should be done before final removal of the immobilization cast. In cases with minimal destruction and deformity, the patient may require only an accommodative inlay in a protective shoe. Such an orthosis may be fabricated from a soft, closed-celled polyethylene (Plastazote), which can be molded to a positive cast or directly to the foot. This Plastazote impression can then be incorporated into a "healing sandal" (Fig. 9–11), a molded shoe, or can simply be used as an inlay in an extra-depth shoe. Initially the Plastazote impression can be fitted to a

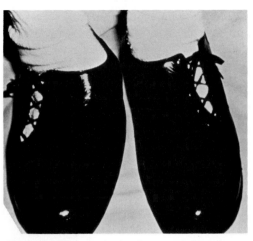

**Figure 9-10** Oxford style of custom-molded shoe.

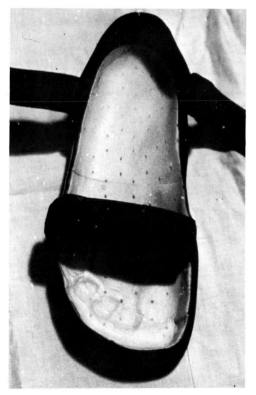

**Figure 9–11** A "healing sandal," fabricated from an impression of the foot, allows the patient to walk comfortably and safely.

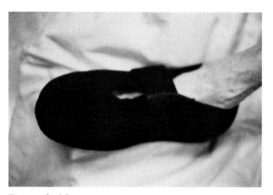

**Figure 9–12** Plastazote healing shoe available over the counter.

wooden sole postoperative shoe; this enables the patient to walk safely while the permanent shoes or sandals are being made. This therapy has been very successful in terms of both patient acceptance and in prevention of further deformity and destruction. A "healing shoe" is commercially available that can accomplish the same goals without the need for impression casting (Fig. 9–12). However, these shoes are also only for short-term usage.

Surgery is rarely indicated. If undertaken during the acute stages marked by hyperemia, resorption, and destruction, surgery is doomed to failure. The potential for postoperative infection is quite high. Therefore, a stabilization procedure should be done only after the quiescent stage has been reached.

Amputation is considered advisable only for those rare patients with severe deformity, ulceration, and infection (osteomyelitis) that prove unresponsive to conservative measures.

## SUGGESTED READING LIST

Frykberg, R. G.: Osteoarthropathy. Clin. Podiatr. Med. Surg. 4:351, 1987.

Frykberg, R. G., and Kozak, G. P.: Neuropathic arthropathy in the diabetic foot. Am. Family Physician 105–113, May, 1978.

Harris, J. R., and Brand, P. W.: Patterns of disintegration of the tarsus in the anesthetic foot. J. Bone Joint Surg. 48B:4, 1966.

Johnson, J. T. H: Neuropathic fractures and joint injuries. Pathogenesis and rationale of prevention and treatment. J. Bone Joint Surg. 49A:1, 1967.

Sanders, L. J., and Frykberg, R. G.: Charcot foot. In Levin, M. E., O'Neal, L. W., Bowker, J. H. (eds.): The Diabetic Foot. 5th ed. St. Louis, Mosby–Year Book, 1993.

Sanders, L. J., and Frykberg, R. G.: Diabetic neuropathic osteoarthropathy: The Charcot foot. In Frykberg, R. G. (ed.): The High Risk Foot in Diabetes Mellitus. New York, Churchill Livingstone, Inc., 1991.

Sinha, S., Frykberg, R. G., and Kozak, G. P.: Neuroarthropathy in the diabetic foot. In Kozak, G. (ed.): Clinical Diabetes Mellitus. Philadelphia, W. B. Saunders Co., 1983, pp. 415–425.

# Chapter 10

# OTHER ARTHRITIC DISORDERS IN THE DIABETIC FOOT

ROBERT C. MELLORS, Jr., M.D.

Rheumatic disorders affecting the foot and ankle may represent local or systemic processes that when combined with a systemic disease such as diabetes mellitus will challenge even the most astute clinician. The variety of structural components of the foot provide the basis for understanding the diversity of rheumatic processes that affect this body area. To begin with, all joint articulations in the forefoot, midfoot, and ankle are synovial in nature and thus the site of synovitis. Many ligaments and tendons insert into and around the bones of the foot in sites referred to as *entheses*. The entheses and adjacent bone are the principal sites of inflammation in certain rheumatic disorders resulting in secondary calcification with periostitis and proliferative new bone formation. With the close proximity of the osseous structures of the foot to the overlying skin that tends to break down over weight-bearing surfaces, the bones and joints of the foot are predisposed to bacterial invasion. Finally, much of the osteoarticular pathology affecting the foot is the result of trauma from the daily impact of supporting the entire body's weight.

This chapter will not attempt to cover the entire clinical spectrum of rheumatic diseases affecting the foot (Table 10–1). It will focus on the major rheumatic diseases of the foot with special emphasis on the clinical approach to the patient. The association of diabetes and certain arthritides will be reviewed, excluding a discussion of neuroarthropathy (Charcot joint), which is discussed in Chapter 9. The multitude of congenital anomalies and static foot disorders are beyond the scope of this review.

## SIGNS AND SYMPTOMS OF RHEUMATIC DISEASE

In most cases, a careful patient history will differentiate the nature of various rheumatic disorders. Pain and stiffness, particularly morning stiffness, and articular dysfunction are the initial reasons that patients seek medical attention. Pain is the most conspicuous symptom and is local or diffuse, depending upon the rheumatic process. Pain of articular origin is generally well localized because of the abundant supply of pain fibers that innervate the joint capsule and periosteum. Pain results when an inflamed synovial joint becomes full of exudative fluid and stretches the normally tight fibrous capsule. In addition, active disease of the vascular subchondral bone or adjacent periostitis contributes to the articular pain, being a deeper and more constant sensation. Painful soft tissue syndromes involving the bursae and tendons are usually but not always well localized, depending upon the degree of associated muscular spasm. When this occurs the painful tissue can often be well localized by reproducing the pain with motion or palpating over the individual bursae and tendons. Contrariwise, radiating pain syndromes from sites deeper in or proximal to the painful region are nearly always diffuse and frequently have a neurological basis. Examples of this in the foot are the tarsal tunnel syndrome, Morton neuroma, and sciatica.

Pain from rheumatic processes also may be characterized by its relationship to activity or rest and time of day. For instance, pain from inflammatory arthritis is generally relieved

## TABLE 10-1.  RHEUMATIC DISEASE OF THE FOOT AND ANKLE

1. Systemic inflammatory diseases
   Rheumatoid arthritis (adult and juvenile)
   Systemic lupus erythematosus
   Scleroderma
   Overlap syndromes
2. Seronegative spondyloarthropathies
   Ankylosing spondylitis
   Psoriatic arthritis
   Reiter's syndrome
   Enteropathic arthritis
3. Metabolic related arthropathies
   Gout
   Chondrocalcinosis
   Endocrinopathies
      (diabetes mellitus, hypothyroidism, acromegaly)
   Hemophilia and hemoglobinopathies
4. Degenerative arthritis (primary and secondary)
5. Infectious arthritis (virus, bacteria, fungi)
6. Nonarticular rheumatism
   Tendinitis and bursitis
   Neuropathic syndromes (tarsal tunnel syndrome,
      Morton neuroma, sciatica)
   Vascular disorders (Raynaud's disease, reflex
      sympathetic dystrophy, vasculitis)
7. Miscellaneous disorders
   Trauma
   Acute rheumatic fever
   Sarcoidosis
   Avascular necrosis
   Hypermobility syndromes
   Neoplasms (primary, metastatic, and related
      disorders)
   Neuroarthropathy (Charcot joint)

after use of the involved joint, but pain from noninflammatory joint disease, such as degenerative arthritis, is nearly always worse with use. The latter is particularly true in the foot with weight bearing. Conversely, rest tends to aggravate inflammatory joint pain but relieves noninflammatory pain, except when there is extensive osteoarticular disease. Nocturnal pain is a frequent complaint of patients with neurological pain, especially in the foot, due to peripheral polyneuropathy. It is also the agonizing consequence of primary or metastatic cancer of the bone.

The history of stiffness is a universal complaint of patients suffering from various types of rheumatic diseases. Morning stiffness in particular forms a valuable diagnostic clue to the presence of inflammatory rheumatic disorders and is one of the essential diagnostic criteria for rheumatoid arthritis (Table 10-2). Stiffness is frequently accompanied by pain and loss of range of motion. However, stiffness is dependent upon joint motion, as

is joint pain, and remits with complete immobility or ankylosis.

Depending upon the mode of onset of certain rheumatic processes, patients will acknowledge a change in their functional capacity. This is particularly true of acute arthritides such as gout or septic arthritis characterized by intense inflammation, which frequently renders the patient immobile. Chronic arthritides are insidious in their impact on joint function, with patients acquiring limitations that are rather easily compensated for in their daily routines. Here careful questioning by the clinician often elicits a history of functional limitation and gross impairments of activities of daily living such as loss of manual dexterity, loss of grip strength, inability of the patient to dress himself, and inability to get up and down from a chair or toilet.

The physical signs of rheumatic disorders center on the inflammatory process, which affects virtually any tissue of the body. Therefore, the physical examination is largely directed at correlating the location and extent of pathology with the underlying anatomy. In the foot, the individual joints—ankle, subtalar, midtarsal, metatarsophalangeal, interphalangeal—are inspected for symmetry and

## TABLE 10-2.  RHEUMATOID ARTHRITIS DIAGNOSTIC CRITERIA (ARA)

1. Morning stiffness
2. Pain on motion or tenderness in at least one joint
3. Swelling of one joint (soft tissue or fluid)
4. Swelling of at least one other joint
5. Symmetrical joint swelling on both sides of the body
6. Subcutaneous nodules
7. Radiographic changes typical of rheumatoid arthritis
8. Positive rheumatoid factor
9. Poor mucin precipitate from synovial fluid
10. Characteristic histological changes in synovial membrane
11. Characteristic histological changes in nodules

To meet criteria 1–5, symptoms present continuously for >6 weeks

| Diagnostic Category | No. Criteria Required |
| --- | --- |
| Classic | 7 of 11 |
| Definite | 5 of 11 |
| Probable | 3 of 11 |

hemochromatosis arthropathy are considered associated states while the other disorders are direct complications of the diabetic state. The relationship between gout and diabetes mellitus appears to be on a clinical basis, although not well defined. Reports have conflicted regarding the association between these two metabolic diseases, and there is evidence suggesting that the prevalence of diabetes in patients with gout is related to obesity or hyperlipidemia or both. Furthermore, although marked hyperuricemia can occur during diabetic ketoacidosis from the inhibition of renal tubular secretion of uric acid by β-hydroxybutyrate, this situation does not account for acute gout in diabetes.

Hemochromatosis arthropathy may occur in patients with diabetes caused by hemochromatosis. In this iron deposition state, mineral may be deposited in the synovial membrane and articular cartilage and is associated with calcium pyrophosphate dihydrate (CPPD) crystal deposition. Thus, in patients with diabetes and joint symptoms, the clinical and radiographic features of CPPD crystal deposition disease secondary to hemochromatosis should be sought and will have the same manifestations in the foot as previously discussed.

Soft tissue ulceration and infection of the ischemic and neuropathic diabetic foot can lead to osteomyelitis and septic arthritis. Most cases of osteomyelitis of the foot in diabetes begin as chronic penetrating ulcers at pressure points beneath the metatarsal heads. The radiographic features of osteomyelitis characterized by irregular and progressive bone resorption and periosteal new bone formation may not be prominent in the diabetic foot, because these changes require an adequate vascular supply. Conversely, the absence of resorptive changes in association with diabetic osteomyelitis supports the inference of the presence of vascular ischemia. Extension of osteomyelitis into the joint space can cause loss of the subchondral bone plate and joint space narrowing associated with septic arthritis. Spontaneous fracture, subluxation, and dislocation of the bones and joints may subsequently supersede; these conditions make the clinical and radiographic distinction between osteomyelitis

and severe diabetic neuroarthrophathy difficult.

Lastly, osteolysis of the forefoot is a unique complication of diabetes mellitus and occurs in the complete absence of infection or neurovascular deficit. It is initially characterized by patchy or generalized osteoporosis of the distal metatarsals and interphalangeal joints associated with pain, which may be quite intense. Progressive osteolysis of the juxta-articular bone of the distal metatarsals and proximal and distal phalangeal joints may then occur, with sparing of the articular surfaces, leading to sharply tapered residual bone ends. The osteolysis may stop at any stage with complete restoration of the bony architecture or progress with complete resorption of the bony anatomy. The etiology of diabetic osteoylsis is uncertain, although it has a similar appearance to diabetic neuroarthropathy and may well be caused by minor degrees of tissue infection or neurovascular disease.

## SUMMARY

It is apparent from this review that a variety of rheumatic processes may affect the foot and ankle. Most are unrelated to diabetes mellitus but sometimes are associated with it. An accurate diagnosis requires a general knowledge of the pathogenesis of these rheumatic processes as well as those related to diabetes mellitus.

## SUGGESTED READING LIST

Bland, J.H., Frymoyer, J.W., Newberg, A.H., et al.: Rheumatic syndromes in endocrine disease. Semin. Arthritis Rheum. 9:1, 1979.

Bluestone, M.B.: Collagen diseases affecting the foot. Foot Ankle 2:311–317, 1982.

Gold, H.R., and Bassett, L.W.: Radiologic evaluation of the arthritic foot. Foot Ankle 2:332–341, 1982.

Guerra, J., and Resnick, D.: Arthritis affecting the foot: Radiographic-pathological correlation. Foot Ankle 2:325–331, 1982.

Katz, W.A.: Rheumatic Diseases: Diagnosis and Management. Philadelphia, J.B. Lippincott Co., 1977.

Kelley, W.N., Harris, E.D., Ruddy, S., and Sledge, C.B.: Textbook of Rheumatology. Philadelphia, W.B. Saunders Co., 1981.

McCarty, D.J.: Arthritis and Allied Conditions. Philadelphia, Lea & Febiger, 1979.

Resnick, D. and Niwayama, G.: Diagnosis of Bone and Joint Disorders. Philadelphia, W. B. Saunders Co., 1981, vol. 1–3.

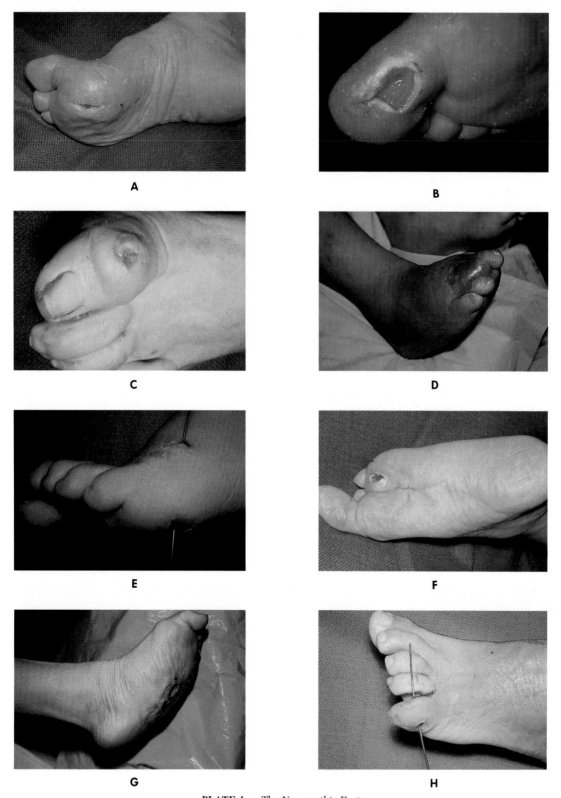

**PLATE 1.** The Neuropathic Foot.

*A,* Neuropathic foot with high arch and cocked-up toes. *B,* Neuropathic ulcer on the great toe, at a pressure point. There is a clean base and good circulation. *C,* Ulcer on top of an insensitive cocked-up toe. *D,* Cellulitis of the third toe and secondary infection. *E,* Septic fifth metatarsophalangeal joint with sinus from ulcer on sole to top of foot. *F,* A transfer ulcer to the adjacent metatarsal head after ray excision of a toe and metatarsal head. *G,* Rocker-bottom Charcot foot. *H,* Osteomyelitis of the proximal interphalangeal joint of the fifth toe.

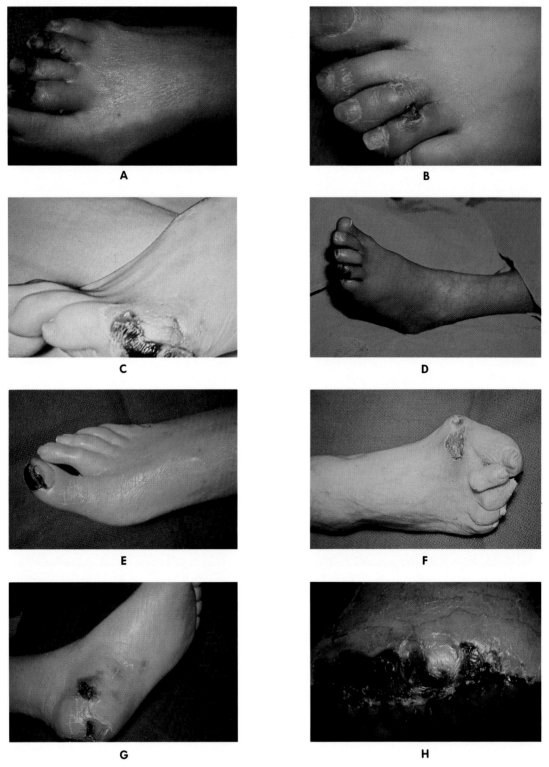

**PLATE 2.** The Ischemic Foot.

A, Dry gangrene of the toes prior to transmetatarsal amputation. B, Ulcers kissing between the toes. C, Gangrene of the toe secondary to an ulcer under the metatarsal head. D, Gangrene of the toe and cellulitis of the foot. E, Gangrene of the toe following an injury to the skin while nails were being trimmed. F, Infected bunion with secondary ulcer and cellulitis. G, Pressure sores on an ischemic heel left unprotected while the patient was hospitalized for another condition. H, A recent transmetatarsal amputation failing to heal because of inadequate circulation.

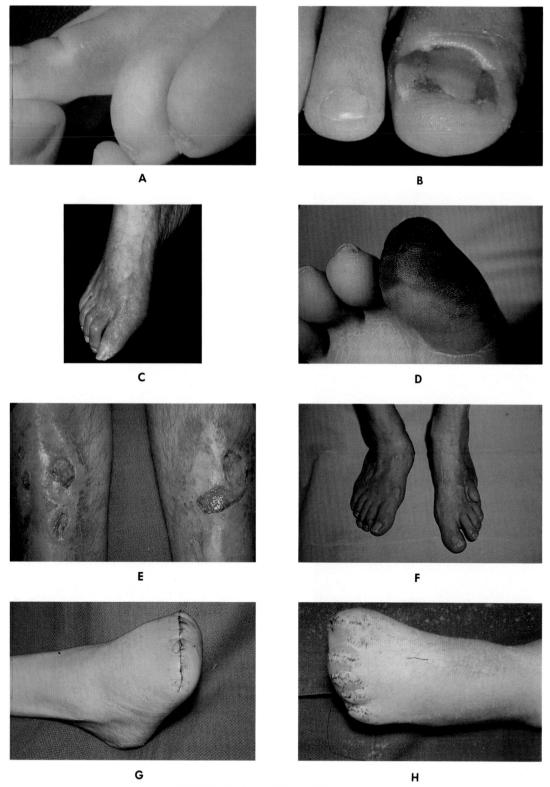

**PLATE 3.** Findings at Physical Examination.

*A*, A blister on a toe, if undetected and untreated, can lead to gangrene. *B*, An infected ingrown toenail. *C*, Dependent rubor in an ischemic foot. *D*, Gangrene of the toe due to trash emboli. *E*, Necrobiosis lipoidica diabeticorum. *F*, Neuropathic feet, and Charcot deformity of the right foot. *G*, A healing transmetatarsal amputation. *H*, Five-toe amputations. Note the lateral flaps. This operation preserves the metatarsal heads.

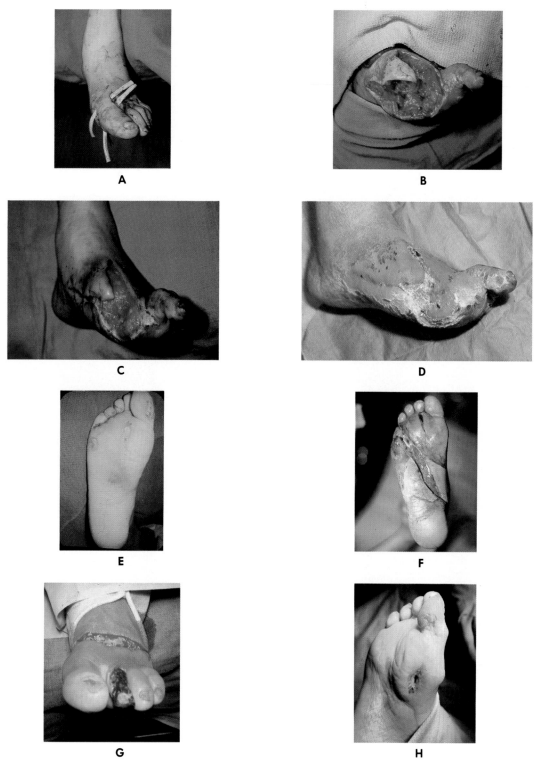

**PLATE 6.** Infection and Complications.

*A* to *D*, Ulcer of the first toe and metatarsal area that has progressed to gangrene and osteomyelitis. *A*, After inadequate debridement and drainage. *B*, Open amputation of the toe and appropriate drainage. *C*, Granulation and healing. *D*, Healed after split thickness skin graft. *E*, Ulcer under the fifth metatarsal head with subfascial extension of infection and abscess pointing in mid-sole. *F*, Proper drainage of the infection shown in *E*. *G*, Gangrene of the second toe. Dorsal incision is for transmetatarsal amputation. *H*, Ischemic foot with osteomyelitis of the first metatarsal head; transmetatarsal amputation will be done.

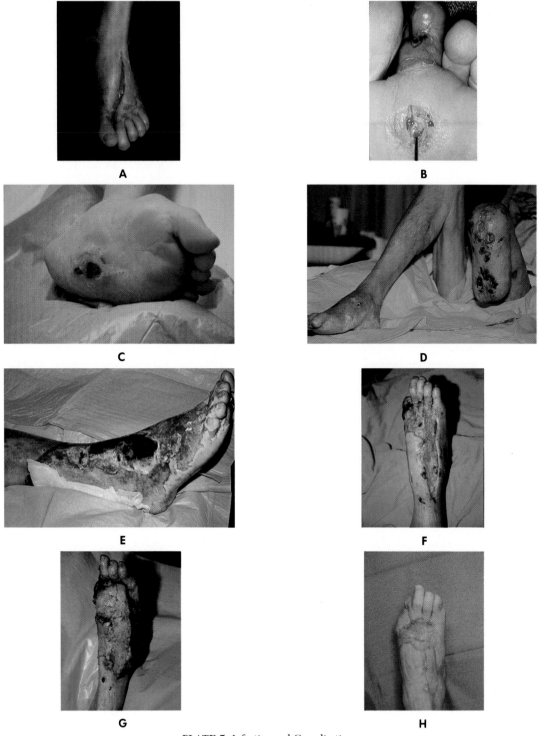

**PLATE 7.** Infection and Complications.

A, Drainage of ulcer in web of the toes and extension of infection into the foot. B, Neuropathic ulcer under the second metatarsal head with extension up the tendon into the toe. Gangrene of the toe is due to infection, not ischemia. C, Neuropathic ulcer under the heel in a Charcot foot with collapsed os calcis. D, While an ulcer of the right foot was being treated, a flexion contracture of the left below-knee amputation stump was forgotten and developed a pressure ulcer from the bed linen. E, First, second and third degree burns caused by hot soaks and a debriding ointment for superficial ulcer on the dorsum of the foot. F to H, Local bunion surgery in an office resulted in severe gas gangrene and septic shock. F, First toe and metatarsal head amputation with wide incision and drainage. G, Removal of two toes and application of a skin graft. H, The foot one year later.

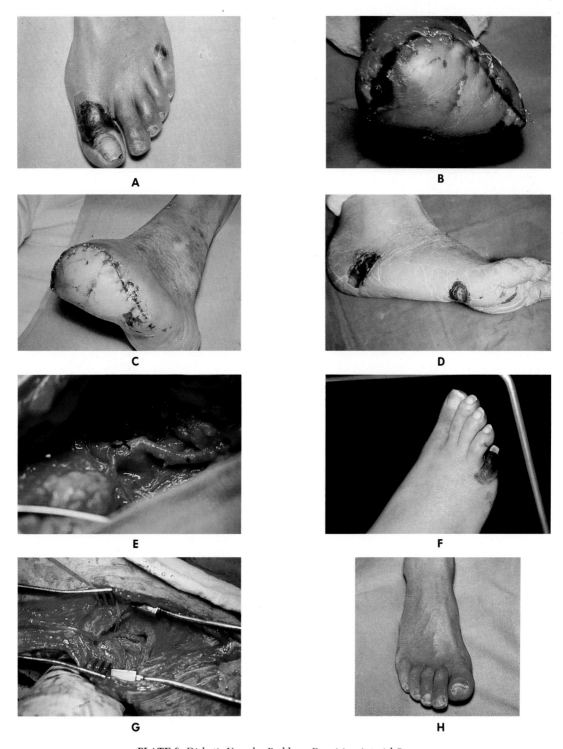

**PLATE 8.** Diabetic Vascular Problems Requiring Arterial Surgery.

A to C, Sequence of events in the same patient. A, Ischemic foot lesions prior to surgery. B, Failing transmetatarsal amputation without revascularization of leg. C, Healing amputation stump after successful femoral-popliteal bypass grafts. D, Superficial gangrene secondary to ischemic fissures in multiple areas; healed after bypass grafting. E, Reversed saphenous vein femoral-popliteal bypass with proximal anastomosis. F, Gangrene of the fifth toe. Toe amputation was successful after in situ vein femoral-popliteal bypass. G, In situ vein femoral-popliteal bypass with distal anastomosis. H, Rubor in an ischemic foot without lesions but with rest pains and intermittent claudication. Vascular surgery should be considered to prevent gangrene and restore function. (A, B, C, D, and H are reprinted from Kozak, G. P.: Clinical Diabetes Mellitus. W. B. Saunders Co., 1982.)

# Chapter 11

# RADIOLOGY IN THE DIABETIC FOOT

HARRY BAILEY, M.D.,
LEONARD CONNOLLY, M.D.,
and HERBERT M. GRAMM, M.D.

Plain film radiographic examination of the foot is the mainstay of diagnosis following clinical detection of a foot abnormality, particularly when infection is present. The neuropathic abnormalities of the foot, in particular, are often revealed only as incidental and often unsuspected findings following radiography in the infected foot or for evaluation of disproportionately severe physical findings following apparently minor trauma.

## TECHNICAL CONSIDERATIONS

It is our practice to obtain views of the foot in the three standard projections. These include an anteroposterior view with additional oblique and lateral projections. The operator must be careful to ensure that the heel is included in the lateral view, together with the full thickness of its soft tissues. The particular shape of the foot poses technical problems because of the relatively greater thickness of the more proximal bones. It may be necessary to obtain supplemental views of the phalanges at a level of penetration approximately 10 kV lower than that used for the tarsals. Standard film and screens are adequate, and it is usually not necessary to use fine grain or nonscreen film if careful attention is paid to technical factors and the nature of the clinical problem being investigated.

The two main clinical problems are infection and osteoarthropathy. Of the two, infection of soft tissues with supervening osteomyelitis is by far the most common, although with the increasing longevity of the diabetic population, osteoarthropathy is becoming a more frequent finding than in the past.

## OSTEOMYELITIS

The exclusion of this entity is the most common indication for radiological examination. The patient usually has soft-tissue swelling and signs of acute or chronic inflammation, usually involving the more distal phalanges or portions of the foot subjected to trauma from badly performed pedicure or from ill-fitting shoes. The proximal portions of the foot are involved with markedly decreasing frequency. Osteomyelitis involving the proximal bones of the foot is so unusual in point of fact that *any destructive process seen proximal to the metatarsals should be considered neuropathic until proven otherwise*. In spite of this axiom, the demonstration of destructive neuropathic changes and the erroneous presumption that these are caused by infection are the most frequent causes of unnecessary and inappropriate laboratory study and surgical intervention (Figs. 11–1 to 11–4).

The soft tissue swelling that is the early sign of infection is apparent clinically as well as radiologically and usually produces no changes in the underlying bone on the radiograph. When ulceration takes place, however, the clinician often has difficulty in deciding whether the underlying bone is involved. When osteomyelitis is present, the radiological changes consist of: (1) early cortical erosion, (2) breakthrough lesions with involvement of cancellous bone that are usually

**109**

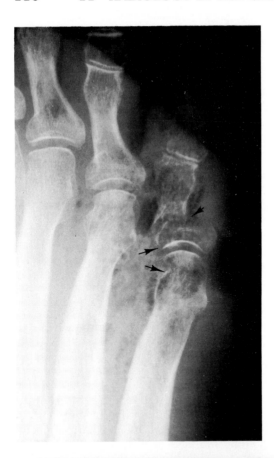

**Figure 11-1** Soft tissue ulcer associated with osteomyelitis and cellulitis with gas formation caused by gas-forming streptococci. Note subarticular bone destruction with involvement of both sides of joint *(arrows)*. (From Kozak, G.P.: Clinical Diabetes Mellitus, Philadelphia, W. B. Saunders Co., 1982.)

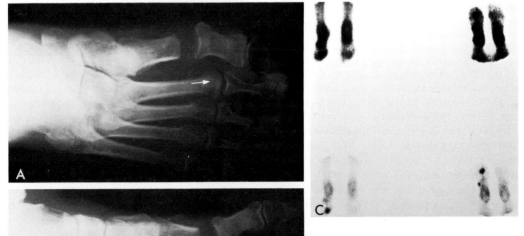

**Figure 11-2** *A*, There is a lytic area in the distal phalanx of the first digit. Note the preservation of the dense cancellous bone of the articular surface with nearly complete destruction of the less compact tuft. The flattening and sclerosis of the base of the second metatarsal is due to aseptic necrosis (Freiberg's infraction) (see *arrow*). This is an early sign of proximal neuropathy. *B*, The osteolytic region is again seen. Incidentally noted is the oblique fracture in the base of the fifth metatarsal (see *arrow*). This can be seen on the AP film as well. *C*, Bone scan demonstrates increased activity in the distal phalanx of the great toe. This corresponds to the site of osteomyelitis clinically. The fifth metatarsal fracture is also hot.

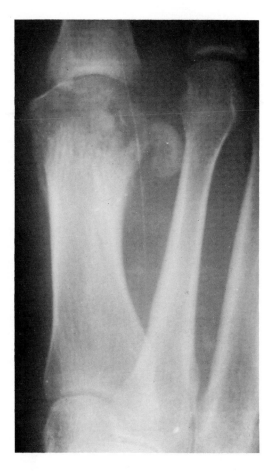

**Figure 11-3** Soft tissue swelling, bony erosion, and periosteal reaction indicate osteomyelitis of first metatarsal head.

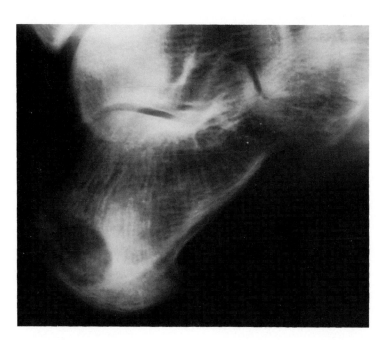

**Figure 11-4** Calcaneal osteomyelitis. One centimeter erosion on the dorsal surface of the calcaneus.

associated with diffuse demineralization, (3) gross destruction of bone involving the cortex and medulla, (4) a further category of infection in which the destructive process invades the joint capsule and leads to the typical changes of septic arthritis (Fig. 11–5A–C). These changes may be accompanied by the presence of gas in the soft tissues. The offending organisms are invariably not clostridial but are usually varieties of gas-forming streptococci. The gas is seen as a collection of very small radiolucent areas often dissecting along soft tissue planes as well as in the subcutaneous and periosseous tissues.

Infection and soft tissue ulceration overlying the weight-bearing surfaces of the calcaneus are also common, but erosion of the underlying one is distinctly unusual because of the extremely dense protective cancellous bone in this location.

An interesting but readily explicable observation is that osteomyelitis is almost never seen in the presence of frank *dry* gangrene of the involved part, since total ablation of

the arterial supply clearly cannot be associated with an inflammatory response. Osteomyelitis *can* be present, however, in "wet" gangrene secondary to veno-occlusive disease.

Finally, it should be pointed out that whereas osteomyelitis shows an overwhelming numerical preponderance in the distal bones of the foot, it can also occur in other areas such as weight-bearing metatarsals and adjacent to fractures and structures made protuberant by neuropathic change (Fig. 11–6).

## SCINTIGRAPHY AND DIABETIC OSTEOMYELITIS

A bone scan may be positive as early as 24 hours after the onset of osteomyelitis; this is a much more sensitive indicator of early changes than the radiograph. The so-called three-phase bone scan is helpful in distinguishing osteomyelitis from cellulitis. A dy-

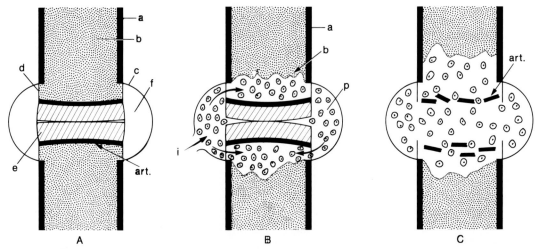

**Figure 11–5** Schema of normal synovial joint *(A)* and evolution of septic arthritis *(B)* and *(C)*.
A, (a) Dense, relatively thick cortical bone of metaphysis.
(b) Cancellous bone with normal degree of mineralization.
(c) Synovium and capsule.
(d) Relatively thin para-articular cortical bone.
(e) Articular cartilage
(art) Dense bone of articular surface.
(f) Synovial fluid.
B, Infection (i)—the breach of the synovium leads to accumulation of pus (p). This attacks the relatively thin para-articular bone and soft vascular subarticular cancellous bone, isolating the dense articular surface and joint cartilage. There is relative demineralization of the cancellous bone because of hyperemia and osteoclastic resorption.
C, Destruction of the subarticular cancellous bone eventually leads to collapse of the articular surface. This usually presents as multiple small compression fractures leaving fragments of articular surface suspended in pus with lysis of cartilage by enzymes.

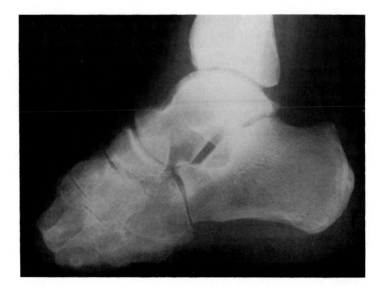

**Figure 11-6** Subcutaneous air and edema of the plantar fibroadipose tissues are fairly characteristic of cellulitis. The infiltration and subsequent blurring of normal soft tissue planes distinguishes these findings from the soft tissue swelling seen with the diabetic neuropathy itself.

namic scan over the region of suspected osteomyelitis is obtained during the first minute following intravenous administration of a technetium 99m phosphate compound. This is followed by an immediate blood pool image and then delayed images at two to four hours. The dynamic and blood pool images reflect vascularity of the lesion and therefore demonstrate increased activity in both osteomyelitis and cellulitis. The delayed images in osteomyelitis reveal persistent and typically more intensely increased activity that localizes to the involved osseous structure. The initial increased activity in cellulitis returns to normal or diminishes and does not localize to bone. The pattern observed in osteomyelitis, however, is nonspecific and may be seen in many conditions, including diabetic neuro-osteoarthropathy. Scintigraphic findings may precede radiographic changes in neuro-osteoarthropathy just as in osteomyelitis. A positive three-phase bone scan is highly sensitive but relatively nonspecific in establishing a diagnosis of osteomyelitis in the diabetic patient. Imaging with agents that localize to sites of infection is therefore frequently employed for this purpose.

Gallium 67 citrate uptake at infected foci is due to many factors, most importantly direct bacterial uptake, direct leukocyte uptake, and binding to local proteins, especially lactoferrin released from leukocytes. Osteomyelitis is distinguished from cellulitis by focal localization to bone with or without a soft-tissue component. Images are obtained 24 to 72 hours following tracer administration. Although this agent may also localize to sites of reactive bone formation, when the degree of gallium 67 citrate uptake exceeds the degree of technetium 99m phosphate uptake, osteomyelitis may be confidently diagnosed in patients with underlying bone disease. A significant percentage of such patients, however, will not demonstrate this pattern but rather will have technetium phosphate uptake exceeding or equaling gallium 67 citrate uptake. For this reason, labeled autologous leukocytes have become the preferred agent for establishing a diagnosis of acute osteomyelitis complicating neuro-osteoarthropathy.

Leukocytes are most often labeled with indium 111 oxine, indium 111 tropolone, or Tc 99m HMPAO (Ceretec, Arlington Heights, Ill). Localization at the site of infection is by direct leukocyte migration. Images are obtained at 4 and 24 hours after administration of indium 111 leukocytes. Imaging is generally completed at four hours after injection of Tc 99m HMPAO leukocytes, although some advocate a 24-hour image in cases of complicating osteomyelitis. Cellulitis is differentiated from osteomyelitis as with gallium 67 citrate imaging. Although sterile reactive bone formation may also cause slightly increased labeled leukocyte uptake, this has been less problematic than with gallium 67 citrate. A diagnosis of osteomyelitis complicating underlying bone disease is made scintigraphically when labeled leukocyte uptake is moderately or markedly greater than uptake in a comparable adjacent or contralateral bone. It is also useful to compare the labeled leukocyte scan with the bone scan in a manner similar to that done with gallium 67 citrate images.

Although a negative bone, gallium 67 citrate, or labeled leukocyte scan militates against a diagnosis of osteomyelitis, a false negative scan may occasionally occur. Peripheral vascular disease and diabetic angiopathy may impair delivery of these agents to a site of osteomyelitis in the diabetic foot. Technetium phosphate bone scans and less frequently labeled leukocyte scans and gallium 67 citrate scans may be falsely negative in patients with chronic osteomyelitis. Renal insufficiency may lessen the target-to-background ratio for bone scans, limiting image quality. Prior antibiotic therapy may result in falsely negative bone and gallium 67 citrate scans, but appears not to adversely affect the results of labeled leukocyte scintigraphy. Severely neutropenic patients are not suitable candidates for labeled leukocyte scanning. The infecting organism's ability to incite a leukocyte response also affects labeled leukocyte migration. Fungal infections may, for example, result in a less significant response.

Patients with suspected osteomyelitis and radiographs revealing either no osseous changes or findings that may be due to neuroarthropathy should initially undergo technetium 99m phosphate bone scanning. This should be performed as the initial scintigraphic examination because of its high sensitivity and rapid time to completion and because the physical characteristics of both gallium 67 and indium 111 effectively preclude bone scanning immediately after imaging with these agents. If the bone scan is normal at the suspected site, further scintigraphic imaging is generally not necessary. When the bone scan is abnormal, a labeled leukocyte or gallium 67 citrate scan will serve a complementary role. Labeled leukocytes are preferable when the condition is acute or the patient has been receiving antibiotic therapy. Gallium 67 citrate imaging may be preferable or equivalent to labeled leukocyte scanning in the diagnosis of chronic osteomyelitis. This combined-method approach is both highly sensitive and specific in establishing a diagnosis of osteomyelitis.

## RADIOLOGY OF DIABETIC NEURO-OSTEOARTHROPATHY

The radiological findings in diabetic neuro-osteoarthropathy are variable and yet somewhat specific. The tarsometatarsal joints are usually the earliest sites of involvement. The ankles and distal joints of the foot follow in frequency. It is unusual to have neuropathic changes in other joints of the body; however, cases of multiple sites of involvement, including the wrist, have been reported.

This predilection for the distal lower extremity tends to separate diabetic neuropathy from the other causes of "neuropathic joints." These other causes are neurosyphilis, congenital insensitivity to pain, spinal cord lesions, syringomyelia, leprosy, and peripheral nerve damage. In some instances, however, the physician would be hard pressed to distinguish between these entities without clinical data.

The pathogenesis of diabetic neuropathy has been a topic of debate essentially since Jordan first described the entity in 1936. Two basic schools of thought concerning the cause of diabetic neuropathy exist. The neurotraumatic theory, based on the data from the studies of Eloesser, states that joint destruction results from a loss of sensitivity to pain resulting in repeated injury to the joints. This theory does not explain the rapidity with which joint destruction, especially bone resorption, can take place.

A neurovascular theory has been reintroduced. The mechanism for this theory involves a neurally incited vascular reflex. This increases blood flow within the bones, and subsequent bone resorption by osteoclasts results. The characteristic fractures, disorganization, and destruction occur as secondary events. In both theories, the degree of "secondary changes" is dependent on the insensitivity of the joint and the continuance of weight bearing on the joint.

The changes seen radiographically range from soft tissue swelling to complete disruption of the joint or bones or both. The follow-

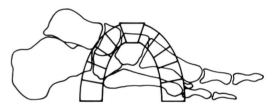

**Figure 11–7** The superimposed gothic arch over the osseous structures of the foot demonstrate the "keystone" of the longitudinal arch. This corresponds to the naviculocuneiform and the cuneiform-metatarsal joints.

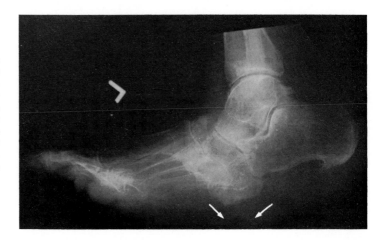

**Figure 11–8** This is the infamous rocker-bottom foot of diabetic arthropathy. Note the normal trabeculation in the tarsal bones and the relatively normal joint spaces. These signify a stable neuropathy. Also note the soft tissue ulcer adjacent to the bony prominence of the rocker deformity (see *arrows*). This is a frequent association and occasionally requires surgical correction.

ing areas within the spectrum of changes will be discussed or illustrated: (1) disorganization, (2) subluxation, (3) demineralization, (4) destruction, (5) osteolysis, and (6) fractures.

**DISORGANIZATION.** This change classically begins with the tarsometatarsal joints, specifically the medial components of the foot. These joints, the naviculocuneiform and the cuneiform-metatarsal, represent the "keystone" of the arch (Fig. 11–7). Once this relationship is lost, the arch rapidly collapses on itself and can progress to the rocker-bottom foot (Fig. 11–8). The end stage of this is Charcot joint.

**SUBLUXATION.** Subluxation is difficult to separate completely from disorganization, as they generally occur together (Figs. 11–9

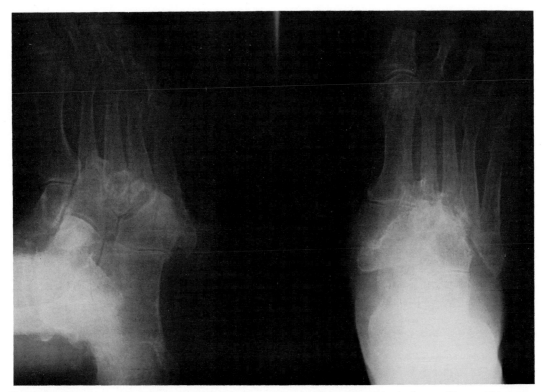

**Figure 11–9** There is a loss of both joint space and normal anatomical relationships in the tarsal bones. This is most evident in the medially located bones. The medial cuneiform is subluxated and there is subluxation and fragmentation of the navicular. Subluxation of the tarsometatarsal and metatarsophalangeal joints is also seen.

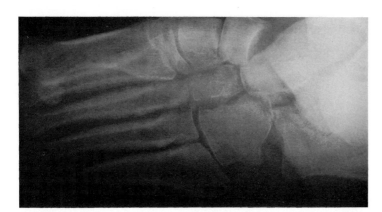

**Figure 11–10** Subluxation at the talonavicular and calcaneocuboid joint (midtarsal joint).

through 11–13). However, in addition to the tarso-metatarsal joints, the distal joints of the foot are frequently involved in this process. The deformity results from early selective loss of anatomical alignment and the stronger pull of the extensor muscle groups.

**DESTRUCTION.** This is manifested by fragmentation of the involved bones along with complete disorganization of the joint. Extensive osteoporosis with varying degrees of sclerosis is usually present. Its appearance mimics osteomyelitis because the involved region can be both painful and warm in spite of the neuropathic basis of the changes. The clinical and radiological picture is therefore frequently misinterpreted as being caused by osteomyelitis, leading to unnecessary biopsies or other forms of inappropriate surgical intervention in an invariably vain attempt to support this diagnosis.

**DEMINERALIZATION.** The mechanism for this aspect of diabetic neuropathy is twofold.

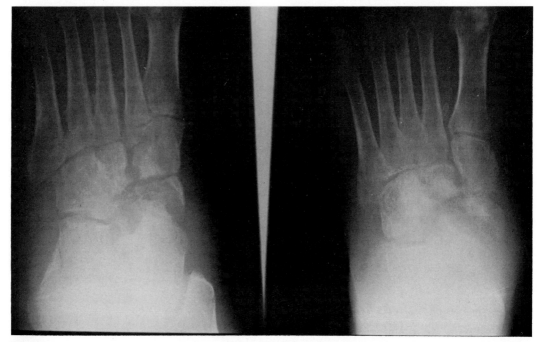

**Figure 11–11** Fragmentation and subluxation of the navicular bone is seen. There is mild to moderate disorganization of all of the tarsal bones with marked soft tissue swelling. Note the vascular calcifications. Once again the fragmentation and subluxation of the navicular are seen. The cuboid and cuneiforms are involved to a lesser extent. Note the considerable blurring and loss of definition of the joint spaces in the proximal bones.

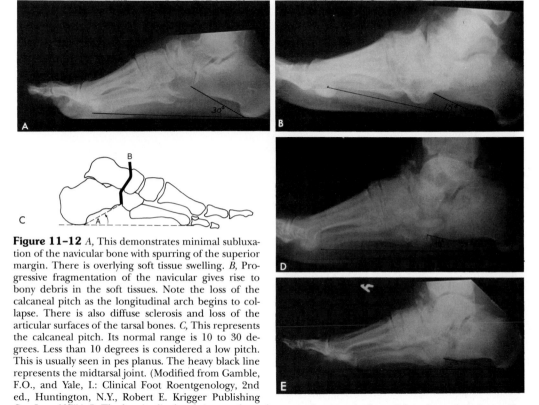

**Figure 11–12** *A,* This demonstrates minimal subluxation of the navicular bone with spurring of the superior
margin. There is overlying soft tissue swelling. *B,* Progressive fragmentation of the navicular gives rise to
bony debris in the soft tissues. Note the loss of the
calcaneal pitch as the longitudinal arch begins to collapse. There is also diffuse sclerosis and loss of the
articular surfaces of the tarsal bones. *C,* This represents
the calcaneal pitch. Its normal range is 10 to 30 degrees. Less than 10 degrees is considered a low pitch.
This is usually seen in pes planus. The heavy black line
represents the midtarsal joint. (Modified from Gamble,
F.O., and Yale, I.: Clinical Foot Roentgenology, 2nd
ed., Huntington, N.Y., Robert E. Krigger Publishing
Co., Inc., 1975.) *D,* The longitudinal arch is now absent because of progressive loss of the calcaneal pitch as well as
the progressive disorganization of the tarsometatarsal joints. Fragmentation of additional tarsal bones is now seen.
The talus is tilted anteriorly, and bone fragments are present within the posterior joint capsule. *E,* Sclerotic changes
in the tarsal bones as well as near reversal of the longitudinal arch are seen. This is in conjunction with the
complete disorganization of the joints. All of these changes often are mistaken for osteomyelitis. The differentiating
point is the absence of soft tissue edema infiltrating tissue planes. Joint effusions, however, are often present. To
further confuse the issue, the foot, in spite of the neuropathic nature of the disease, can be warm and painful.

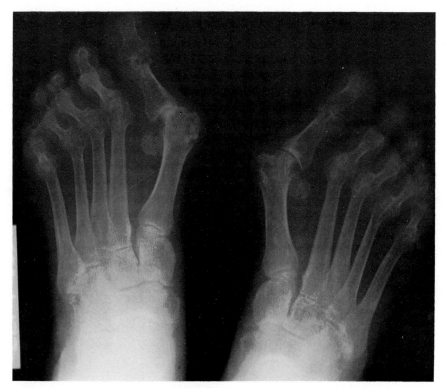

**Figure 11-13** Marked subluxation of the metatarsophalangeal joints.

There is the increased bony metabolism secondary to an increased blood flow. This is augmented by a relative disuse of the joint because of the nature of the neuropathy. The input of the second part is related to the relative degree of insensitivity. There is an overall osteopenia present in the diabetic state. The demineralization is a subjective finding and difficult to evaluate by standard radiographic techniques because of the wide variation in bone mineralization throughout the population by age group and sex. Radiographic assessment of bone mineralization requires sophisticated controlled techniques not widely available. Therefore, pictorial examples of demineralization will not be provided.

**OSTEOLYSIS.** This refers to the "sucked

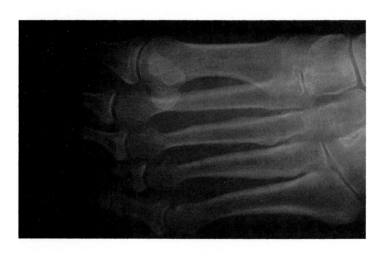

**Figure 11-14** This patient has had no operations on the feet. The distal portion of the fourth digit is absent, a result of autoamputation.

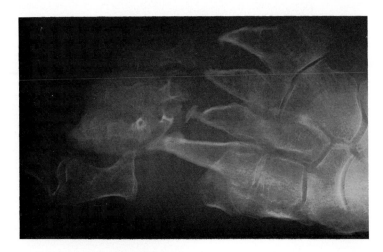

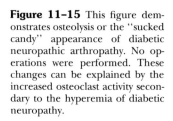

**Figure 11-15** This figure demonstrates osteolysis or the "sucked candy" appearance of diabetic neuropathic arthropathy. No operations were performed. These changes can be explained by the increased osteoclast activity secondary to the hyperemia of diabetic neuropathy.

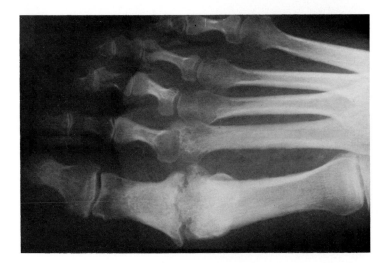

**Figure 11-16** Impacted fracture of the first metatarsal head with involvement of the base of the proximal phalanx. Note the relative sclerosis of the involved bones.

**Figure 11-17** Fracture of the proximal phalanx with extension into the joint. No recollection of trauma and minimal symptoms (edema of the toe) were the history and physical findings for this patient.

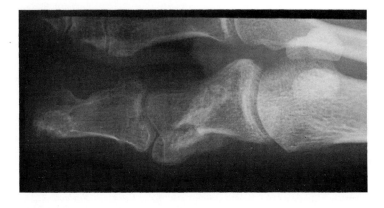

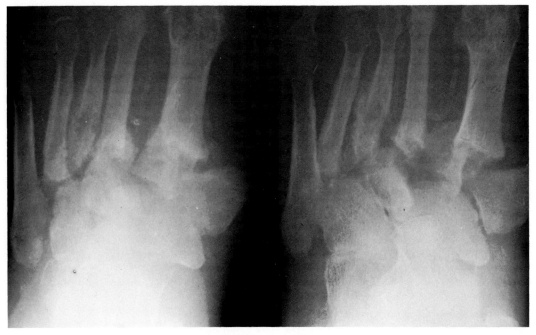

**Figure 11-18** Multiple metatarsal fractures and gross disorganization of the tarsal bones are seen in this example.

candystick'' appearance in the involved bones. The metatarsals are the most frequently involved bones. The cause of this has long been a topic of discussion. As previously mentioned, the neurovascular mechanism best explains this process (Figs. 11–14 and 11–15).

**FRACTURES.** These are characterized by often bizarre-appearing fractures in unusual locations, often with a history of minimal or no recollectable trauma to the involved area. Bones involved include the calcaneus, shafts of the metatarsals (especially the first), and the phalanges, which may sustain impacted fractures (Figs. 11–16 through 11–18).

## SUGGESTED READING LIST

Brower, A.C., and Allman, R.M.: Pathogenesis of the neurotrophic joint: Neurotraumatic versus neurovascular. Radiology 139:349, 1981.

Clouse, M.E., Gramm, H.F., Legg, M., and Flood, T.: Diabetic osteoarthropathy—clinical and roentgenographic observations in 90 cases. Am. J. Roentgenol. Radium Ther. Nucl. Med. 121:22, 1974.

Colwell, J.A., Halushka, P.V., Sarji, K.E., et al.: Vascular disease in diabetes; pathophysiological mechanisms and therapy. Arch. Intern. Med. 139:225, 1979.

Eymott, M.J., Alavi, A., Dalinka, M.K., and Kyle, G.C.: Bone scintigraphy in diabetic osteoarthropathy. Radiology 140:475, 1981.

Feldman, M.J., Becker, K.L., Reefe, W.E., and Longo, A.:

Multiple neuropathic joints including the wrist, in a patient with diabetes mellitus. JAMA 209:1690, 1969.

Frykberg, R.G., and Kozak, G.P.: Neuropathic arthropathy in the diabetic foot. Am. Fam. Physician 17:105, 1978.

Gamble, F.O., and Yale, I.: Clinical Foot Roentgenology, 2nd ed. Huntington, N.Y., Robert E. Krigger Publishing Co., Inc., 1975.

Gondos, B.: The pointed tubular bone—its significance and pathogenesis. Radiology 105:541, 1972.

Heath, N. III., Melton, L.J., III., and Chu, C.: Diabetes mellitus and risk of skeletal fracture. N. Engl. J. Med. 303:567, 1980.

Kozak, G.P.: Clinical Diabetes Mellitus. Philadelphia, W. B. Saunders Co., 1982.

Kraft, E., Spyropoulos, E., and Finby, N.: Neurogenic disorders of the foot in diabetes mellitus. Am. J. Roentgenol. Radium Ther. Nucl. Med. 124:17, 1975.

Kristiansen, B.: Ankle and foot fractures in diabetes provoking neuropathic joint changes. Acta Orthop. Scand. 51:975, 1980.

McCarthy, K., Velchik, M. G., Alavi, A., et al.: Indium-111 labeled white blood cells in the detection of osteomyelitis complicated by a pre-existing condition. J. Nucl. Med. 29:1015, 1988.

Schanwecker, D. S., Park, H-M., Mock, B. H., et al.: Evaluation of complicating osteomyelitis with Tc-99m MDP, In-111 granulocytes and Ga-67 citrate. J. Nucl. Med. 25:849, 1984.

Al-Sheikh, W., Sfakianakis, G. N., Mnaymneh, W., et al.: Subacute and chronic bone infections: Diagnosis using In-111, Ga-67, and Tc-99m MDP bone scintigraphy and radiography. Radiology 155:501, 1985.

Newman, J.H.: Noninfective disease of the diabetic foot. J. Bone Joint Surg. 63B:593, 1981.

Reinhardt, K.: The radiological residua of healed diabetic arthropathies. Skeletal Radiol. 7:167, 1981.

# Chapter 12

# INFECTION OF THE DIABETIC FOOT: MEDICAL AND SURGICAL MANAGEMENT

GARY W. GIBBONS, M.D.,
and GEORGE M. ELIOPOULOS, M.D.

In the first edition of this text in 1984 the lead sentence in this chapter was "More in-hospital days are spent treating diabetic foot infections than any other complication of diabetes." Unfortunately, despite all of our advances in medical care and technology, this statement remains true. Diabetes affects 6 per cent of (14 million) people in the United States, and 25 per cent of diabetic persons will seek the advice of a health care professional for a foot- or leg-related problem at some point during the course of their diabetes. Diabetic foot problems account for 20 per cent of all hospital admissions for diabetic patients. The medical, social, and economic impact of foot problems is enormous with attendant cost of hospitalization alone running over $600 million per year. A review of a 12-month period, 1987 through 1988, at the New England Deaconess Hospital and the Joslin Clinic revealed that lower-limb infections in diabetics constituted 7.3 per cent of all admissions and 13 per cent of all in-patients' stays.

The fact that the risk of amputation is 15 times greater in diabetic patients than in their nondiabetic counterparts led the American Diabetes Association to set as a goal a 50 per cent reduction in the number of major amputations in diabetics by the end of 1991. This is significant since two thirds of all non-traumatic amputations performed in the United States (50,000 per year) are performed on diabetics. It is our feeling that many of these continue to be performed needlessly because of misconceptions that still persist regarding the appropriate treat-ment of diabetic foot or leg problems. For the most part, therapeutic strategies have relied strongly upon microbiological studies of diabetic foot lesions, knowledge of the in vitro antimicrobial activity of various antibiotics, and the clinical expertise of physicians in the therapy of diabetic foot infections. This chapter reviews the etiology, discusses the misconceptions, and presents strategies for optimal management of patients with foot or leg ulcerations. The major amputation rate at the New England Deaconess Hospital has been reduced to less than 5 per cent (from 28 per cent in the early 1980s) by an aggressive team approach devoted to salvaging the diabetic foot.

## HOST CONSIDERATIONS

While minor trauma leading to cutaneous ulceration is the actual culprit, it is the trio-pathy of neuropathy, vascular insufficiency, and an altered response to infection that either singularly or more often in combination makes the diabetic uniquely susceptible to foot problems. Neuropathy not only results in sensory loss to pain and pressure, but also loss of position sense of the foot, while motor neuropathy affects all of the muscles of the foot, leading to the deformities one characteristically sees. Add to this an autonomic neuropathy that results in a falsely warm foot secondary to altered blood flow. This also impairs sweating manifested by dry cracking skin susceptible to fissures, cracks,

121

and callous formation. The result of neuropathy is a foot highly susceptible to even a small amount of trauma or injury.

Peripheral vascular disease and its treatment are discussed in Chapters 19, 20, and 21. In two of our studies examining diabetic patients with limb-threatening foot infections, neuropathy was present in more than 98 per cent, but ischemia was identified as severe in 50 per cent. One has to remember that ischemic necrosis has other causes besides peripheral vascular disease, including pressure necrosis and/or uncontrolled infection. Unrecognized ischemia, however, is a common reason diabetic foot ulcerations fail to respond to conservative treatment.

There is question whether infections in general occur with increased frequency in diabetic patients. Infection is not usually the direct cause of an ulceration. Rather, an open ulcer serves as a portal of entry for pathogenic bacteria. The diabetic has an altered response to infection with certain defects in leukocyte function and wound repair identified. Diabetic patients tolerate infection poorly: Infection adversely affects diabetes control, and uncontrolled diabetes adversely affects infection. Clinically the most significant fact is that clinical manifestations of infection may be subtle or absent because systemic signs and symptoms (such as temperature elevation or increased heart rate) of a serious limb- and life-threatening infection are frequently absent or occur late. The only evidence of local infection initially may be disturbance of blood glucose control and/or a flu-like syndrome.

## PREVENTION

Prevention of ulceration and recurrence once ulceration has occurred are the ultimate goals of any modern team approach to the diabetic foot. The risk of developing severe foot problems and how well such problems are treated are directly influenced by the degree to which the patient, physician, and other health care professionals understand properly the basic principles of foot care. Minor trauma resulting in loss of skin integrity and the interplay of neuropathy, ischemia, and infection must never be forgotten. The role of proper footwear and hygiene therefore cannot be overemphasized. Patients with severe neuropathy and ischemia can live and function without ever developing a foot ulceration or problem. The diabetic patient and his family must establish a routine for daily foot and shoe inspection and hygiene. Proper footwear is often a major problem because the most attractive shoes are not necessarily the best fitting. Changing shoes during the day can relieve high-risk pressure areas and allow for the reaccumulation of edema. Every patient must be taught to shake his shoes out and inspect them prior to wearing. The frequency of injury that can be avoided by this simple maneuver is amazing.

Proper hygiene must become a religion. Washing the feet every day with mild soap and rinsing and drying thoroughly especially between the toes are advised. Moisture-restoring cream should be applied everywhere, except between the toes, daily and more often when needed. Socks must be clean, intact, and appropriate for particular shoeing. Diabetic patients should avoid the use of all astringents as well as most over-the-counter preparations for calluses, nails, and the like. Self-"bathroom" surgery must be avoided at all costs and nails trimmed with a slightly rounded edge. There are just some objects and situations all diabetics should avoid. Diabetics should never soak their feet or use heat—such as heating pads—in any form or sleep next to space heaters or stoves. The hot and cold sensations that diabetics often get are related to neuropathy and not to poor circulation. It should be understandable to all why diabetics should never go barefoot.

The physician or health care provider must always set the example: Controlling blood glucose, weight, and blood pressure; eliminating smoking; and encouraging daily exercise are important. The patient's legs and feet, including the heels and between the toes, must be examined at regular intervals, and any patient whose blood glucose suddenly becomes difficult to manage should be carefully inspected for an occult limb-threatening infection. Periodic neurological and vascular examinations are important, as are noting any skin changes, callous formations, or foot deformities that should be further evaluated. If the health care professional inspects the shoes for appropriateness, excessive wear, and foreign bodies, the patient learns its importance. Early recognition and prompt reporting of a problem, no matter what time of day, are encouraged. Neuropathy and an overwhelming fear of amputation may delay early reporting of a problem by some diabetics. In the interest of maximizing limb salvage, the physician caring for a diabetic patient with a foot problem should not hesitate to consult a specialist when there is any doubt about the appropriate management of the problem.

## MICROBIOLOGY

In the last decade, several studies have called attention to the fact that most (70 to 80 per cent or more) foot infections severe enough to require hospitalization of the diabetic patient are polymicrobial. In various reports, the mean number of different microbial species isolated from an infected site has ranged from two to six. Cultures frequently reveal a mixture of gram-positive and gram-negative aerobic (and facultative) organisms, as well as one or more strictly anaerobic isolates in 30 to 80 per cent of cases.

*Staphylococcus aureus* features prominently among the gram-positive cocci recovered, being found in approximately one third to one half of the cases. However, coagulase-negative staphylococci and various streptococci also are isolated in a substantial percentage of infections. Enterococci are encountered in about 25 to 30 per cent of patients, almost always as part of a mixed microbial flora. Among the aerobic (or facultatively anaerobic) gram-negative bacteria, Proteus species and *Escherichia coli* are typical isolates, but a wide variety of other Enterobacteriaceae are represented. *Pseudomonas aeruginosa,* while present in only a minority of cases, is important to recognize because these organisms may be resistant to antimicrobials active against many other gram-negative bacilli. Anaerobic isolates from foot infections include various gram-positive cocci (peptococci, peptostreptococci) or bacilli (Clostridia) as well as several gram-negative bacteria, the most important of which are the Bacteroides species. When anaerobic bacteria are present, their absolute numbers determined by quantitative colony counts of deep tissues may exceed those of the aerobes isolated.

The bacteriology of ulcer-associated foot infections may potentially be influenced by a number of factors. For example, anaerobes and gram-negative bacilli may play a less prominent role in relatively superficial ulcerations with non–limb-threatening infection. Prior antimicrobial therapy may also influence the microbiology of a given infection. First, in patients with persistent or progressive infection despite initial empirical therapy targeted at common pathogens, infection with less common but more antibiotic-resistant organisms such as enterococci or *P. aeruginosa* must be considered. Next, local epidemiological factors must be kept in mind. For example, in most regions of the United States, methicillin resistance among community isolates of *S. aureus* would be uncommon. In contrast, the risk of infection with methicillin-resistant *S. aureus* might be substantially greater in an environment where such strains are more prevalent.

Finally, it must be noted that the ultimate value of bacteriological evaluation still depends upon the degree to which the specimen provided to the laboratory is a representative sample of the active site of infection. There is often incomplete correlation between bacterial species isolated from superficial swabs of an open ulcerative process and those recovered at surgery from deep tissues or even by scraping of the ulcer base after removal of superficial debris. Superficial cultures may thus occasionally fail to detect organisms later proven to exist more deeply within an infected area or, more commonly, may reveal multiple organisms, including some that are primarily colonizers with little role in the active infectious process.

## PRINCIPLES OF ANTIBIOTIC THERAPY

Because patients with potentially limb-threatening infections require hospitalization, it is most prudent initially to administer antibiotics parenterally to ensure adequate serum levels. Thus, potential uncertainties about the adequacy of drug absorption, in this population known for disorders of gastrointestinal function, are avoided. Establishment of good initial serum levels of antimicrobials seems intuitively important when local host factors (edema, devitalized tissue, altered tissue pH, and the like) might impede delivery or impair efficacy of drug(s) at the site of infection.

Selection of an initial empirical antibiotic regimen is influenced by several factors, including the expected pathogens as discussed above, prevailing local antibiotic resistance patterns, and various host factors, including history of allergic reactions or coexisting medical conditions (e.g. renal or hepatobiliary dysfunction) that might make more complicated the use of some agents. Prior culture data are often of great help, which is why even seemingly minor ulcers should be cultured, even if there is every expectation these would heal with careful outpatient management.

It is important to realize that no one antimicrobial regimen, no matter how broad spectrum or well tolerated it would appear, will guarantee optimal treatment of all possible pathogenic microorganisms in a given individual. Therefore, initial empirical therapy should always be viewed as a temporary measure subject to modification based on either culture results or clinical response, or both. Such modifications may result in broadening of the antimicrobial spectrum to cover previously unsuspected organisms, in focusing antibiotic activity against specific pathogens isolated, or even in selection of alternative agents that may be better tolerated during a full course of therapy. In many cases, of course, the initially selected regimen will prove perfectly appropriate for continued therapy.

The availability of a wide variety of excellent antimicrobial agents over the last decade has, on the one hand, greatly facilitated the selection of treatment regimens for diabetic patients with foot infections. At the same time, however, balancing the sometimes subtle differences of activity or toxicity can certainly make selection of a regimen potentially more complicated than when just a few agents were available. At the heart of this complexity is the polymicrobial nature of these infections, and the fact that, while many of the newer agents have some activity against a fairly broad range of microorganisms, activity against specific bacteria may be substantially lower than that of the best specifically targeted drugs. This situation often leads us to use multidrug regimens in the empirical treatment of serious infections, while in less serious infections the relatively broad coverage of some single agents (even with only modest activity against some likely pathogens) may be deemed perfectly acceptable.

For a number of years, combinations of clindamycin with an aminoglycoside (tobramycin or gentamicin) have been used effectively in the management of serious infections because of broad activity against most S. aureus, streptococci, anaerobes, and gram-negative bacilli. In some cases, ampicillin was added to the regimen for added activity against clostridia and for coverage of enterococci. Although the latter organisms are frequently encountered, successful treatment of mixed infections with agents ineffective against enterococci has shown that targeting these bacteria specifically is not always necessary. However, their importance in some cases is unequivocal; therefore they cannot be ignored. Whether specific therapy aimed at enterococci is needed in any one situation remains, therefore, a matter of clinical judgment.

While such regimens are still occasionally useful, the significant toxic potential of aminoglycosides has stimulated the growing use of other regimens. In principle, such alternative regimens are constructed around a "core" antibiotic active against many of the expected pathogens. For example, a third-generation cephalosporin (e.g. cefotaxime, ceftizoxime, ceftriaxone, ceftazidime) or extended-spectrum penicillin (e.g. piperacillin or mezlocillin) might serve as a core drug. In the case of the former, one could add more potent staphylococcal activity with an antistaphylococcal penicillin (e.g. oxacillin, nafcillin) or with vancomycin, which would also provide activity against enterococci. Clindamycin would provide supplemental anaerobic (as well as antistaphylococcal) coverage, as would metronidazole, which has no antistaphylococcal activity. The extended-spectrum penicillins mentioned would provide good gram-negative and anaerobic activities at most institutions, as well as excellent activity against streptococci (and enterococci). However, supplemental antistaphylococcal coverage would be necessary, as would, in some cases, broader activity against gram-negative bacteria and anaerobes.

Three beta-lactam/beta-lactamase-inhibitor combination drugs are currently available for parenteral use: ampicillin/sulbactam, ticarcillin/clavulanate, and piperacillin/tazobactam. The beta-lactamase inhibitors extend the spectrum of the penicillin components to include S. aureus and additional gram-negative bacilli (e.g. Klebsiella). Anaerobic activities of the three drugs are excellent. Ampicillin and piperacillin provide activity against enterococci, while ticarcillin and piperacillin provide coverage against *P. aeruginosa*. Given their relatively broad antimicrobial spectra, these drugs have the potential for use as single agents; however, variable numbers of strains, even within generally susceptible bacterial species, may be resistant at any one institution.

By virtue of its extremely broad spectrum of activity against expected pathogens (staphylococci, streptococci, enterococci, gram-negative bacilli including *P. aeruginosa*), imipenem has an obvious appeal as an empirical choice. Nevertheless, resistant organisms are occasionally encountered (some enterococci, methicillin-resistant *S. aureus,* and coagulase-negative staphylococci, some Pseudomonas species), and resistance can emerge during therapy (Pseudomonas). The drug is expensive on a per gram basis, although compared with multidrug regimens it may be cost-effective. Severe renal insufficiency substantially complicates use of this drug because of the risk of adverse central nervous system reactions (seizures).

Although the oral formulations have been available for some time, intravenous ciprofloxacin and ofloxacin are now also available. As a core drug, ciprofloxacin or ofloxacin would provide excellent activity against most gram-negative organisms and would be expected to inhibit most *S. aureus* and *P. aeruginosa* isolates. Anaerobic activity is poor, however, and streptococci would probably not be optimally covered. In several institutions in which fluoroquinolones have been used widely, resistance to this group of compounds among methicillin-resistant *S. aureus* and coagulase-negative staphylococci and among some gram-negative organisms has been encountered at significant rates. Because of these factors, we usually prefer to use fluoroquinolones only after control of the acute process has been achieved, microbiology ascertained, and the patient can tolerate oral antibiotic therapy. In selected circumstances use of these agents in this manner can be very rewarding. An important consideration in the use of any oral quinolones is that oral antacids, sucralfate, and other substances (iron, some mineral-supplemented vitamins) may substantially impair absorption of this class of antimicrobial. One must also remember that diabetic gastroparesis may prevent orderly absorption of any oral medications.

Other antimicrobials are very useful in special circumstances. For example, trimethoprim-sulfamethoxazole (oral or intravenous) is active against some relatively resistant gram-negative bacteria. It has also been helpful in penicillin-cephalosporin–allergic patients. Likewise, aztreonam, which is a monobactam antibiotic, may be tolerated by some individuals allergic to other beta-lactams (although serious allergic reactions can potentially occur). When this drug is used, it is important to realize that it lacks activity against gram-positive bacteria and anaerobes, so suitable supplementary coverage must be provided as appropriate.

Discussion of dose selection and adjustment in the presence of renal insufficiency, of therapeutic drug level monitoring, and of potential adverse drug reactions is beyond the scope of this chapter. Physicians unfamiliar with the use of these drugs or therapies should seek expert advice to ensure their safe and effective application.

## PRINCIPLES OF SURGICAL MANAGEMENT

Certain basic management principles applicable for all diabetic foot ulcers and infections are outlined in Table 12–1, and treatment considerations and misconceptions most responsible for failure in Table 12–2.

### Inspection

The severity of the infected foot ulcer will determine the proper course of treatment. The first major decision is whether the patient can be initially treated as an outpatient

### TABLE 12–1. BASIC MANAGEMENT PRINCIPLES

Early recognition and prompt intervention
Control of blood glucose
Complete rest of injured area
Careful but complete debridement and drainage of *all* involved areas
Appropriate antibiotic coverage
Wound care and dressings
Appropriate vascular reconstructions
Careful follow-up, including podiatric appliances and modified footwear
More experienced consultation as necessary

made in it, whereas in the ischemic foot, a wound left open seldom heals unless a vascular reconstructive operation is possible to improve the flow of blood to the affected limb.

## Dressings

Most foot infections do not require extensive incisions and debridement, yet the principles must always be remembered. The surgeon who inspects the infected wound with a pair of sharp sterile scissors, a smooth forceps, and a probe will seek and expose infected areas that might otherwise be undetected and untreated. Dressings are used to serve the following purposes:

1. Contain wound drainage
2. Debride a wound
3. Protect an area from trauma
4. Protect a wound from contamination
5. Promote proper wound healing

The vascular nurses and doctors follow established guidelines to treat the patient and reduce the risk of additional trauma.

The basic equipment necessary for bedside foot care is:

1. Sterile debridement set containing:
   a. Sharp scissors for debriding
   b. Blunt-ended needle wound probe
   c. Smooth forceps
2. Sterile toenail clippers
3. Sterile gauze dressings:
   a. 2×2 inch sponges
   b. 4×8 inch sponges
   c. 4 inch roller gauze (Kling)
   d. 5×9 inch abdominal pads (Combine Dressing)
4. Tube gauze (No. 1 Surgitube)
5. Paper tape (1 inch Micropore)
6. Culture tubes (aerobic and anaerobic)
7. Medicines:
   a. Povidone-iodine 2.5 per cent
   b. Chlorazene 0.25 per cent (Dakin's solution 0.3 gm/30 ml water)
   c. Bacitracin ointment
   d. Lanolin, Eucerin
   e. Vaseline gauze
   f. Bismuth tribromophenate gauze 3 per cent (Xeroform)
   g. Normal saline
   h. Coly-Mycin 75 mg/50 cc NS (colistin)
   i. Calcium alginate dressing (Kaltostat)

The medicines we use routinely in daily foot care have proved to be effective and safe. The topical solutions are made isotonic. There are no debriding ointments, and *no* caustic agents such as salicylic acid are used.

Betadine is bactericidal. It acts upon surface bacteria and helps to debride a necrotic wound. Dakin's solution is a chlorine-releasing agent that is both bactericidal and active in loosening necrotic tissue to aid in local debridement. Dakin's also helps control fetid odors from severely infected wounds.

Bacitracin, a mild antibacterial ointment, is used to soften calluses and fissures. Ointment is sometimes used to soften eschar to facilitate mechanical debridement. The need for ointment must be evaluated with each dressing change to avoid macerating the area. Often ointment dressings are alternated with Betadine or Dakin's solution to provide a correct balance of moisture.

Vaseline gauze makes a sterile nonadhering bandage for new scar or grafted areas. Xeroform does the same and protects blisters or breaks in the skin that might become infected if left uncovered. Gauze moistened with normal saline is applied to clean granulating wounds and preoperative skin graft sites to promote healing. The mild antibiotic solution of colistin, 75 mg/50 cc NS, is effective on wounds harboring Pseudomonas and/or anaerobic organisms.

Calcium alginate (seaweed) dressings have been tested and successfully used in Great Britain since the early 1980s. Our experience shows these dressings work best when used on skin graft donor sites, clean granulating wounds, and venous stasis ulcers.

With few exceptions, a full foot dressing is applied each time a foot lesion is treated (Figs. 13–1 to 13–3). Every wound is inspected, gently probed to disclose unexpected sinuses, debrided by cutting away any necrotic tissue, and then treated with an appropriate dressing.

Open wounds require packing using an unfilled gauze moistened with a therapeutic solution. Changing packing two or three times a day is recommended for debridement of a necrotic wound. Allowing sufficient time between dressing changes gives the packing time to begin to dry and therefore provide gentle debridement as the packing is removed from the wound. Unfilled gauze is recommended for packing wounds. The loose weave of the gauze absorbs drainage and adheres to the necrotic material. The

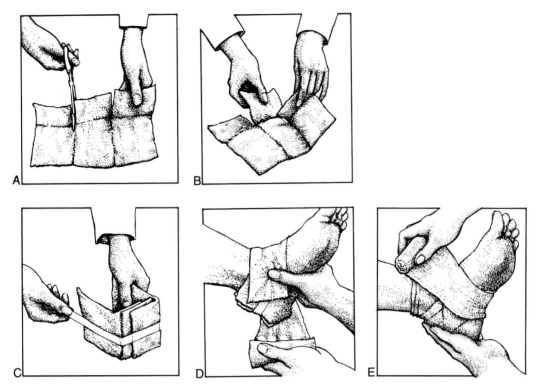

**Figure 13–1** A heel dressing to cover a heel ulcer or simply to provide a soft heel pad for bedridden patients to help prevent heel blisters or ulcers. Supplies are the same as for the full foot dressing (Fig. 13–3), plus a soft 5 × 9 inch abdominal pad. An abdominal pad is cut as shown (*A*) and then folded with overlaps (*B*) to make a four-sided cap-like dressing held with a piece of ½ inch adhesive (*C*). The heel cap (or cup) is placed on the heel and secured (*D, E*) with a figure-of-eight roller gauze, wrapped three times for security. This heel dressing may be incorporated into a full foot dressing.

gauze remains intact as it is removed, without leaving bits of cotton filler or lint in the wound. When used as a wick, an open sponge is elongated and twisted so that one corner of the gauze is threaded into the depth of the open wound, and the remaining gauze is then gently fed into the wound. Care must be taken not to pack the wound too tightly. Packing the wound too tightly obstructs drainage and acts only as a stopper instead of facilitating wound healing from the inside out. Ribbon-like gauze strips (Nu-gauze) are sometimes used as wicks in wounds with narrow openings. These packing strips are made of finely woven gauze and have been found to be less absorbent than the loosely woven 2 by 2 inch gauze.

To minimize trauma to the incision, closed incision lines are not cleansed routinely. Any moisture or exudate along the incision line is

**Figure 13–2** A bandage to hold a small dressing on a single toe. Supplies: Tubular gauze size No. 1 for small toes. No. 2 for great or large toes. Paper tape, size 1 inch. Method: A piece of tubular gauze is cut to 6 or 8 inches. One end is stretched and pulled over the toe. *A*, The long end of the gauze is twisted and turned back over the toe again and secured with a short piece of hypoallergenic tape.

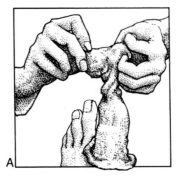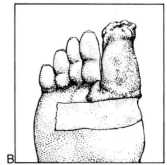

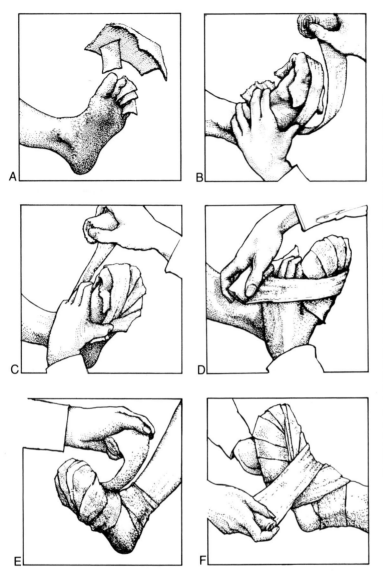

**Figure 13–3** A full foot bandage covers the toes and forefoot and holds a medicated dressing on or between the toes, or on any part of the forefoot. A protective heel dressing may be incorporated into it to cover the whole foot. Supplies: Sterile 2 × 2 inch gauze sponges; sterile 4 × 8 inch gauze sponges; 4 inch sterile soft roller gauze; and 1 inch hypoallergenic "paper" tape. Method: *A*, A sterile 2 × 2 gauze pad is placed between each toe, and an opened 4 × 8 gauze pad is placed over the end of the foot. *B*, The foot is grasped with one hand while a roller gauze is applied over the end of the foot, from instep to heel, and *C*, fanned out from side to side to cover the entire forefoot. *D*, The roller gauze is next carried around the sides of the foot, advancing ½ to 1 inch with each wrap. *E* and *F*, The ankle is incorporated with *three* figure-eight wraps to hold the bandage securely to the foot. The bandage is held with three long pieces of tape, placed (1) from instep to heel, (2) from side heel to inner heel around the front and (3) encircling the midfoot.

gently wiped away with a Betadine swab. The incision is then covered with sterile gauze and secured with paper tape.

Dressings on single digits are secured with tube bandage and paper tape. A heel "cup" is often fashioned from a 5 by 9 inch surgical pad cut and folded to fit over the heel and hold on a gauze dressing and/or to protect the heel from rubbing on the bed sheets. The heel cup also serves as a soft cushion to help reduce external pressure and is easily incorporated into a full foot dressing.

When enclosing the foot in a full bandage, the digits must be separated by dry gauze to absorb the skin moisture and to reduce the pressure of one digit on another. After plac-

ing 2 by 2 inch gauze between each toe, fluff at least two 4 by 8 inch sponges over the toes and forefoot. The primary dressing is held in place with a 4 inch roller gauze. Beginning on the dorsum, unroll the roller gauze over the toes to the plantar surface, fan-fold the roller gauze, overlapping to the left and then to the right. Continue a spiral wrap toward the ankle, enclosing the heel in a figure-eight fashion, ending the roller gauze back on the dorsum of the foot. Secure the dressing with paper tape. A properly applied dressing will not constrict the foot or leg or slip, possibly causing wound trauma or exposure. Spiraling or wrapping the roller gauze in a figure-eight fashion is the best way to prevent a tourniquet effect and will decrease the risk of compromising the circulation to the foot.

### Routine Foot Dressing

1. Moisten gauze with appropriate solution. If packing a wound, always unfold the gauze. Beginning with a corner, slide the moistened gauze into the deepest part of the wound. Using a wound probe, gently feed the rest of the gauze packing into the wound. As previously mentioned, it is important not to stuff a wound. Packing should always act as an aid to healing by helping to debride a necrotic wound or to act as a wick for a granulating wound. Proper wicking will assist in secondary healing from the inside out.
2. Place 2 by 2 inch gauze between the toes.
3. Fashion a heel cup from a cut, folded, and taped abdominal pad.
4. Fluff two 4 by 8 inch gauze sponges over toes and/or forefoot.
5. Secure the primary dressing, including heel cup, with 4 inch roller gauze. Beginning on the dorsum of the foot, unroll the gauze over the end of the foot to the plantar surface. Spiral the roller gauze toward the ankle and include the heel pad by wrapping in a figure-eight fashion, ending the roller gauze back on the dorsum of the foot.
6. Apply paper tape to secure the roller gauze.

### Casts/Splints

A cast or splint may be applied to immobilize a limb after a skin graft or to protect the incision and reduce contractures after a below-knee amputation.

Applying a rigid plaster cast or splint to any neuropathic extremity can be hazardous and may cause pressure sores. The patient may not feel or suspect undue pressure until after a sore has developed. Casts should be well padded and bivalved to allow daily removal and inspection of all skin surfaces. If a patient *ever* complains of a painful spot under a cast, the surgeon must promptly remove the cast or cut a window in it to expose the suspicious area. A pain beneath a cast means a problem until proven otherwise. Sniffing the open end of a cast is sometimes the first (and best) way to know if an infection lies beneath. This is a simple, satisfactory, and noninvasive way to know whether or not all is well under the plaster.

The soft commercially made splints with adjustable straps can and should be removed daily to permit wound and skin inspection and to change the position of the leg within the splint.

### Amputation-Stump Dressings

The dressing applied to any amputation stump is fashioned to meet the needs of the wound. Since most amputation wounds do not have drains, the dressing is put on more for wound protection than to collect and contain blood and secretions. Obviously, at times some infected amputation wounds are left open for drainage. Such wounds need to be encompassed in bulky dressings that will contain the excretions and protect the environment from contaminated matter.

The following are special requirements for fresh amputation stump dressings:

Toe amputation incisions, single or multiple, are covered with the standard foot bandage, care being taken to place several 2 by 2's over the incision itself and to place 2 by 2's between the remaining toes. Unless there is unexplained bleeding, fever, or pain in the amputation site, the initial dressing may be left unchanged for two or three days.

A first transmetatarsal amputation (TMA) dressing is a bulky standard foot dressing. A posterior splint may be applied to prevent plantar flexion and thus avoid tension on the delicate suture line. The time the splint is used depends upon the patient's circulatory status and reliability in protecting the foot. Depending on surgical preference, the original TMA dressing may remain unchanged for one to five days.

A below-knee amputation (BKA) requires an extra bulky initial dressing to contain the initial expected bleeding. BKA's are managed with a posterior splint that extends from the crease of the buttocks to beyond the end of the stump. A well-padded knee immobilizer is the splint of choice. It is applied while the patient is anesthetized to prevent knee flexion that occurs almost at the time the anesthesia ends. Knee flexion is a natural pain-relieving action or reflex that, if allowed to occur, can lead to a serious contracture. Overcoming such a contracture can take weeks of physical therapy and can greatly delay the use of a prosthesis. It is customary to have a patient with a BKA measured for a prosthesis on the third or forth postoperative day. Depending on the progression of stump healing, a patella-bearing prosthesis may be fitted and the patient begin ambulation eight to ten days postoperatively.

The initial dressing for an above-knee amputation (AKA) is bulky and similar to the BKA dressing. Splints are not used for our AKA despite the tendency for patients to hold up and flex the painful thigh. The stump usually falls down with muscle fatigue, thus decreasing the tendency for a hip contracture. If such a contracture occurs, having the patient lie face down in bed for an hour several times a day is usually sufficient to correct the flexion tendency. A hip contracture will greatly interfere with a patient's being able to use a prosthesis.

Arterial reconstruction commonly involves extensive incisions originating on the abdomen and extending distally across the inguinal ligament in the groin, along the inner thigh, past the knee, down the calf, and onto the dorsum of the foot. The incision is dressed with dry gauze, with special attention being paid to the groin where moisture in the skin folds can lead to maceration and secondary wound infection. This area is cleaned with a Betadine swab and kept covered with dry gauze for at least five days postoperatively. The remaining bypass incision is covered with a dressing only if drainage is present.

Skin graft dressings are usually applied in accordance with the surgeon's preference. Mesh grafts are the most common split-thickness skin graft. The mesh graft has proven to be the most successful because the open mesh allows adequate wound drainage. Postoperatively some grafts are left open to air and are simply protected with surrounding padding. The majority of skin graft dressings are composed of nonadherent gauze—bulky fluffed gauze securely wrapped with roller gauze and an Ace wrap. A posterior splint is applied to further immobilize and protect the grafted area. The vascular nurse is prepared to care for each skin graft in accordance with the specific surgeon's practice.

## SPECIAL NEEDS AT THE BEDSIDE

Bed rest is the first item in the care of a diabetic foot lesion. Bed rest must be absolute and continuous. A patient with diminished circulation who has a painful ischemic foot lesion may be helped by having the head of the bed elevated 6 to 8 inches. This elevation allows gravity flow of blood to the feet and is known as the arterial position or modified reverse Trendelenburg position. Patients in this position tend to drift slowly down to the foot of the bed. They may be at increased risk for developing abrasions or pressure sores from friction on the sheets and the pressure of the footboard or base of bed. This position should be used only if it helps the symptoms and does not adversely affect any peripheral vascular problems.

Raising the feet, as is done with the gatch bed, is often comfortable, but is ill advised for those with ischemia because of the increased pressure exerted on the popliteal area. While elevation of any infected part is the traditional position, it is felt that the disadvantages outweigh any advantages. Elevation to the horizontal level is the best way to position an infected foot, whether neuropathic or ischemic. The most significant factor about the patient's position in bed is having the patient *off the foot entirely.* In the presence of severe edema, the legs should be elevated above the horizontal until the edema subsides.

Bed rest for the ill, fragile, or immobile patient puts increased pressure on the backs of the heels and other bony prominences. Anyone in bed for more then a few days is at risk of developing heel or other pressure ulcers. All patients with a foot problem are provided with a foam rubber foot pillow that is placed under the calves to raise the extended legs off the bed and reduce the pressure to the heels. The foot pillow is 24 × 12 × 2 inches, and although it gets continually kicked around the bed, it does help to keep the heels off the bed most of the time. Patients at increased risk for skin breakdown are placed on special decubitus or therapeutic mattresses.

The weight of the bed clothes on the feet can be annoying and troublesome and can also cause pressure sores. A foot cradle (Fig. 13–4) is provided with every bed. This is a heavy wire metal or plastic tubing frame with the base held in place under the end of the mattress while the remainder of the frame arches up off the end of the bed, holding the covers off the end of the bed and thus off the extended feet in the bed. It is simple, effective, and usually not bumped by the patient turning in bed.

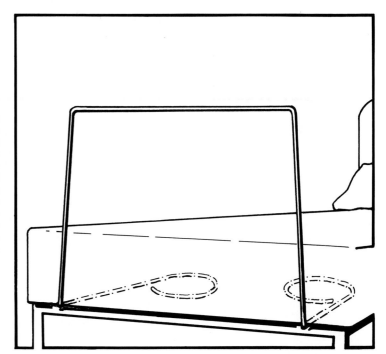

**Figure 13–4** A foot cradle. This is used to hold bed clothes off the feet at the foot of the bed, to keep pressure off the toes, and to permit easy foot motion in bed. The cradle is fashioned from a piece of steel wire or metal tubing, bent to form an arch 18 inches above the bed, and bent to allow a wide circle at each end of the structure to fit and be secured under the mattress by the weight of the mattress.

An overhead trapeze is essential for every patient confined to bed. It is indispensable to anyone pulling up in bed, getting onto a bedpan, or turning over when a leg is immobilized by a splint. A trapeze may be the only device enabling the bedridden patient to exercise and to maintain some semblance of muscle tone while otherwise being totally incapacitated. An effort is made to see that all bedridden foot patients have a trapeze unless their cardiac status prohibits its use.

A bedside commode is another essential for most patients at bed rest. The physician will most often allow patients to use a commode as long as they are able to keep the affected limb elevated.

Prevention of skin and respiratory problems is a challenge in caring for a patient with a diabetic foot problem who is usually confined to bed. Only with continual assessment and supportive physical and emotional nursing care by the vascular nurses, doctors, and other care givers can these patients be restored to health.

# Chapter 14

# NONINVASIVE EVALUATION OF THE ARTERIAL SYSTEM IN THE DIABETIC LOWER EXTREMITY

FRANK B. POMPOSELLI, Jr., M.D.

Diabetic patients with foot lesions frequently have associated arterial occlusive disease in the lower extremity. In simplest terms, if the foot pulses are not palpable, it can be assumed that occlusive disease is present. The mere presence of occlusive disease, however, tells nothing about its significance with regard to the presenting foot problem or how it might affect the likelihood of successful treatment. A careful history and physical examination for peripheral vascular disease often give the experienced clinician a good impression of how important a role ischemia is playing in a particular foot problem. It is hardly foolproof, however, since it relies upon subjective interpretation and is difficult to quantify. Clinical interpretation can be particularly difficult in patients with neuropathy when there is absence of foot pulses and foot lesions. Neuropathic pain may be mistaken for ischemic rest pain when circulation is adequate, and totally insensate patients may have no circulatory symptoms in the face of apparently advanced and limb-threatening ischemia.

When a patient with missing pulses has a foot lesion that requires a minor amputation or podiatric procedure, the surgeon is faced with the often difficult decision whether to proceed directly to the foot procedure, which may result in partial or complete foot loss if primary healing does not occur, or correcting the circulatory deficit before foot surgery, which often requires vascular reconstruction with its attendant risks. Quantitative data supplied by the noninvasive laboratory can provide the clinician with added information about the adequacy of the circulation for primary healing and whether or not angiography and vascular surgery are needed first. Following vascular reconstruction, the noninvasive vascular laboratory quantifies the degree of improvement in ischemia. Deterioration in noninvasive vascular laboratory parameters following vascular reconstruction may precede the onset of recurrent symptoms, heralding the need for repeat angiography and revision of the vascular reconstruction to prevent graft thrombosis.

It is in these circumstances that the noninvasive vascular laboratory has added greatly to the evaluation of diabetic patients with foot problems and ischemia. With current technology, hemodynamic measurements can be performed painlessly in an outpatient setting at no risk to the patient. Moreover, the extensive data collected in the screening, diagnosis, and follow-up of these patients has greatly added to our understanding of the evolution and impact of atherosclerotic occlusive disease on diabetic foot problems.

In this chapter the commonly used noninvasive vascular tests to evaluate ischemia in the diabetic patient are described. The data derived from these tests and how they complement the clinical evaluation and treatment of these patients will be discussed.

## DOPPLER-DERIVED PRESSURES

The simplest noninvasive procedure to perform is measurement of the ankle systolic

**138**

pressure. A continuous-wave Doppler device is placed over the dorsalis pedis or posterior tibial artery on the foot, with an appropriate-sized pneumatic cuff around the ankle. The cuff is inflated until the flow signal disappears and then is slowly deflated. The pressure at which the signal returns is the ankle systolic pressure.

Normally the ankle systolic pressure should slightly exceed arm systolic pressure. Significant (greater than 50 per cent) proximal stenoses or occlusions will reduce the ankle pressure. In most diabetic patients, absolute ankle pressures of less than 55 mm Hg suggest critical ischemia threatening limb viability. Because the ankle pressure fluctuates with changes in blood pressure, more consistent results can be obtained by comparing the ankle pressure with the brachial artery systolic pressure. This ratio is obtained by dividing the ankle pressure by the brachial pressure and is commonly referred to as the ankle/brachial index, or ABI. A normal ABI is usually 1.0 or slightly higher. Studies have shown that the ABI correlates well with degrees of ischemia, especially in nondiabetic patients. Generally, an ABI of less than 0.8 is seen in patients with claudication and less than 0.5 in patients with rest pain or tissue loss. Moreover, in patients with clinically successful arterial reconstruction, the ABI will usually increase by at least 0.3. A reduction of the ABI of 0.15 or more following successful revascularization had been shown to be a reliable predictor of worsening vascular occlusive disease.

Further information can be obtained from segmental limb pressures. Appropriately sized cuffs are placed around the thigh, calf, and ankle. Some centers use a high-thigh and a low-thigh cuff. Each cuff is separately inflated and the pressure measurement obtained from the Doppler signal heard in the foot. A pressure reduction of greater than 10 mm Hg between two adjacent cuffs suggests significant stenosis or occlusion in the corresponding arterial segment between the cuffs. Normally the high-thigh pressure is about 30 mm higher than the arm pressure. Values substantially below this suggest aortoiliac or proximal femoral arterial occlusive disease. Unfortunately the thigh pressure does not reliably distinguish between aortoiliac and femoral occlusive disease, especially when combined superficial femoral and deep femoral disease is present.

While Doppler-derived pressures have proven to be generally reliable in nondiabetic patients, significant problems occur in many diabetic patients. Most errors of measurement with Doppler pressures result from spuriously high values obtained because of medial calcification of the vessels that renders them incompressible. Diabetic patients are particularly prone to medial calcification; it occurs in approximately 30 per cent of our patients. Medial calcification should be suspected whenever the ankle pressure greatly exceeds arm pressure or when the Doppler signal cannot be obliterated with greater than 250 mm Hg ankle pressure. Medial calcification may also give inaccurate segmental pressures. It should be suspected whenever an inverse gradient is found between two corresponding cuffs (i.e. the distal cuff has a higher pressure than the more proximal one).

One proposed method of overcoming incompressible vessels is measurement of toe pressure. A small pneumatic cuff is placed around the base of the toe and a flow sensor placed distally. Since Doppler signals are difficult to obtain from the distal toe, a photoplethysmograph is used on the distal toe as a flow sensor. Normal patients usually have toe pressures of greater than 50 mm Hg, while ischemic patients generally have toe pressures of less than 40 mm Hg. As with Doppler-derived pressures, a toe/brachial index (TBI) can be obtained by dividing the toe pressure by the brachial artery pressure. The normal TBI ranges from .7 to 1.0. In claudicants the TBI is usually in the range of .35 to .45 and in patients with ischemic rest pain or tissue loss it is less than .25. Several investigators have shown little difference in toe pressure measurements from diabetic and nondiabetic patients, suggesting that medial calcification rarely affects toe pressure measurements. Consequently, toe pressures should be obtained whenever ankle indices are artifactually high.

Toe pressure measurements can also be used to determine the presence of ischemia in the pedal circulation. Occasionally a diabetic patient with advanced forefoot ischemia will have normal or near-normal ankle pressures and pulse volume tracings (see below) and abnormal toe pressures, suggesting the presence of occlusive lesions at the ankle level or proximal aspect of the foot. Identification of these patients is important, since bypass to the pedal vessels is technically possible and has been shown to be efficacious in foot salvage.

The accuracy of toe pressures is affected by room temperature, hypertension, and cuff size. In addition, we have seen an occasional patient in our practice who has noncompressible digital arteries. Nonetheless, toe pressures appear to be a valuable addition to the evaluation of foot ischemia, especially in diabetic patients.

Occasionally, patients will have apparent symptoms of claudication with palpable foot pulses and normal pressures at rest. Exercising the lower extremity increases blood flow by reducing resistance in the vascular bed. In the presence of occlusive lesions, blood flow cannot appropriately increase, causing a reduction in ankle pressure that will make lesions apparent that were not obvious at rest. The patient is instructed to walk on a treadmill at the rate of 1½ mph on a 10 per cent grade for five minutes or until symptoms occur. Ankle pressures are then obtained at one, three, six, and ten minutes following exercise. Patients with normal circulation can usually exercise for five minutes with no drop in ankle pressures. Patients with significant proximal occlusive disease frequently cannot exercise for five minutes and will always demonstrate a drop in ankle pressure and prolonged recurrence time to baseline pressures. A patient who can exercise for five minutes with no reduction in ankle pressure does not have significant proximal occlusive disease, and another cause should be sought.

It is important to realize that stress testing adds nothing to the evaluation when there are obvious signs and symptoms of ischemia at rest or when abnormal resting pressures are present. Moreover, exercise stress testing may be impossible in patients with significant foot lesions or severe cardiopulmonary disease. The value of stress testing in diabetic patients with ischemic foot lesions is therefore limited.

## WAVE FORM ANALYSIS

In measuring lower extremity pressures with the Doppler flow probe, recognition of the presence of the arterial signal is all that is required. Additional important information can be obtained, however, by examining the changes in blood flow velocity that occur

with occlusive disease. Disturbances in the flow pattern due to occlusion cause recognizable changes in blood flow velocity. The experienced observer can recognize the typical auditory changes in the flow signal that occur with alterations in flow. Visual interpretation is possible by creating a wave form of the flow velocity signal on a strip chart recorder. The normal Doppler wave form is triphasic. With proximal occlusive disease, the shape of the wave form becomes monophasic (Fig. 14–1). Unlike Doppler-derived ankle pressures, wave form analysis gives no quantitative information and is usually used in conjunction with other tests. In our laboratory, we have used Doppler wave form analysis to determine the presence of aortoiliac occlusive disease, which may be difficult to distinguish from femoral disease by segmental limb pressures or pulse volume recording (see below). If a triphasic Doppler wave form is obtained from the common femoral artery, the presence of significant aortoiliac disease is unlikely. The converse is not necessarily true, however, since a monophasic signal may be obtained even when the aortoiliac segment is normal, if the common femoral artery is insonated near a superficial femoral artery occlusion.

## PULSE VOLUME RECORDING

The pulse volume recorder is a segmental plethysmograph that measures and records the changes in volume that take place in an extremity with arterial pulsation. Standard-size cuffs are placed around the extremity at the thigh, calf, ankle, and forefoot levels, which are inflated with a known quantity of air until a preset pressure is reached (45 mm Hg). Analog tracings of the pulsatility of flow are then obtained at all levels with a sensitive recorder, usually in conjunction with and immediately prior to segmental limb pressures.

The normal pulse volume recording (PVR) trace has a steep upward deflection, narrow peak, and dicrotic notch (Fig. 14–2A). Changes in the pulse volume trace, contour, and amplitude can be graded from mildly to severely abnormal, with increasing degrees of arterial insufficiency (Fig. 14–2B). Pulse volume measurements have proven to be particularly valuable in diabetic patients, since they are unaffected by medial calcification. When noncompressible vessels give falsely elevated

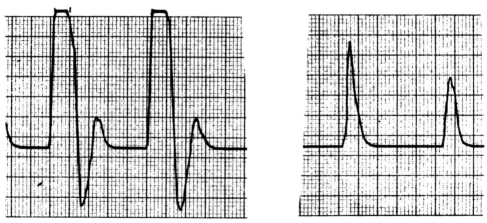

**Figure 14–1** Doppler wave form analysis: The example to the *left* shows the typical triphasic wave form of unimpeded arterial flow. The monophasic wave form to the *right* suggests significant stenosis or occlusion proximal to the artery being insonated.

**Figure 14–2** *A,* Sequential pulse volume recordings of a normal left lower extremity. Characteristics of a normal pulse volume tracing are steep upward and downward deflection with a dicrotic notch. *B,* Abnormal pulse volume tracing. Mild abnormality is seen at the level of the thigh due to loss of the dicrotic notch. Significant abnormalities are noted at the level of the calf with significant loss of amplitude and blunting of the wave form. The ankle and forefoot tracings show the most severe abnormalities where the wave form is essentially flat.

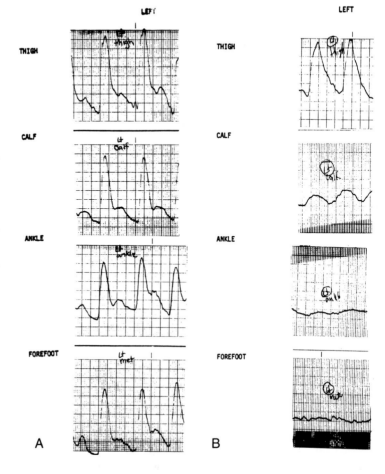

Doppler pressure, they are important in evaluating ischemia in the presence of foot pain and ulceration. In general, forefoot PVR tracings with abnormal contours and amplitude less than 10 mm are seen in the presence of ischemia. Pulse volume amplitudes less than 5 mm suggest severe ischemia.

Incorrectly sized cuffs, obesity, peripheral edema, and congestive heart failure can all cause erroneous PVR measurements. We have also noted that PVR tracings tend to underestimate the degree of ischemia when compared with arteriograms. They have also been poor in differentiating aortoiliac and femoral occlusive disease. In spite of these shortcomings, when used in conjunction with a careful clinical evaluation they have proved to be extremely useful in assessing ischemia in diabetic patients.

## DUPLEX ULTRASONOGRAPHY

Duplex scanners employ a real-time B-mode and ultrasound imager to locate the blood vessel being studied with a pulse Doppler flow detector and spectrum analyzer to obtain velocity information from the same location. Unlike other noninvasive methods that indirectly ascertain the degree of ischemia by evaluating the circulation at a point remote from the occlusive lesion, duplex scanning directly interrogates the diseased arterial segment, thereby giving the precise location in addition to the hemodynamic significance of the lesion being studied.

The path of the Doppler beam is indicated by a white line on the B-mode image. Unlike continuous-wave Doppler, which summates blood flow velocity from the entire lumen of the blood vessel, pulse Doppler can measure velocity from specific locations within the flow stream, known as the sample volume. A small line crossing the Doppler beam indicates the location of the sample volume and can be aligned with the path of blood flow. This allows measurement of the angle of incidence of the ultrasound beam (Doppler angle) within the artery. Velocity can then be calculated using the Doppler equation.

Using dedicated software (fast Fourier transform analysis), the spectrum analyzer determines the frequency and amplitude of the Doppler signal as it is reflected from the flowing blood. These data are displayed graphically in real time with frequency on the x-axis, time on the y-axis, and amplitude depicted by gradations in the gray scale of the image. These collected data over time create a spectral wave form. The normal spectral wave form has a brisk upward deflection in systole, indicating flow toward the probe, followed by a rapid downward deflection, indicating flow away from the probe in early diastole followed by a small upward and downward deflection, indicating forward flow in late diastole. Normally, undisturbed arterial flow is laminar, which gives the wave form a narrow frequency spectrum with a clear "window" (Fig. 14–3). Systolic and diastolic flow velocity are also calculated. With narrowing of the arterial lumen, due to atherosclerotic plaque, laminar flow becomes more disordered or turbulent, resulting in a wider frequency spectrum (spectral broadening) and loss of the window. Diastolic forward flow is lost. Both systolic and diastolic flow velocity are increased within the stenosis and reduced more distally. The type and magnitude of these changes in the spectral wave form have been related to four categories of increasing luminal stenosis and total occlusion (Table 14–1). The duplex scanner's capability of locating atherosclerotic lesions and determining their hemodynamic significance and being able to differentiate near-total from total occlusion has proven valuable in following the progression of occlusive disease, without having to subject the patient to the potential risks of repeated arteriography. Some centers have performed intraoperative duplex scanning at the completion of the vascular reconstruction to evaluate grafts for technical errors that may result in graft thrombosis. It has also been used to follow vascular reconstructions over the long term to uncover stenotic graft lesions from intimal hyperplasia and the progression of atherosclerosis, which may result in sudden graft thrombosis.

Although several centers have reported impressive sensitivity and specificity rates in diagnosing arterial occlusive lesions with the duplex scanner used by experienced technologists, significant errors are common in improperly performed tests. Duplex scanning is also time comsuming, with complete examinations of the lower extremities taking upward of an hour. The recent development of color duplex scanners allows the technician to rapidly identify stenotic segments of arteries and vein grafts. Flowing blood is displayed in different colors, depending on the

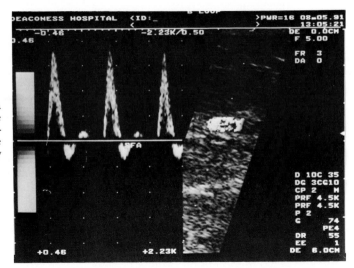

**Figure 14-3** Duplex scan taken from a normal superficial femoral artery. Note the steep upward and downward deflection in systole and reversal of flow in late diastole. There is also a narrow frequency spectrum with a clear "window" noted.

direction of flow, either toward or away from the probe, making the differentiation of veins and arteries and occluded vessels easier. Areas of increased velocity indicating stenosis are also rapidly identified by an increase in the "brightness" of the color image. These improvements have shortened the examination time, making it more practical for periodic follow-up examinations.

## TRANSCUTANEOUS OXYGEN TENSION

Use of the modified Clark electrode to measure the partial pressure of oxygen diffusing through the skin adds another dimension to noninvasive vascular testing. Because the amount of oxygen diffused through the skin is dependent upon the amount of oxygen supplied through the capillary circulation and not extracted by the tissue, it gives a physiological, as opposed to a hemodynamic, assessment of tissue circulation at the level being studied. The relationship between tissue perfusion and oxygen diffusion is complex, however, and nonlinear. In general, the amount of oxygen supplied so far exceeds the demand that oxygen diffusion does not change significantly until perfusion is greatly impaired. As a result, changes in $TcPO_2$ are found only with significant arterial occlusion. Moreover, in situations of marginal perfusion in which demand equals or exceeds the supply, all available oxygen is extracted by the tissue, causing the $TcPO_2$ value to be 0, even though blood flow may still be detectable by other methods. Many observers have noted that the $TcPO_2$ values in normal extremities tend to be lower distally than more proximally on the leg. Older patients also tend to have lower values than younger patients, even when both have normal circulation. Fluctuations in cardiac output or concomitant pulmonary disease may also affect measurements. To overcome these problems, one group has advocated the use of a regional perfusion index (RPI), which is obtained by dividing the limb $TcPO_2$ by the value obtained on the anterior chest wall. In general, in older patients, the normal $TcPO_2$ is 60 mm Hg and the normal RPI is 0.9.

Many investigators find $TcPO_2$ measurements particularly attractive for diabetic patients, since they are not affected by medial

## TABLE 14-1. CRITERIA FOR CLASSIFICATION OF ARTERIAL STENOSIS BY DUPLEX SCANNING

| | |
|---|---|
| Normal | Triphasic signal with minimal spectral broadening and narrow spectral band |
| 1–19% | Normal wave form and normal peak systolic velocity with spectral broadening |
| 20–49% | Peak systolic velocity increases 30 to 50% with marked spectral broadening |
| 50–99% | Monophasic wave form with systolic peak velocity increases by at least 100% with marked spectral broadening |
| Occlusion | No detectable flow in the imaged artery |

calcinosis. It is also possible to measure $TcPO_2$ levels in proximity to nonhealing ulcers and at proposed levels of amputation. To optimize capillary blood flow and facilitate diffusion, it is necessary to heat the skin to 45°C prior to obtaining measurements, which has occasionally resulted in burns. There are also a host of factors that can result in erroneous measurements, including poor adherence of the probe to the skin, edema, cellulitis, and hyperkeratosis.

Although enthusiasm for $TcPO_2$ measurements has been growing, wide variability in observations from different laboratories and lack of equipment standardization have made comparisons difficult. In addition, there appears to be a wide overlap between values obtained where wound healing is likely or not likely to occur. The large "gray area" makes it difficult to rely solely on $TcPO_2$ measurement in making judgments about amputation level or the likelihood of ulcer healing.

## OTHER METHODS

### Laser Doppler

The laser Doppler measures the velocity of capillary blood flow by shifts in frequency of monochromatic laser light reflected from moving red cells. The principle is analogous to the one used in ultrasonic measurements, but the problems are more complex, since the capillary bed is a network of vessels running in multiple directions and light is scattered by surrounding tissues.

The laser Doppler can also be used under a pneumatic cuff to estimate skin blood pressure. In this application, the laser Doppler is used simply as a probe to sense capillary blood flow. Preliminary investigations have shown that laser Doppler measurements reliably identify ischemia. Its ability to predict ulcer healing and amputation levels is less clear. Since much of the information it provides is already supplied by other methods, its future role in the noninvasive vascular laboratory remains uncertain.

### Radioisotope Clearance

A variety of radioisotope clearance techniques have been developed to directly measure skin blood flow and to measure skin perfusion pressure. Skin blood flow is determined by injecting xenon 133 gas dissolved in saline into the muscle or dermis. This is removed from the site of diffusion across the capillary cell membrane by a diffusion gradient. The rate of diffusion is determined by the rate of capillary blood flow, which, in turn, is determined by degree of arterial insufficiency. By using a scintillation counter and rate meter, blood flow can be measured in milliliters per 100 gm of tissue per minute. One group found that skin blood flow rates greater than 2.6 ml per 100 gm per minute at a proposed amputation site predicted successful healing.

Skin perfusion pressure is measured by injecting a radioactive isotope into the dermis and applying a blood pressure cuff over the depot. Once a steady state of clearance has been reached, the cuff is incrementally inflated until clearance stops. The pressure at which clearance stops is the skin perfusion pressure. A variety of radioisotopes have been used in this method. Several investigators have reported that skin perfusion pressure greater than 40 mm Hg is usually predictive of healing, while pressure less than 20 mm Hg suggests failure of healing.

The physiological nature of isotope clearance techniques is attractive, and it is unaffected by medial calcinosis. However, several problems exist. It is a relatively invasive procedure involving injection of a radioactive isotope. Infection and cellulitis can affect measurements. Measurements can be inconsistent in the same patient tested at different times. Large overlap between predictive values for healing and nonhealing puts many patients in the "gray area." Moreover, amputations have been reported to heal with values that have predicted failure and not healed when success was deemed likely. While several groups have reported that use of isotope clearance techniques has improved amputation results, other groups, including our own, have reported comparable results relying on surgical judgment alone. In comparison to the data obtained from other methods such as Doppler-derived pressures and pulse volume recordings, it is unclear if the more invasive and complex isotope clearance methods add much information for the majority of patients.

### Magnetic Resonance Angiography

The ability of magnetic resonance to image flowing blood led to the development of techniques to image the circulation in the 1980's that became known as magnetic resonance angiography or MRA. The most common application of MRA in peripheral vascular surgery has been evaluation of the aorta and carotid arteries, but recently this technique has also been used to image the arteries of the lower extremity.

MRA is particularly attractive in evaluating diabetic vascular disease, since it obviates the need for potentially nephrotoxic contrast agents routinely used in standard arteriography. Other advantages include the ability to obtain cross-sectional images of arteries and measurement of blood flow velocity, which makes it a single method capable of obtaining both three-dimensional anatomical and physiological information.

## CLINICAL APPLICATIONS

The diabetic patient with a nonhealing foot ulcer or who requires a minor amputation often presents a challenge to the clinician. In the absence of palpable pulses, the surgeon is faced with the often perplexing decision of whether to attempt the amputation or to first correct underlying ischemia with a revascularization procedure. In patients requiring a major limb amputation, preserving the knee joint is preferable, since the functional result and chance for successful rehabilitation are far superior with below-knee amputations. Unfortunately, the converse is true of healing potential—amputations above the knee heal much more readily than those below the knee. Thus, if there is no chance for a below-knee amputation to heal, the need for a second procedure can be avoided by proceeding directly to an above-knee amputation.

Because of these difficulties in clinical decision making, most centers have attempted to establish criteria for predicting healing in ischemic patients based on noninvasive laboratory data. Results of cumulative data on the use of ankle pressures ranging from 60 to 80 mm Hg demonstrate that they correctly predicted healing (sensitivity) from 68 to 87 per cent of the time and correctly predicted nonhealing (specificity) from 40 to 63 per cent of the time. In our own experience, we have found that 30 to 50 per cent of diabetic patients have falsely elevated ankle pressures. In one study of predicting forefoot amputation healing, ankle systolic pressures predicted failure in 38 per cent of patients who had healing and success in 11 of the 18 patients whose amputation sites failed to heal. Had we relied solely on ankle pressures to make the clinical decision whether or not amputations would have healed, 20 patients would have undergone higher amputation than necessary. As a result, we feel that surgical judgment is superior to ankle pressure alone in determining a likelihood of healing of forefoot amputations.

Pulse volume tracings also must be used cautiously in predicting healing of ulcers or amputation at the forefoot level. In our study, a flat or nearly flat forefoot trace incorrectly predicted failure of minor amputation in 53 per cent that ultimately healed. Although strongly positive PVR forefoot tracings were associated with uniform healing in this study, we have since had an occasional patient in whom an ulcer has not healed in spite of near-normal PVR traces, who, when studied with arteriography, was found to have significant correctable distal arterial occlusions (Fig. 14–4).

The unreliability of ankle level measurements in diabetic patients may partially be due to the occurrence of occlusive lesions in the very distal tibial and peroneal circulation. This has prompted several investigators to rely on toe pressure values. Unfortunately, similar problems have been found in attempting to predict the likelihood of ulcer or forefoot amputation with this method. Although most investigators have found that healing nearly uniformly occurs with toe pressures greater than 55 mm Hg, no absolute pressure measurement has been found below which healing will never occur.

We have encountered similar difficulties in determining the level of successful major limb amputation healing. When using the criteria for successful healing of below-knee amputation of 80 mm Hg at the thigh, 65 mm Hg at the calf, and 30 mm Hg at the ankle, but determining amputation level on clinical judgment alone, we found that systolic pressures were falsely elevated or predicted incorrectly in greater than 50 per cent of cases. Pulse volume tracings also correlated poorly with healing in this series. In a separate retrospective review of 100 consecutive below-knee amputations in which the decision to perform below-knee amputation was determined by clinical judgment alone, no

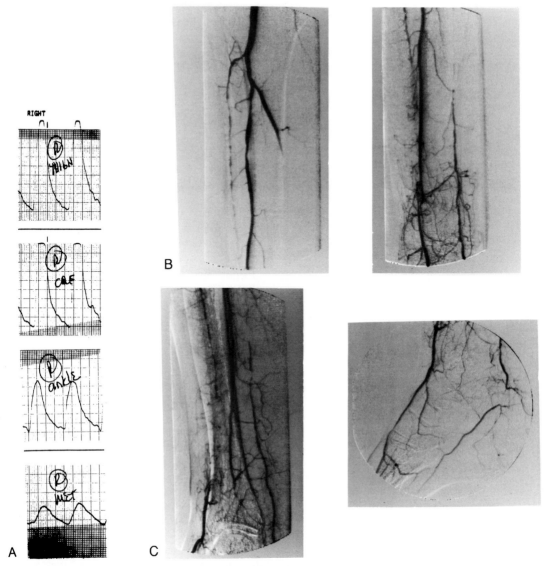

**Figure 14-4** Pulse volume recordings and corresponding lower extremity arteriogram in a 65-year-old diabetic man with right foot ischemia. *A*, Pulse volume recordings showed only mild abnormalities at the forefoot level. *B*, Intra-arterial digital subtraction arteriogram of the below-knee arteries. The popliteal artery is widely patent. The anterior and posterior tibial arteries are occluded proximally. The peroneal artery is moderately narrowed proximally and occludes just proximal to the ankle joint. *C*, Lateral view of the distal area of the leg and foot. The peroneal artery is occluded proximal to the ankle joint. The posterior tibial artery reconstitutes proximal to the ankle, but then occludes again at the level of the plantar bifurcation. The anterior tibial artery reconstitutes at the ankle joint and flows into a patent dorsalis pedis artery and tarsal arch. The patient underwent a below-knee popliteal to dorsalis pedis artery bypass with nonreversed saphenous vein.

amputation failed, although 18 per cent had wound complications that required delay of rehabilitation until they were successfully treated. These results compare favorably with those of other series that have endorsed the use of criteria for amputation level based on a variety of noninvasive vascular surgical methods, including TcPO$_2$ measurements and xenon clearance techniques.

As previously described, wide variability and often contradictory results have been reported with TcPO$_2$ measurements and radio-isotope clearance studies. As with other methods, normal or near-normal results are usually reliable in predicting success of wound or amputation healing; however, an absolute value below which healing will never occur has not been found.

These findings emphasize the continued importance of clinical judgment in determining amputation level or the likelihood of ulcer healing. Attempting to apply rigid guidelines based on noninvasive vascular assessment will result in some patients being subjected to an amputation in whom healing might otherwise have occurred. As a general principle, we have used the vascular laboratory data to confirm initial clinical impressions about the patient's vascular status. When the tests are indicative of significant ischemia, the high degree of success and safety of modern vascular surgical techniques generally justifies an attempt at vascular reconstruction first, if possible, prior to an amputation or foot surgery. If vascular reconstruction is not possible or appropriate, lesser amputations will be attempted first, when the patient has any chance for rehabilitation, even if the noninvasive studies suggest a low probability of healing. This gives the patient the "benefit of the doubt," preventing loss of potentially salvageable limbs and, in our experience, rarely results in increased morbidity.

Although experience with MRA in imaging the tibial, peroneal, and pedal arteries most commonly bypassed in patients with diabetes has been limited until recently, initial reports on its use in this area have been encouraging. In one study, MRA of the infrapopliteal arteries proved to be superior to conventional arteriography in imaging these arteries. One problem with this study was an unusually high failure rate of standard contrast arteriography to demonstrate patent distal arteries (17 per cent). This may have been due to the very limited use of intra-arterial digital subtraction angiography, which many centers have found superior to conventional arteriography in imaging distal arteries. In our own practice where intra-arterial digital subtraction arteriograms are routinely obtained in all evaluations for lower extremity arterial reconstructive surgery, a patent distal artery for bypass has been demonstrable in greater than 95 per cent of patients studied. Moreover, our preliminary results with MRA show that resolution of images of distal arteries is inferior to that routinely obtained with intra-arterial digital subtraction angiography. Nev-

ertheless, MRA is an exciting development in noninvasive vascular assessment that may revolutionize the evaluation of the ischemic diabetic lower extremity. As experience with this technique increases and technology improves, it may well supplant contrast arteriography in preopertive assessment of these patients. Further studies are required comparing MRA to both standard and digital subtraction angiography techniques.

## CONCLUSIONS

The noninvasive vascular laboratory has a proven role in the assessment of arterial insufficiency in diabetic patients with foot problems. The currently available tests can reliably identify ischemia with a high degree of accuracy and add greatly to the clinician's initial clinical evaluation. Newer techniques, such as color duplex scanning and magnetic resonance angiography, may revolutionize the evaluation of ischemia in these patients in the future.

The role of the vascular laboratory in predicting wound healing or amputation level remains adjunctive to the surgeon's clinical judgment. Application of rigid guidelines based on test results is inappropriate and may result in a more proximal amputation than necessary, which may deny some patients a chance for successful rehabilitation.

## SELECTED READING LIST

Carter, S. A.: Response of ankle systolic pressure to leg exercise in mild or questionable arterial disease. N. Engl. J. Med. 287:578, 1972.

Castronuovo, J. J., Pabst, T. S., Flanigan, D. P., et al.: Non invasive determination of skin perfusion pressure using a laser doppler. J. Cardiovasc. Surg. 28:253, 1987.

Faris, I., and Duncan, H.: Skin perfusion pressure in the prediction of healing in diabetic patients with ulcers or gangrene of the foot. J. Vasc. Surg. 2:536, 1985.

Fearon, J., Campbell, D. R., Hoar, C. S., et al.: Improved results with diabetic below-knee amputations. Arch. Surg. 120:777, 1985.

Fronek, A., Johansen, K. H., Dilley, R. B., et al.: Non-invasive psysiologic tests in the diagnosis and characterization of peripheral arterial occlusive disease. Am. J. Surg. 126:205, 1973.

Gibbons, G. W., and Wheelock, F. C.: Problems in the non-invasive evaluation of peripheral circulation in the diabetic. Practical Cardiol. 8:115, 1982.

Gibbons, G. G., Wheelock, F. C., Siembieda, C., et al.: Noninvasive prediction of amputation level in diabetic patients. Arch. Surg. 114:1253, 1979.

Karanfilian, R. G., Lynch, T. G., Zirul, V. T., et al.: The value of laser doppler velocimetry and transcutaneous oxygen tension determination in predicting healing of ischemic forefoot ulcerations and amputations in diabetic and non-diabetic patients. J. Vasc. Surg. 4:511, 1986.

Kohler, T. R., Nance, D. R., Cramer, M. M., et al.: Duplex scanning for diagnosis of aortoiliac and femoro-popliteal occlusive desease: A prospective study. Circulation 76:1074, 1987.

Malone, J. M., Anderson, G. G., Lalka, S. G., et al.: Prospective comparison of noninvasive techniques for amputation level selection. Am. J. Surg. 154:179, 1987.

Moore, W. S., Henry, R. E., Malone, J. M., et al.: Prospective use of xenon 33 clearance for amputation level selection. Arch. Surg. 116:86, 1981.

Ouriel, K., and Zarins, C. K.: Doppler ankle pressure. Arch. Surg. 117:1297, 1982.

Strandness, D. E., Schultz, R. D., Sumner, D. S., et al.: Ultrasonic flow detection: A useful technique in the evaluation of peripheral vascular disease. Am. J. Surg. 113:311, 1967.

Vollrath, R. D., Sulles-Cuhna, S. X., Vincent, D., et al.: Non-invasive measurement of toe systolic pressures. Bruit. 4:27, 1980.

White, R. A., Nolan, L., Hanley, D., et al.: Non invasive evaluation of peripheral vascular disease using transcutaneous oxygen tension. Am. J. Surg. 144:68, 1982.

Owen, R. S., Carpenter, J. P., Baum, R. A., et al.: Magnetic resonance imaging of angiographically occult runoff vessels in peripheral arterial occlusive disease. N. Engl. J. Med. 326:1577, 1992.

# Chapter 15

# ARTERIOGRAPHY

KENNETH R. STOKES, M.D., FRANK B. POMPOSELLI, Jr., M.D.,
and H. ESTERBROOK LONGMAID, III, M.D.

## PERIPHERAL ARTERIOGRAPHY

Lower extremity atherosclerosis represents a major cause of morbidity in the diabetic patient. Overall, 16 per cent of diabetic patients have peripheral vascular disease, 20 times more than nondiabetics, and as many as 20 per cent of these patients have gangrene. The degree of atherosclerotic occlusive disease is related to the duration of diabetes: 15 per cent have involvement at 10 years after initial diagnosis and 45 per cent at 20 years. The severity of diabetes also correlates with the severity of tibial-peroneal atherosclerotic disease, but not with large vessel disease. Other risk factors (such as smoking, hypertension, and obesity) further increase the severity of atherosclerosis. The incidence in women is nearly equal to that in men; the disease affects both premenopausal and postmenopausal women. Diabetics are also affected at a younger age.

Peripheral vascular disease in diabetic patients is often diffuse with involvement of both the large arteries, including the aorta, and the peripheral arteries of the calf and foot. The tibial and peroneal arteries may be severely affected without involvement of more proximal vessels, a distribution rarely seen in nondiabetic patients. Atherosclerosis involves the arteries of the foot in 40 per cent of diabetic patients. Vascular disease is also more prevalent in the deep femoral artery and geniculate arteries, and the ability to develop collateral circulation is reduced. For this reason, stenoses or occlusions produce more serious symptoms in the diabetic than in the nondiabetic patient. A solitary severe stenosis or multiple relatively mild stenoses in the iliac, femoral, popliteal, or calf arteries can lead to frank gangrene.

Atherosclerotic plaques in diabetic patients show an increased propensity for ulceration and cracking; otherwise they are indistinguishable from lesions in nondiabetic patients. The arteries have extensive calcification in up to 25 per cent of patients with adult-onset diabetes. This calcinosis involves the media and results in the typical radiographic *pipe stem* or *trolley track* appearance (Fig. 15–1). Calcification is not associated with arterial occlusion, but its distribution is important to evaluate because dense vascular calcifications may prevent arterial bypass

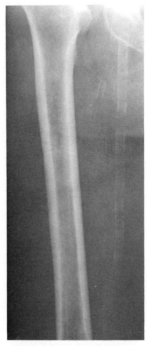

**Figure 15–1** Medial calcinosis of the superficial and deep femoral arteries showing pipe stem or trolley track calcification.

anastomosis or may alter the choice of bypass procedure.

## Indications

Peripheral arteriography is performed in diabetic patients for disabling claudication, ischemic rest pain, ischemic ulceration, and gangrene. Because atherosclerotic occlusive disease is frequently diffuse, pedal arteries may be patent even when the pedal pulses are not palpable and noninvasive examination shows no evidence of flow. At the same time, the presence of palpable foot pulses does not exclude significant proximal vascular disease. If the symptoms are present, therefore, arteriography should be performed regardless of the status of peripheral pulses. As a general rule, a patient should not have an amputation before arteriographic evaluation.

## Technique

Preprocedure orders for peripheral arteriography in diabetic patients are similar to those in nondiabetic patients. Because of the increased incidence of renal impairment in diabetes, renal status should be carefully evaluated. Before, during, and after the procedure, all patients should be well hydrated (e.g. 5 per cent dextrose and ½ normal saline at 75 to 100 ml/hour), preferably starting the night before the procedure. Overhydration, however, must be avoided, because many of these patients have coronary artery disease and are prone to congestive heart failure.

Oral diabetes medication is withheld on the day of the procedure, and any morning insulin injection is reduced by half. Patients in whom the procedure is scheduled for the afternoon may receive a liquid breakfast. All patients may eat after completion of the procedure. Blood glucose levels are followed closely at all times and adjusted by sliding-scale insulin administration as necessary.

For catheterization, the common femoral artery is preferable to the axillary or proximal brachial artery. Whether the common femoral artery is punctured ipsilateral or contralateral to the more severely diseased lower extremity is a matter of preference. With the use of 4 F or 5 F catheters, the incidence of hematoma or arterial injury after catheteriza-

tion of the ipsilateral femoral artery is small and, if present, does not significantly hinder peripheral bypass.

When the contralateral artery is catheterized, iliac angioplasty can be readily performed by crossing over the aortic bifurcation with either a cobra or Simmons catheter. Furthermore, a superficial femoral angioplasty can be performed with this approach without a second antegrade puncture in the ipsilateral femoral artery.

When the femoral arteries cannot be catheterized or when a femoral bypass graft is present, we prefer to gain access through the proximal left brachial artery or, if necessary, the right brachial artery. The brachial vessel is catheterized using the standard Seldinger technique at the junction of its proximal one third and distal two thirds. Because of the vessel's relatively small size, a 4 F pigtail catheter is preferred. The catheter can easily be placed in the abdominal aorta even if the thoracic aorta is tortuous. By placing the pigtail tip in the direction of the descending aorta, a guide wire can be advanced into the distal aorta without difficulty. After catheterization, 1000 units of intravenous heparin helps prevent pericatheter thrombosis. When catheterization is difficult or the artery is believed to be small, a vasodilator such as nifedipine (Procardia 10 mg sublingual) is administered to prevent spasm. Any dampening of the left brachial pulse or decrease in the left arm blood pressure indicates subclavian artery disease and contraindicates brachial catheterization.

When transbrachial or transfemoral catheterization is not possible, translumbar arteriography is used. This technique, especially the low (L-2) puncture, is otherwise avoided because catheterization of a severely atherosclerotic distal aorta may cause aortic occlusion or distal embolization. Selective iliac injection and angioplasty are also more difficult or may not be possible from this approach.

When aortoiliac disease is suspected clinically or by noninvasive examinations, the aorta and iliac arteries are best evaluated by routine arteriographic filming. When aortoiliac disease is not suspected or when the patient has compromised renal function, digital subtraction arteriography may be performed with less than half the contrast volume of routine arteriography. For digital aortography, we typically inject 30 ml of Conray-30 rather than the 40 ml of Conray-60 or the equivalent used for routine aortography.

Depending upon the patient's clinical symptoms and renal status, peripheral arteriography may be unilateral or bilateral. Routine bilateral iliofemoral arteriography provides the best delineation of the iliac and femoral arteries. When the atherosclerotic disease is limited, a single aortic injection may visualize both lower extremities. Because of the diffuse nature of diabetic atherosclerosis and poor collateral flow, however, delineation of the tibial and pedal arteries is often suboptimal, requiring selective catheterization and additional injections of contrast medium. For these reasons, we initially use DSA by selective external iliac injection to evaluate the lower extremities (Fig. 15–2).

Anteroposterior and lateral views of the foot are routinely obtained to visualize the dorsalis pedis and tibialis posterior arteries below the ankle (Figs. 15–3 and 15–4). The patency and quality of these vessels must be known when severe tibial vascular disease necessitates pedal bypass. Evaluation of the arterial anatomy in the foot is also important because the long-term patency of distal bypass grafts depends on patency of the pedal arch.

With diffuse atherosclerosis, patent distal arteries, especially the pedal arteries, may not be delineated even with selective injection and DSA. Further, because of poor inflow, pedal arteries that appear to be small on arteriography may in fact only be constricted and at surgery may be found to be quite large (Fig. 15–5). To better delineate these vessels, intra-arterial nitroglycerin (200 to 400 $\mu$g) can be injected to dilate the arteries and improve opacification. Papaverine (30 mg) or tolazoline (Priscoline 25 to 40 mg) can also be used. Because extensive medial calcinosis and poor flow to the distal calf are often present, however, effects of these drugs may be somewhat limited. A thigh tourniquet used to cause reactive hyperemia has proven to be unreliable in our experience and in diabetic patients appears to be less effective than intra-arterial vasodilators.

Limited flow distal to multiple levels of occlusion may make the distal vessels appear smaller on the arteriogram, and patent pedal arteries may not be opacified even when all of the aforementioned techniques are used. With limb-threatening ischemia or when amputation is considered, the suitability of

a pedal vessel for bypass should be based on surgical exploration and not on the arteriographic appearance. We have successfully bypassed 6 of 12 patients in whom a weak Doppler signal was present over the dorsalis pedis artery although this vessel was not visible on arteriography.

## Digital Subtraction Arteriography

In digital subtraction arteriography (DSA), televised fluoroscopic images of the arteriogram are first digitized for computer processing. A noncontrast mask image is then electronically subtracted from postinjection images. The resulting images contain only contrast-agent-filled structures free of background detail. This image is then enhanced by a computer and displayed on a video monitor for evaluation.

DSA has been much maligned because of poor early equipment, but the image quality of DSA now approaches that of routine arteriography. Because of the advantages in patients with severe atherosclerotic disease, DSA has largely supplanted routine arteriography in our institution. The advantages of DSA over routine arteriography are:

1. High-contrast resolution in DSA provides improved delineation of peripheral arteries with a lower volume of contrast medium than required for conventional arteriography. With DSA, minimally opacified pedal arteries can be identified that would not be evident on routine arteriography. This improved arterial visualization may eliminate the need for more selective arterial catheterization and further large-volume injections of contrast medium.

2. Less contrast-medium-related discomfort occurs with the less-concentrated ionic contrast medium used in DSA. The lower volume also reduces the necessity of using less painful but significantly more expensive nonionic contrast agents.

3. Reduced cost of examination with DSA results from eliminating the cost of nonionic contrast material and from reducing the quantity of radiographic film required. Film processing and storage costs are also reduced. The disadvantage of DSA is the decrease of spatial resolution from the 5 to 6 lines/mm of routine arteriography to the 2 to 3 line pairs/mm of DSA.

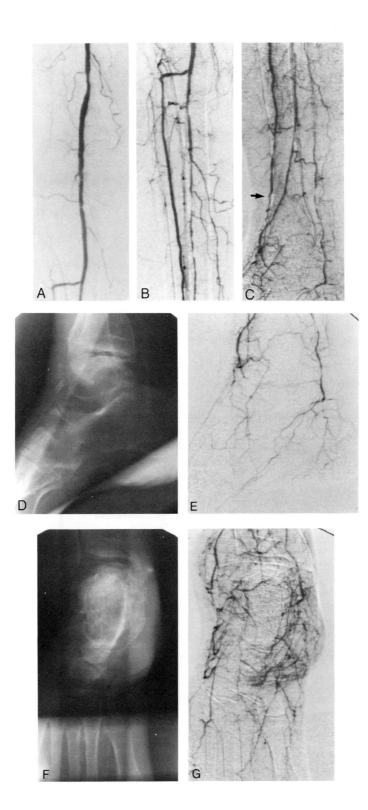

**Figure 15–4** Use of DSA to evaluate pedal vasculature. The iliac and superficial femoral arteries are not unusual. The popliteal artery is patent (A). AP proximal calf film (B) reveals the proximal anterior tibial artery to be patent. The posterior tibial and peroneal arteries are severely diseased. Lateral distal calf DSA (C) shows occlusion of the distal anterior tibial artery (arrow) and severely diseased posterior tibial and peroneal arteries. Lateral foot scout view (D) and DSA (E) and AP scout (F) and DSA (G) disclose occlusion of the dorsalis pedis artery at the ankle with minimal filling distally. The posterior tibial artery is severely diseased below the ankle with poor filling of the plantar arch. Amputation was eventually required.

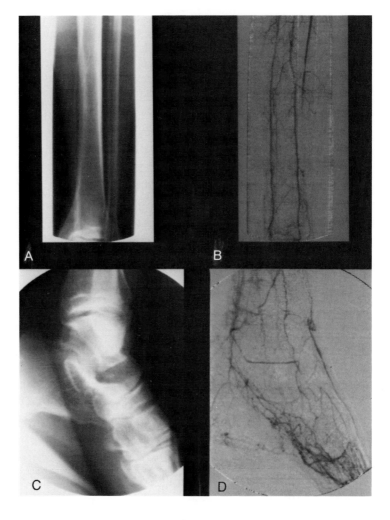

**Figure 15–5** Evaluation of distal vasculature. AP nonsubtracted view *(A)* and DSA *(B)* of the calf disclose anterior tibial artery occlusion with patent but severely diseased posterior tibial and peroneal arteries. Lateral scout view of the foot *(C)* and DSA *(D)* reveal posterior tibial occlusion at the ankle. The dorsalis pedis artery is reconstituted at the ankle and appears small. At surgery, this artery was found to be larger and of better quality than its radiographic appearance suggests, and an insitu vein graft was placed into the dorsalis pedis artery.

The consequences are as follows:

1. Although arteries less than 1 mm can be delineated, the images are not adequate for diagnostic evaluation.

2. Reduced edge sharpness in larger vessels compromises their measurement and eliminates fine detail. The combined effects of decreased spatial resolution and image subtraction can result in underestimation of the degree of atherosclerosis, especially in large vessels such as the aorta and iliac arteries. Consequently, we prefer routine arteriography of the aorta and iliac arteries over DSA. When DSA is performed, intra-arterial pressures are a useful aid in the evaluation of any questionable aortoiliac atherosclerotic disease.

## Complications

Complications of arteriography are principally the result of arterial catheterization, reaction to contrast medium, and contrast-agent–induced renal failure. Other problems are usually related to the cardiovascular system, such as congestive failure and vasovagal reactions. Hessel et al. reported a complication rate of 1.73 per cent and a mortality rate of 0.03 per cent for arteriography performed by femoral catheterization. The complication rates for axillary artery catheterization (3.29 per cent) and translumbar catheterization (2.89 per cent) were higher than for the femoral approach.

Problems at the femoral catheterization site included significant hematoma formation (0.26 per cent), occlusion or thrombosis (0.14 per cent), false aneurysm (0.05 per cent), arteriovenous fistula (0.01 per cent), and distal embolization (0.10 per cent). The incidence of limb amputation was 0.01 per cent.

In our experience, hematoma formation and thrombosis are more common with the high brachial or axillary approach than with the femoral approach. In our series of 600 brachial catheterizations, six brachial arterial occlusions occurred immediately, but all responded to full heparinization. None of these patients received the initial 1000-unit intravenous heparin bolus we now routinely employ. Since we initiated administration of this heparin bolus after brachial arterial catheterization, thrombosis has not occurred. Over the entire series, five patients required evacuation of a large hematoma that was causing brachial nerve compression. One patient with arteritis experienced distal embolization to the hand. No vertebral neurovascular complications occurred.

In the literature, true reactions to contrast material are cited in 0.14 per cent of patients and involve urticaria, bronchospasm, laryngospasm, laryngeal edema, and cardiopulmonary arrest. Fatal reaction occurs in 0.02 per cent of instances of conventional arteriography. If a patient has a history of reaction, we premedicate with prednisone (50 mg by mouth every 6 hours for 24 hours), diphenhydramine (Benadryl, 50 mg intramuscularly or intravenously), and cimetidine (300 mg orally or intravenously). We also use nonionic contrast material, which may cause fewer reactions.

Patients with diabetic nephropathy have an increased incidence of contrast-agent–induced renal failure, varying from 9 per cent to 22 per cent. Defining contrast-medium–induced renal failure as an increase of 25 per cent in the serum creatinine, Parfrey et al. found an 11.8 per cent incidence in well-hydrated diabetic patients with pre-existing renal failure (baseline creatinine concentration of 1.7 to 5.0 mg/dl). No patients, however, required dialysis. Creatinine increase occurred in 2 per cent of the diabetic patients without pre-existing renal failure, but this elevation was frequently mild and transient. This rate is comparable to that in nondiabetics with normal renal function. Acute renal failure occurs in nearly all patients with baseline creatinine levels greater than 5.0 mg/dl and may be irreversible. Other factors that increase the incidence of contrast-medium–related renal failure include congestive heart failure, hyperuricemia, proteinuria, advanced age (greater than 60 years), dehydration, myeloma, and concomitant nephrotoxic medication.

To limit nephrotoxicity, the quantity of contrast material injected should be kept to a minimum. In high-risk patients (creatinine greater than 2.0 to 2.5 mg/dl), aortoiliac arteriography can be omitted in the presence of strong femoral pulses and normal noninvasive examinations. Selective injection of the involved limb (instead of bilateral leg arteriography) and the use of DSA can greatly reduce the quantity of contrast medium injected. At this time, nonionic contrast material has not been shown to reduce the incidence of renal failure induced by contrast medium.

The patient should be well hydrated with overnight intravenous fluids depending upon cardiac status. The patient should be further hydrated following the examination. It may be beneficial for patients with serum creatinine levels greater than 2 to 2.5 mg/dl to receive 500 ml of 25 per cent mannitol infused at 20 ml/hr starting one hour before the arteriography and continuing for six hours afterward. In addition, 100 mg of furosemide is injected for each milligram per deciliter above 2.0 attained by the creatinine level. The patient is well hydrated before the procedure and urinary output is replaced with 5 per cent dextrose in 0.45 per cent saline with 30 mEq of potassium chloride per liter.

## SUGGESTED READING LIST

Andros, G., Harris, R.W., Dulauna, L.B., et al.: The need for arteriography in diabetic patients with gangrene and palpable foot pulses. Arch. Surg. 119:1260, 1984.

Berkseth, R.A., and Kjellstrand, C.M.: Radiologic contrast-induced nephropathy. Radiol. Clin. North Am. 68:351, 1984.

Cochran, S.T., Wong, W.S., and Roe, D.J.: Predicting angiography-induced acute renal function impairment: Clinical risk model. AJR 141:1027, 1983.

Dardik, H., Ibrahim, I.M., Sussman, B., et al.: Morphologic structure of the pedal arch and its relationship to patency of crural vascular reconstruction. Surg. Gynecol. Obstet. 152:645, 1981.

D'Elia, J.A., Gleason, R.E., Alday, M., et al.: Nephrotoxicity from angiographic contrast material: A prospective study. Am. J. Med. 72:719, 1982.

Gibbons, G.W., and Freeman, D.: Vascular evaluation and treatment of the diabetic. Clin. Podiatr. Med. Surg. 4:377, 1986.

Harrington, D.P., Boxt, L.M., and Murray, P.D.: Digital subtraction angiography overview of technical principles. AJR 139:781, 1982.

Hessel, S.J., Adams, D.F., and Abrams, H.L.: Complications of angiography. Radiology 138:273, 1981.

Janka, H.V., Standl, F., and Mehnert, H.: Peripheral vascular disease in diabetes mellitus and its relation to cardiovascular role factors: Screening with the Doppler ultrasonic technique. Diabetes Care 3:207, 1980.

Kahn, P.C., Boyer, D.N., Moran, J.M., et al.: Reactive hyperemia in lower extremity arteriography: An evaluation. Radiology 90:975, 1968.

Kaufman, S.L., Chang, R., and Kadir, S.: Intraarterial digital subtraction angiography in diagnostic arteriography. Radiology 151:323, 1984.

Kinnison, M.L., Powe, N.R., Steinberg, E.P.: Results of randomized controlled trials of low- versus high-osmolarity contrast media. Radiology 170:381, 1989.

Kozak, B.E., Bedell, J.E., and Rosch, J.: Small vessel leg angiography for distal vessel bypass grafts. J. Vasc. Surg. 8:711, 1988.

Kruger, R.A., and Riederer, S.J.: Basic Concepts of Digital Subtraction Angiography. Boston, G. K. Hall Medical Publishers, 1984.

McGill, H.C., Jr.: Diabetes and vascular lesions. In Moskowitz, J. (ed): Diabetes and Atherosclerosis Connection. New York, Juvenile Diabetes Foundation Medical Series, 1981.

Melton, L.J., Macken, K.M., Palumbo, R.J., and Elveback, L.R.: Incidence and prevalence of clinical peripheral vascular disease in a population-based cohort of diabetic patients. Diabetes Care 3:650, 1980.

Moore, R.D., Steinberg, E.P., Powe, N.R., et al.: Frequency and determinants of adverse reactions induced by high-osmolarity contrast media. Radiology 170:727, 1989.

O'Mara, C.S., Flinn, W.R., Neiman, H.L., et al.: Correlation of foot arterial anatomy with early tibial bypass patency. Surgery 89:743, 1981.

Ovitt, T., and Newell, J.D., II: Digital subtraction angiography: Technology, equipment and techniques. Radiol. Clin. North Am. 23:177, 1985.

Parfrey, P.S., Griffiths, S.M., Barrett, B.J., et al.: Contrast material-induced renal failure in patients with diabetes mellitus, renal insufficiency, or both. N. Engl. J. Med. 320:143, 1989.

Pomposelli, F.B., Jepsen, S.J., Gibbons, G.E., et al.: Efficacy of the dorsalis pedis bypass for limb salvage in diabetic patients: Short term observations. J. Vasc. Surg. 11:745, 1990.

Schwab, S.J., Hjatky, M.A., Pieper, K.S., et al.: Contrast nephrotoxicity: A random controlled trial of a nonionic and ionic radiographic contrast agent. N. Engl. J. Med. 320:149, 1989.

Shehadi, W.H.: Contrast media adverse reactions: Occurrences, recurrences, and distribution patterns. Radiology 143:11, 1982.

Shehadi, W.H., and Toniolo, G.: Adverse reactions to contrast media. A Report from the Committee on Safety of Contrast Media of the Interventional Society of Radiology. Radiology 137:299, 1980.

Sternby, N.H.: Atherosclerosis and diabetes mellitus. Acta. Pathol. Microbiol. Scand. 194 (Suppl.):152, 1968.

Wolf, G.L., Arenson, R.L., and Cross, A.P.: A prospective trial of ionic vs nonionic contrast agents in routine clinical practice and comparison of adverse effects. AJR 152:939, 1989.

# Chapter 16

# PREOPERATIVE EVALUATION OF THE DIABETIC PATIENT

MICHAEL A. SASSOWER, M.D., STUART W. ZARICH, M.D.,
O. STEVENS LELAND, M.D., and STANLEY M. LEWIS, M.D.

The presence of cardiovascular disease is the major risk factor for perioperative complications in patients undergoing surgery. The diabetic patient who is about to undergo peripheral vascular surgery is at particularly high risk for cardiovascular complications because of the great prevalence of significant coronary artery disease and left ventricular dysfunction in this population. The evaluation of the status of diabetic patients is complicated by diminished awareness of cardiac symptomatology and functional limitations impeding provocative testing. In addition, anesthesia is frequently lengthy, and significant blood loss and volume repletion may be required. The diabetic population requiring surgery therefore poses a major challenge to the diabetologist, cardiologist, and surgeon. This chapter will deal with the preoperative cardiac evaluation, operative risk, and subsequent management approach to this high-risk group.

## OPERATIVE RISK FACTORS

### Angina

Diabetic patients, especially those with peripheral vascular disease, have a high likelihood of concomitant coronary artery disease. However, the symptomatic assessment of angina may be difficult because of impaired sensory perception and the physical limitations imposed by vascular disease.

The presence of stable angina was recently evaluated in a study of diabetics undergoing peripheral vascular surgery. Diabetic patients with a clinical history of angina carried the same preoperative risk as those patients with two or more areas of reversible ischemia determined by dipyridamole-thallium scanning. In this same series, diabetics with a history of angina had a greater number of reversible thallium segments than those without angina. These findings are in contrast to previous studies that found stable angina to be a relatively minor predictor of perioperative morbidity, despite its known importance in the ambulatory population. Given the fact that stable exertional angina may represent a significant factor in the assessment of preoperative risk, it is also important to note that the goal of peripheral vascular surgery is not only limb salvage, but also maximizing functional capacity. Additionally, debilitating exertional angina pectoris may well affect postoperative recuperation and subsequent rehabilitation, prompting evaluation for determination of appropriate therapy.

The presence of unstable angina, or rest angina, is felt to be prognostically important, requiring preoperative evaluation for either aggressive medical therapy or revascularization procedure.

### Silent Ischemia

The presence of silent (asymptomatic) ischemia is an important issue in the preoperative assessment in all patients, but is especially important in the diabetic population. A number of studies using either Holter monitoring with ST segment analysis or thallium studies have shown a high prevalence of asymptomatic ischemia in diabetics. Utilizing dipyridamole-thallium 201 scintigraphy in diabetic patients with peripheral vascular disease, 57 per cent of these patients without a clinical suspicion of coronary artery disease had thallium abnormalities. Of these patients, 47 per cent had reversible thallium defects compatible with ischemia, and 37 per cent had evidence of prior, clinically silent, myocardial infarction.

Silent ischemia and symptomatic ischemia have a similar perioperative and long-term risk. This difficult problem will be discussed further in the section on preoperative evaluation.

## Myocardial Infarction

One of the most important factors in the assessment of operative risk is the presence of a recent (less than 6 months) myocardial infarction. Patients with a history of prior myocardial infarction have a markedly increased risk of perioperative infarction.

The time interval from the initial infarction to the time of the perioperative period is the most crucial variable. Patients with a Q wave myocardial infarction undergoing general anesthesia within six months of infarction are at a particularly high risk. Reinfarction rates of 30 per cent in patients undergoing surgery within three months of their myocardial infarction, 15 per cent between three and six months postinfarction, and approximately 6 per cent after six months have been noted (Fig. 16–1).

The high operative morbidity and mortality associated with a recent infarction contraindicate *elective* surgery in any patient less

than three months following myocardial infarction. If possible, surgery should be delayed for at least six months. In those patients in whom operation cannot be delayed because of excessive morbidity and mortality from their primary condition, aggressive perioperative management guided by invasive hemodynamic monitoring can markedly reduce reinfarction rates. Using this approach, Rao et al. noted a reinfarction rate of only 5.8 per cent in patients with a myocardial infarction within three months (Fig. 16–2).

## Congestive Heart Failure

Congestive heart failure (CHF) represents a major risk factor for surgery in the diabetic patient. The prevalence of CHF is markedly increased in diabetics, especially in female patients. CHF is a predictor of perioperative morbidity, and the risk may be proportional to the severity of symptoms. It is important to remember, however, that CHF is a manifestation that may reflect either systolic or diastolic dysfunction. Perioperative risk seems to be largely confined to those with systolic dysfunction. In a series from Seattle using radionuclide ventriculography preoperatively to evaluate postoperative outcome in patients undergoing revascularization of an extremity, patients with an ejection fraction of 50 per cent or less had a lower overall survival rate than those with an ejection fraction greater than 50 per cent. In this study, both diabetes and smoking were also associated with significantly diminished overall survival.

Although cardiac dysfunction is associated with coronary atherosclerosis in many diabet-

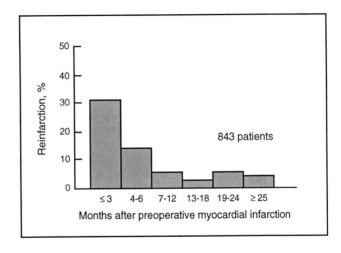

**Figure 16–1** Inverse relationship of risk of perioperative myocardial reinfarction during noncardiac surgical procedure and time since prior preoperative myocardial infarction in 843 patients. (From Rao, T. L. K., Jacobs, K. H., El-Etr, A. A.: Reinfarction following anesthesia in patients with myocardial infarction. Anesthesiology 59:499, 1983.)

mize the occurrence of these arrhythmias by ensuring good pulmonary care, by aggressively treating infections with both antibiotics and antipyretics, by maintaining optimal hemoglobin levels, and by careful assessment of intravascular volume both clinically and with invasive monitoring equipment when appropriate.

Regurgitant lesions may also be present in the diabetic patient. Again the major concerns are the degree of left ventricular dysfunction present and the patient's current volume status. Appropriate adjustment of inotropic agents, diuretics, and vasodilators preoperatively is the key to success.

## FEATURES PECULIAR TO DIABETIC PATIENTS

In the previous sections, the cardiac risk factors common to all patients undergoing noncardiac surgery were reviewed. Although there is no evidence of higher operative mortality in diabetic patients, complicating features are frequently found in diabetics that represent potential sources of morbidity.

### Autonomic Neuropathy

Autonomic neuropathy occurs with high frequency in patients with long-term diabetes, and it is frequently found in association with peripheral neuropathy. In addition to peripheral neuropathy, important symptoms associated with underlying cardiac autonomic neuropathy are orthostatic hypotension and impairment of hypoglycemia awareness. However, neither impotence nor gastroparesis alone has a high association with underlying cardiac autonomic neuropathy. Autonomic neuropathy frequently coexists with renal failure in diabetics.

Perhaps the most important feature of autonomic neuropathy is the masking of anginal discomfort, likely contributed to in part by the destruction of afferent nerve fibers. Atypical anginal symptoms are not infrequent in diabetics—for example, nausea, vomiting, lightheadedness, and general malaise and awareness of coexisting autonomic neuropathy should alert the physician to the possibility of silent myocardial ischemia. It is therefore important to obtain objective evidence of both myocardial ischemia and left

ventricular function in the preoperative assessment, since these patients' symptomatic perception may be grossly impaired.

A particularly high index of suspicion is also indicated in the postoperative period, because myocardial ischemia and infarction may be symptomatically subtle. Since the likelihood of myocardial infarction is greatest within three days postoperatively, rather than intraoperatively, particular vigilance during this period is warranted. Frequently the only symptoms of infarction in this group of patients will be nausea, diaphoresis, transient hypotension, or vague gastrointestinal symptoms, all of which are frequently ascribed to routine noncardiac postoperative problems. Frequent electrocardiography and heightened clinical awareness are necessary perioperatively to recognize myocardial ischemia and infarction in patients with altered sensory perception.

In addition to the loss of sensory afferent fibers, autonomic neuropathy is frequently complicated by the loss of parasympathetic tone. The lack of vagal innervation to the heart results in a higher resting heart rate and leaves the sympathetic acceleratory fibers relatively unchecked. Without the modulating tone of the vagal fibers, therefore, the heart rate has a higher set point and potentially is more responsive to sympathetic stimulation. During periods of stress this theoretically could result in a greater degree of tachycardia that is less responsive to heart rate–slowing medications, such as beta-adrenergic blocking agents.

### Renal Insufficiency

Although not specifically evaluated in studies of operative risk factors, renal failure most likely is associated with perioperative morbidity and mortality. Although the presence of a chronic disease state does necessarily increase perioperative risk, renal failure poses a unique problem. In diabetics there is an increased prevalence of renal dysfunction that ranges from mild proteinuria to nephrotic syndrome and from mild azotemia to chronic renal failure requiring dialysis.

The major complicating feature of diabetic renal disease is azotemia and chronic renal failure, which limits the concentrating and excretory function of the kidney. In addition, those patients with long-standing chronic renal failure frequently have concomitant hypertension and left ventricular hypertrophy, resulting in a noncompliant ventricle that is dependent on maximum end-diastolic volume for adequate performance. In addition, anemia and bleeding diatheses frequently complicate chronic renal failure and add to the operative risk by limiting cardiac reserve and by increasing the likelihood of blood loss with resultant hypotension. Certain recommendations are warranted in the operative management of diabetics with renal failure. Adequate preoperative dialysis should be performed to normalize clotting mechanisms, and transfusions to reach a hematocrit of at least 30 per cent are necessary to allow for cardiac reserve should volume depletion occur. The recent advent of erythropoietin administration to patients with renal failure may lessen the prevalence and degree of anemia in this population.

Preoperative radiological evaluation for surgery may also adversely impact upon renal function. Radiographic contrast media should be severely limited, since the diabetic patient with mild azotemia is at high risk to develop superimposed acute renal failure that may not be recognized for two to three days following the radiographic procedure, just as the patient's operative procedure may be completed. A number of series have revealed a higher than usual incidence of contrast-medium-induced renal failure in patients with diabetic azotemic nephropathy undergoing cardiac catheterization. A prospective Canadian study revealed little risk of nephrotoxicity in diabetic patients with normal renal function or nondiabetic patients with pre-existing renal insufficiency undergoing computed tomography or abdominal imaging procedures. However, the risk for patients with both diabetes and renal insufficiency was 8.8 per cent compared to 1.6 per cent for the controls. Other studies have shown that the presence of proteinuria is a predictor of adverse renal effects of radiocontrast media in diabetics. This is especially relevant for peripheral vascular procedures when large volumes of radiographic contrast media are frequently employed. This problem is best dealt with by preventive measures, including limitation of contrast media usage to a minimum and adequate hydration. Some of the newer lower osmotic compounds used in radiographic procedures may reduce the changes of nephrotoxicity, although this has not been proven as yet. In addition, mannitol given intravenously prior to the arteriographic procedure may diminish the risk of subsequent acute renal failure.

Diabetics with renal failure often require perioperative hemodynamic monitoring to minimize the changes of hypervolemia with resultant CHF or hypovolemia with hypotension with its risk of myocardial infarction or peripheral artery bypass graft occlusion. Optimal volume status is critical in the management of these patients, and right heart catherization and arterial lines may help guide management in this respect.

## Regulation of Blood Glucose

No evaluation of perioperative risk factors has ever conclusively documented hyperglycemia itself as a significant risk factor. Coronary artery disease, prior myocardial infarction, and CHF are the major risks associated with diabetes rather than any metabolic abnormality. Nevertheless, there are compelling reasons to optimize glucose control in the perioperative period. Hyperglycemia results in intravascular volume expansion and can thereby result in decompensation of left ventricular function in patients with marginal cardiac performance. Healing, especially of an amputated limb, is frequently marginal because of jeopardized perfusion. Failure to optimize blood glucose control can result in impairment of white cell function that is necessary for normal healing and control of potential infection.

## THE SURGICAL PROCEDURE

The magnitude of the surgical procedure is an important component of operative risk. Additionally, the type and duration of anesthesia need to be considered. In general there appears to be little difference in perioperative risk between general and regional types of anesthesia. However, in the patient with CHF, regional anesthesia alleviates the risk of myocardial suppression occurring with general agents and is preferred.

To evaluate the risk of procedures in diabetic limb surgery, three general levels of risk are outlined below.

1. Low risk. These are procedures that

have very low likelihood of accompanying blood loss, hypotension, myocardial infarction, or exacerbation of CHF regardless of the type of anesthesia used. This group is composed of toe amputations, transmetatarsal amputations, and below-knee amputations. Extensive preoperative cardiac evaluation need rarely be initiated with these procedures, given the low associated risk, and they may be considered when the cardiac risk of a more extensive operation appears prohibitive.

2. Moderate risk. This group consists of femoral-politeal, femoral-tibial, and axillofemoral bypass procedures and above-knee amputations. This type of surgery poses major risks, and most patients should undergo preoperative cardiac evaluation, or if the instability of the clinical situation warrants, consideration of a less stressful operation.

3. High risk. All procedures involving either the aorta or iliac artery comprise the high-risk group. These procedures involve major abdominal surgery and frequently the anastomosis of synthetic grafts, both of which can result in a high incidence of significant blood loss and hypotension. Therefore, careful preoperative cardiovascular evaluation is indicated in all patients undergoing a high-risk operation. In select patients, cardiac catheterization for evaluation for a possible revascularization procedure, either percutaneous or coronary artery bypass grafting, is warranted as a prelude to major aortic and iliac surgery.

## PREOPERATIVE EVALUATION

### Initial Assessment

The status of the diabetic patient about to undergo surgery should be assessed according to the presence and severity of underlying cardiovascular disease and the degree of risk associated with the particular operative procedure.

The major cardiac risks for noncardiac surgery include advanced age, signs of CHF, previous myocardial infarction, the presence of angina, valvular heart disease, general medical status, and severity and urgency of the operative procedure. Recent studies have attempted to separate vascular surgical procedures from other forms of noncardiac surgery. By totaling the allotted points for each

risk factor, a relative estimate of operative risk is obtained (Table 16–1). These protocols, however, must be used only as a guide with respect to decision making in various clinical situations.

The initial evaluation should consist of a careful history and physical examination to determine symptomatic and functional limitations. This is frequently inadequate, however, as many diabetics with peripheral vascular disease limit their exercise and also have diminished sensory perception of myocardial ischemia. The next stage is careful analysis of the electrocardiogram, with a specific search for evidence of previous infarction. Silent infarction is more common in the diabetic and, if present on the electrocardiogram, substantially increases the operative risk.

## Evaluation of Left Ventricular Function

Assessment of left ventricular function preoperatively in diabetics is important because

### TABLE 16–1. PREOPERATIVE CARDIAC RISK INDEX FOR NONCARDIAC SURGICAL PROCEDURES

| VARIABLE | POINT SCORE |
|---|---|
| History: | |
| Age >70 yr | 5 |
| Preoperative MI within 6 mo | 10 |
| Physical examination: | |
| $S_3$ gallop or increased JVP (>12 cm $H_2O$) | 11 |
| Significant valvular aortic stenosis | 3 |
| Electrocardiogram: | |
| Rhythm other than sinus, or atrial ectopy | 7 |
| Documentation of >5 VPC/min at any time | 7 |
| General medical status: | |
| $PaO_2$ <60 mm Hg or $PaCO_2$ >50 mm Hg | |
| $K^+$ <3.0 mEq/L or $HCO_3^-$ <20 mEq/L | 3 |
| BUN >50 mg/dl or creatinine >3.0 mg/dl | |
| Chronic liver disease or debilitation | |
| Operation: | |
| Intraperitoneal, intrathoracic, or aortic | 3 |
| Emergency | 4 |
| Total possible points | 53 |

Modified from Goldman et al.: Multifactorial index of cardiac risk in noncardiac surgical procedures. N. Engl. J. Med. 297:845, 1977.

BUN, blood urea nitrogen; JVP, jugular venous pressure; MI, myocardial infarction; VPC, ventricular premature contractions.

it can confirm and quantitate any degree of left ventricular dysfunction and can indirectly estimate left ventricular reserve, which may be important during times of perioperative stress. In addition, cardiac performance can deteriorate dramatically if the left ventricle is functioning at either less than or greater than its optimal filling pressures. The inability of an impaired ventricle to compensate for changes in preload (volume status) and afterload highlights the need for careful fluid status monitoring in all patients with severe pre-existing left ventricular dysfunction.

Noninvasive evaluation of left ventricular function is obtained by either radionuclide ventriculography or echocardiography. Radionuclide ventriculography is superior to echocardiography in quantitating overall left ventricular function, but is limited in terms of identifying regional wall motion abnormalities and valvular abnormalities. A major advantage of radionuclide ventriculography is the ability to obtain high-quality studies in virtually all patients, whereas echocardiography requires a technically adequate "window" to the heart. In addition to identifying regional wall motion abnormalities, echocardiography, two-dimensional and Doppler, is superior in affording a view of the cardiac valves, pericardium, wall thickness, and great vessels. In general, radionuclide ventriculography and echocardiography are complementary techniques, and the decision as to which procedure to be used should depend on the question being asked, overall quantitation of left ventricular function versus regional wall motion abnormality or valvular dysfunction.

## Evaluation of Coronary Artery Disease

The presence of significant coronary artery disease, whether symptomatic or silent, could complicate an episode of perioperative hypotension or hamper postoperative rehabilitation. In the evaluation of myocardial ischemia, it is important to consider the magnitude of risk of a particular operation. As noted in the previous section describing risk categories, those diabetic patients undergoing either moderate-risk or high-risk procedures should, when appropriate, undergo preoperative cardiac evaluation.

Methods for assessing coronary artery disease and myocardial ischemia have changed recently, especially with respect to the diabetic population. When possible, exercise stress testing by treadmill is an excellent way of assessing myocardial ischemia and allowing risk stratification based on functional capacity in exercise. When a patient has a likelihood for a false positive test, for example an abnormal electrocardiogram based on left ventricular hypertrophy or previous infarction, the addition of thallium scintigraphy allows a higher specificity and sensitivity for the detection of coronary artery disease. Intravenous thallium will only be taken up by myocardium with adequate perfusion. By injection of thallium immediately after exercise and scanning the patient initially and after a period of rest, the two sets of images are compared to assess if any area of hypoperfusion on the stress images has revealed reperfusion during rest (redistribution). These areas represent regions of myocardial ischemia. Areas of hypoperfusion at stress and at rest (fixed lesions) may represent regions of previous infarction. However, up to 40 per cent of regions of hypoperfusion with stress and at rest may not represent areas of fixed lesions but may represent profoundly ischemic regions. Delayed images after repeat thallium injection may allow these areas of severe coronary artery disease to take up thallium and show up as reversible ischemia. Similarly, reinjection of thallium prior to the rest imaging may reveal viable, yet ischemic, myocardium (Fig. 16–3).

Of course, exercise stress testing with or without thallium would be preferable in all patients, allowing both risk stratification and anatomical localization of possible ischemic myocardium. This is not always possible, however, especially with diabetics undergoing peripheral vascular surgery whose functional limitations may be based on symptoms of claudication or previous operative procedures. In these patients, dipyridamole-thallium scintigraphy has been shown to be comparable to treadmill exercise testing in its ability to assess the presence and severity of coronary artery disease. Dipyridamole, with its vasodilating effects, induces dilation of normal arteries, causing a relative redistribution of coronary blood flow. Thallium is then preferentially taken up by adequately perfused myocardium, with immediate and delayed scintigraphic images obtained looking for areas of reversible ischemia or infarction.

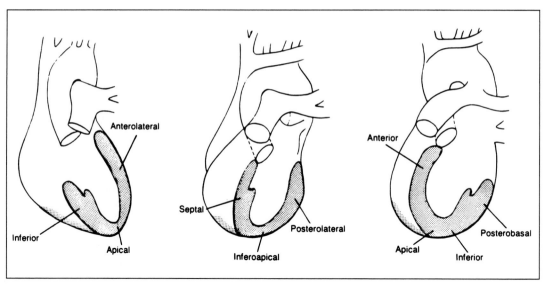

**Figure 16–3** Views and segments analyzed during thallium imaging. (From Lane, S. E., Lewis, S. M., Pippin, J. J., et al.: Predictive value of quantitative dipyridamole-thallium scintigraphy in assessing cardiovascular risk after vascular surgery in diabetes mellitus. Am. J. Cardiol. 64:1275, 1989.)

Although a high incidence of abnormal dipyridamole-thallium scans is seen in the diabetic population, many of these patients do not suffer postoperative cardiac events. The simple demonstration of a defect by dipyridamole-thallium scintigraphy in diabetics is thus of limited usefulness in predicting risk of postoperative cardiac complications. In a recent study of 101 diabetics undergoing peripheral revascularization, those with five or more areas of thallium reversibility, those with reversibility in the vascular distribution of the left anterior descending coronary artery, and those patients with angina were found to be at higher risk. At least one thallium defect was documented in more than 80 per cent of patients, but this did not correlate with clinical markers of coronary disease or complications of surgery. Overall only 11 per cent of patients suffered cardiovascular complications. Thus, patients with multiple reversible thallium defects or reversibility in the left anterior descending distribution should be considered for preoperative coronary angiography. Similarly, clinical variables (history of angina or myocardial infarction) when combined with thallium scintigraphy can markedly improve the predictive value of preoperative screening. Diabetics without clinical suspicion of coronary artery disease rarely have positive thallium scans unless other cardiac risk factors are present (Fig. 16–4). Ambulatory monitoring of ST segments for asymptomatic ischemia may also be useful to assess cardiac risk prior to peripheral vascular surgery.

## Overall Preoperative Assessment and Management

It can be seen that preoperative cardiac evaluation of the diabetic patient starts, as with all patients, with a full history and physical examination. Then, based on this initial assessment, involving evaluation of age and coexisting morbidity, additional noninvasive information may be obtained by electrocardiography.

With the above information in hand, a scoring protocol such as the one by Goldman et al. may be used in the assessment of preoperative risk. In the presence of appropriate risk factors, for example previous infarction or symptoms of congestive heart failure, appropriate noninvasive testing may continue. This may involve echocardiography, radionuclide ventriculography, or both, based on findings on history, physical examination, or electrocardiography.

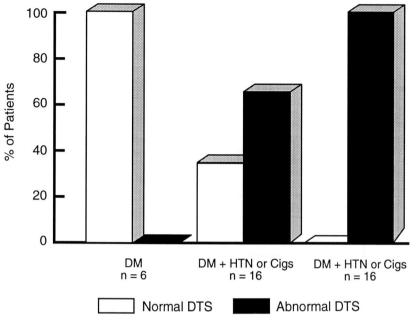

**Figure 16-4** Comparison of the percent of patients with normal (*light columns*) and abnormal (*dark columns*) dipyridamole-thallium scans according to associated coronary artery disease risk factors ($P = 0.001$). *Cigs*, history of cigarette smoking; *DM*, diabetes mellitus; *DTS*, dipyridamole-thallium scintigraphy; *HTN*, hypertension. (From Nesto, R. W., Watson, F. S., Kowalchuk, G. J., et al.: Silent myocardial ischemia and infarction in diabetics with peripheral vascular disease: Assessment by dipyridamole thallium 201 scintigraphy. Am. Heart J. 120:1023, 1990.)

Although convenient, preoperative risk scoring may be of little benefit in the diabetic undergoing peripheral vascular surgery. Functional limitations in spite of significant prevalence of coronary artery disease render ischemia frequently asymptomatic. Dipyridamole-thallium scintigraphy or ambulatory Holter monitoring of ST segments provides an excellent assessment of cardiac risk in these instances.

In patients with angina, segmental wall motion abnormalities, or those with evocable ischemia, assessment of the degree of coronary artery disease preoperatively may be appropriate. This may be either by exercise stress testing with or without thallium scintigraphy or by dipyridamole-thallium scintigraphy, looking for patients with significant findings. Significant findings would include (1) a positive exercise stress test, (2) the presence of angina, or (3) exercise-thallium or dipyridamole-thallium scanning with five or more reversible segments or reversibility in the vascular distribution of the left anterior descending artery. These patients may then be considered for preoperative coronary angiography for contemplation of a possible revascularization procedure, either by percutaneous transluminal coronary angioplasty or coronary artery bypass grafting.

Patients with symptoms of unstable angina, those with recent myocardial infarctions, or those with recurrent or continuing symptoms of CHF may be considered for immediate preoperative coronary angiography without the noninvasive ischemic evaluation described above. Indeed, exercise testing is contraindicated in patients with unstable angina. These patients would then also be evaluated for possible valvular dysfunction or coronary artery disease.

After all the above are considered, the impression whether the patient can tolerate the procedure is formed. A decision for coronary revascularization, valvular repair, or performance of a lower-risk surgical procedure can then be made. The usefulness of aggressive hemodynamic monitoring and therapy, including pulmonary artery catheterization, arterial catheterization, or intravenous anti-anginal therapy, is then decided upon. However, prospective data available on the benefits of either invasive hemodynamic monitoring or prophylactic use of intravenous nitroglycerin are somewhat limited.

## CONCLUSIONS

It is apparent that the evaluation of the diabetic patient about to undergo surgery,

# Chapter 17

# MANAGEMENT OF DIABETES DURING SURGERY

E. JAMES BUSICK, M.D.,
and GEORGE P. KOZAK, M.D.

The patient with diabetes has a high probability of requiring surgery during his lifetime—50 per cent of diabetics has been the estimation. This number may be higher today with surgical advances making possible a number of procedures that may not have been done in the past, such as coronary artery bypass grafts, newer vascular techniques, vitrectomy. The necessity for surgical intervention in most areas approximates that in the nondiabetic population. One major exception is vascular problems involving the feet and lower limbs, in which ischemia or neuropathy or both frequently lead to serious infection, ulcerations, and gangrene. In caring for diabetic patients through surgery, the physician, surgeon, and anesthesiologist must work together as a well-coordinated team.

In order to best manage diabetes and the metabolic and nutritional status of the diabetic patient undergoing surgery, it is necessary to understand the hormonal and metabolic homeostatic mechanisms that occur through the operative and postoperative periods. These mechanisms are similar to the homeostatic mechanisms that occur in response to trauma. Indeed, surgery may be considered a controlled injury to the body involving skin, fascia, and muscle incision and major fluid shifts within the body. The body's response to trauma is a series of neural and endocrine alterations that has been evolved to allow survival. The initial events cope with blood loss, shifts of fluid from intravascular and exchangable extravascular spaces to injured tissues, and decreased delivery of oxygen to tissues caused by impaired circulation. After adequate circulation has been ensured, the adaptive responses make available to the damaged tissue substrates needed for tissue repair.

In the surgical patient, this may need to be accomplished at the time when the injury itself prevents efficient mobilization of substrates. The repair of damaged tissue must therefore be accomplished at the expense of other body tissues, such as the breakdown of muscle protein to supply healing tissue with amino acids for protein synthesis and glucose as a source of energy. The supply of glucose is initially maintained through glycogenolysis in the liver and muscles. Glycogen is quickly depleted and the body then turns to hepatic gluconeogenesis, using muscle protein substrates for its source of glucose. Once repair of tissue has been accomplished, the protein used for gluconeogenesis must be replenished. Weight is regained and the body returns to its uninjured state.

Although this series of events is a continuum, Sir David Cuthbertson has divided them into several distinct phases. The initial phase, in which blood loss and fluid shifts may lead to circulatory impairment, has been termed *ebb* phase. The second phase, in which catabolic events occur to supply substrates to the healing tissue, has been termed the *flow* phase. The next phase, when depleted protein is restored, is called the *anabolic* phase. The final phase, in which weight is regained and body energy stores replenished, has been referred to as the *fat* phase. Most studies have involved the initial two phases and it is these two phases that will be discussed. If the neuroendocrine response to surgery is viewed by this schema, many of its features become more comprehensible. This view makes it possible to intervene in ways

170

that will help the body through each of the recovery phases.

The neuroendocrine response to surgery may be initiated through several pathways. These involve hypovolemia or hypotension, hypoxia, and painful or other noxious sensory stimulation. Hypoxia or hypotension is sensed by baroreceptors located in the atria, aorta, and carotid bodies. Sensory input from these receptors is then transmitted to the brain stem and on to the hypothalamus. Hypoxia is sensed by chemoreceptors in the carotid bodies and in the medulla, and afferent pathways ascend to the hypothalamus. Stimulation of pain fibers even in the unconscious or anesthetized patient may result in afferent signals that ascend in the spinothalamic tracts to the thalamus and on to the hypothalamus. The final common pathway therefore is the hypothalamus. If tracheal intubation is difficult with resulting sensory stimulation or if the pharmacological effects of anesthetic agents result in hypotension, the induction of anesthesia may be the triggering event for the neuroendocrine response. However, good anesthesia technique minimizes these effects so that little or no response is usually seen.

The next surgical event that is significant in regard to the neuroendocrine response is the surgical incision. This usually is the major stimulus that triggers the body's response to surgery. The fact that the response is mediated neurally via peripheral nerves to the spine and then centrally is confirmed by the blunting of the hormonal response when spinal anesthesia blocks the pathway of stimulation.

The hypothalamus then initiates two major responses. One is mediated through the autonomic nervous system, the other through hormonal release from the pituitary gland. Sympathetic nerve stimulation of the chromaffin cells in the adrenal medulla leads to release of epinephrine. A generalized increase in sympathetic nervous activity will increase the release also of norepinephrine from sympathetic nerve endings. Most of this is taken up by pre- and postsynaptic cells, but some of the norepinephrine will reach the circulation. A measure of changes in sympathetic activity can be obtained by measuring plasma norepinephrine levels. The catecholamines may have a direct effect on pancreatic beta cells, with a marked inhibition of insulin release and at the same time an effect on

alpha cells that increases the release of glucagon. Insulin levels have been shown to be significantly depressed acutely during surgery. In a nondiabetic patient, insulin, however, rises postoperatively and remains elevated for a number of days. Glucagon levels have been variably reported but have generally shown little to no change during the day of surgery despite adrenergic stimulation, but they rise substantially on the days following surgery. If followed through the surgical period, the insulin-to-glucagon ratio will show a fall the day of surgery entirely caused by the fall in insulin. The ratio then returns to a preoperative value on the days following surgery secondary to the parallel rise in both insulin and glucagon levels. The reason for the failure of glucagon to rise on the day of surgery when adrenergic stimulation is high is unclear. The mechanism of rise on subsequent days may be related to the effects of cortisol levels on glucagon secretion.

The second major response initiated by the hypothalamus is stimulation of the pituitary to release a variety of hormones. ACTH is released and in turn stimulates the adrenal gland to release cortisol in near maximal amounts. Growth hormone is released and exerts a modest diabetogenic effect.

Prolactin release is also stimulated. This response is greater in women than in men, reaching levels of 150 to 200 ng per ml and 60 to 70 ng per ml, respectively. The levels return to baseline by the first postoperative day. The mechanism of increased prolactin output by the pituitary is probably not through thyrotropin-releasing hormone release, because thyroid-stimulating hormone release is not stimulated. A fall in dopamine levels in the pituitary would remove inhibition of prolactin secretion, but peripheral dopamine levels rise with surgical stress, being released from the adrenal gland. The level of dopamine in the pituitary itself remains uncertain. Opiate receptors on pituitary (lactotrophs) are now known to stimulate prolactin release. It has been shown that naloxone, an opiate antagonist, administered during surgery inhibits (though incompletely) prolactin release, making it likely that opiate receptors are active in this mechanism.

Antidiuretic hormone (ADH) is released in response to surgery. This can be mediated by hypotension and baroreceptors in the atria, aorta, and carotid bodies but has been observed in situations in which hypotension was absent. The afferent signal responsible for triggering release in the absence of hypotension is the skin incision and other painful stimulation. It is blocked by spinal anesthesia and is absent in paraplegic patients operated on in an anesthetic area. It is also increased with incision through layers of fascia, muscle, and peritoneum and also with manipulation of viscera. Peak ADH levels were seen during the operation itself, when levels averaged 25 times greater than preoperative. These levels dropped quickly following surgery to five to six times baseline and remained one to two times baseline for several days postoperatively. Increased ADH accompanying surgery will help maintain vascular volume at that time, although sometimes at the expense of serum osmolality.

Results of gonadotropin changes with surgery have shown variations. Follicle-stimulating hormone (FSH) has generally shown little change. However, luteinizing hormone (LH) has been reported to be elevated in males but unchanged in pre- and postmenopausal females. Testosterone levels have been reported to fall postoperatively. It has been suggested that this may be caused by a reduced sensitivity of the testis to LH with stress but may also be caused by changes in binding to sex hormone binding globulins or to the level of this protein in the blood postoperatively.

Thyroid hormone levels are affected by surgery. $T_4$ (thyroxine) levels have been reported to be elevated in some circumstances, but this appears to be related to the effects of some anesthetic agents in which $T_4$ is released from storage in the liver, while other agents do not produce this effect. $T_4$ levels actually fall slightly during surgery done with epidural anesthesia. $T_3$ (triiodothyronine) levels fall during surgery and remain low at least six days postoperatively. This is associated with concomitant rises in reverse $T_3$. $T_3$ resin uptake is also elevated at least acutely with surgery. The reason for this change is unclear. The rise in reverse $T_3$ does not appear to be related to afferent neural responses to surgery, because it occurs both in general anesthesia and with epidural anesthesia. Cortisol elevations are known to cause a rise in reverse $T_3$, but this does not appear to be the cause of the response, because the rise occurs even when cortisol levels have been documented to be normal following epidural anesthesia.

These complex hormonal changes may be better understood if they are divided into those that predominate during the ebb and flow phases. The ebb phase is characterized by the acute sympathetic response that occurs during the surgery and immediately postoperatively. It is generally not more than 24 hours in length in uncomplicated situations. Sympathetic discharge is evidenced by the norepinephrine rise that occurs and results in an inotropic and chronotropic cardiac response. Peripheral vascular resistance increases and coronary perfusion increases. This sympathetic discharge also causes release of epinephrine into the circulation. ADH (antidiuretic hormone) is released acutely, but this quickly falls again. All of these responses can be viewed as attempts by the body to maintain intravascular fluid and adequate circulation.

In addition, release of epinephrine has several metabolic effects. These include stimulation of glycogenolysis in liver and muscle. This results in an increase in release of glucose from the liver and an increase in G-6-P (glucose-6-phosphate) and F-6-P (fructose-6-phosphate) in muscles as a result of muscle glycogen breakdown. These in turn lead to hyperglycemia and inhibition of muscle hexokinase, which is inhibited by G-6-P and F-6-P. Epinephrine does not inhibit the uptake of glucose by muscle tissue but blocks phosphorylation of glucose, thus blocking utilization of blood glucose by muscle. Increased uptake of glucose in hind limb preparations during shock may then be the result of increased uptake of glucose by fat rather than muscle. Once glycogen stores in muscles are depleted, levels of G-6-P will fall and inhibition of phosphorylation of glucose may decrease, allowing utilization of peripheral glucose again. Whether this actually occurs remains to be demonstrated. If circulation becomes impaired, there will be reduced availability of oxygen, which may explain the shift in metabolism toward anaerobic glycolysis with increased production of lactate and pyruvate. These products are taken up by the liver and may be recycled as an energy source via the Cori cycle (lactate→glucose in the liver). The inhibition of insulin release during this phase may then be a benefit in promoting release of this recycled glucose from the liver for peripheral use. If the circulation is well maintained by proper fluid management through the operative and postoperative period, the duration of the ebb phase may be minimal and the patient is brought rapidly into the flow phase.

In flow phase, hormonal changes are influenced mainly by the increased cortisol levels. Growth hormone and glucagon levels are also elevated. Sympathetic nervous activity decreases and insulin release is no longer inhibited. Hyperinsulinism occurs in the nondiabetic patient.

The hormonal and metabolic changes during the ebb phase are needed to maintain circulation and provide energy sources that can be used during the anaerobic period of impaired circulation. The flow phase changes make available substrates for healing tissue. The formation of granulation tissue requires glucose as the main energy source. Amino acids are needed for protein synthesis in healing tissues. This explains the catabolic response that has long been noted in response to injury. The catabolism takes the form of proteolysis of muscle protein and leads to an increase in amino acids in muscle cells. The amino acids are then deaminated and the amino group is transferred to pyruvate-forming alanine. The alanine is released into the circulation and taken up by the liver where it is converted via the Cori cycle to glucose.

Despite the rise in insulin levels in nondiabetics, the hyperglycemia seen in the ebb phase persists into the flow phase, probably because of the increased level of glucagon and other hormones opposing insulin's action. Some investigators have believed that the increased levels of cortisol and glucagon seen during this time were insufficient to explain the hyperglycemia. It is now thought, however, that extrahepatic glucose oxidation is normal or increased and that the hyperglycemia is secondary to increased hepatic gluconeogenesis.

In the initial phase of fasting there is an obligatory need for glucose production to supply those tissues such as nervous tissue and red blood cells that cannot utilize any other fuel source than glucose. This obligatory glucose production amounts to about 100 gm of glucose per day. Glycogen supplies this initially but is rapidly depleted and the glucose must then be supplied by increased gluconeogenesis from peripheral protein. A similar situation exists in injured patients and patients undergoing surgery. In fasting, however, the gluconeogenesis can be suppressed by the infusion of glucose. In studies of injured patients, the gluconeogenesis was found to be nonsuppressible when glucose infusion rates were about 150 gm per day (levels that are known to suppress gluconeogenesis in normal subjects). More recent studies, however, in burn patients have shown that wound areas utilize glucose at high rates, 130 to 300 gm per day. Reparative tissues that participate in the inflammatory response to injury and wound healing use glucose predominantly, thus raising the obligatory need for glucose during this period several times to the range of 300 to 400 gm per day. In earlier studies an insufficient supplement of glucose may simply have been supplied to demonstrate a response. In severely injured patients who are supplied glucose at a rate comparable to their raised metabolic rate (700 to 800 gm per day), gluconeogenesis is affected. Glucose output from the liver remains at a high level, but a greater proportion is presumably from glycogen formed from exogenous glucose infusion and a lower proportion is from gluconeogenesis from lactate (12 per cent as opposed to 30 per cent). Despite the increased gluconeogenesis by the liver and glucose uptake by healing and granulation tissue, measurement of the respiratory quotient yields values in the range of 0.70 to 0.76, indicating that fat remains the primary fuel for the body. The availability of free fatty acids through lipolysis of triglycerides in adipose tissues is increased by catecholamines, ACTH, and cortisol rises produced by the neuroendocrine response.

## MANAGEMENT OF DIABETIC PATIENTS ON THE DAY OF SURGERY

If at all possible, surgery should be done early in the day so as to minimize the extent to which insulin therapy must be modified. The patient will usually be fasted overnight before operation. To maintain glycogen stores and to help avoid hypoglycemia, 5 per cent dextrose should be started intravenously early in the morning. A minimum of 100 to 150 gm of carbohydrate intake should be planned over the next 24 hours unless the patient is able to begin eating after the operation. This will require that the IV be run about 100 ml per hour.

A number of different regimens have been

proposed for insulin adjustment the day of surgery. The main choices are between regimens using subcutaneous insulins and those in which insulins are given in intravenous infusions at fixed, pulsed, or variable rates. One of the most commonly used regimens is that of administering one half of the usual insulin dose before operation and one half after. This is done by dividing both the short-acting insulin such as regular in half as well as the intermediate insulin NPH or lente. This allows for the release of needed insulin activity into the bloodstream during the morning to help utilize the glucose infused during this time (if the ebb phase is minimized).

If the operation is delayed until midmorning or afternoon, the blood glucose should be rechecked prior to the induction of anesthesia to adjust the insulin dose or the glucose infusion rate.

The blood glucose is then measured when the patient reaches the recovery room. At this time the second half of the insulin can be administered or the dose may be adjusted according to the postoperative blood glucose obtained. The blood glucose is then frequently monitored from that time on. If the patient has been taking two injections a day, this should be continued. It is also very likely that patients receiving glucose infusions will require additional doses of insulin through the night even if they did not require this prior to surgery. During long surgical procedures the insulin regimen may be further monitored intraoperatively. With modern technology, blood glucose determinations are much easier and readily available. On occasion, continuous blood glucose monitoring can be done. With such follow-up, tighter control of blood glucose should be possible. Anesthesiologists are becoming increasingly interested in control of blood glucose during surgery, and in fact some anesthesiologists have recommended that blood glucose be evaluated every two hours through the course of the operation, with appropriate adjustment of insulin treatment and glucose infusion rates, and that intensive follow-up be carried out postoperatively.

Patients whose diabetes is controllable by diet alone may need only close following of the blood glucose postoperatively along with routine perioperative fluid management. In the case in which postoperative blood glucose becomes elevated to values greater than 250, or ketones appear in the urine in large quantities, a short course of insulin therapy can be helpful in preventing acute problems with hyperglycemia. This is usually necessary for only a few days following surgery. In such circumstance, highly purified pure pork insulin or human insulin should be used to lessen the possibility of insulin allergy developing at a later date. With the technology available enabling continuous monitoring of blood glucose, intravenous administration of insulin is likely to be used more frequently. Studies have shown that variable-rate intravenous insulin governed by algorithms utilizing blood glucose levels has produced significantly better blood glucose control than subcutaneous or fixed-rate intravenous infusions. This same regimen can be used immediately preoperatively, intraoperatively, and postoperatively. One caution should be noted. The short half-life of intravenous insulin (a matter of minutes) can result in a trough in the insulin level if intravenous insulin is stopped and subcutaneous insulin restarted. There should be overlap between the treatments to avoid this gap—one to two hours if regular insulin is part of the subcutaneous regimen and five to six hours if immediate-acting insulins alone are used.

Diabetics being treated with oral hypoglycemia agents prior to surgery can be managed by withholding the oral agent the day of surgery. Again, intravenous glucose infusion should be started the morning of the operation. If the oral intake can be restarted the day of operation, the oral hypoglycemia agent can be reinstituted as well. The blood glucose should be monitored until oral agent is reinstituted and blood glucose response noted. If the blood glucose becomes markedly elevated, the patient can be managed the same way as the patient whose diabetes is diet controlled and who experiences elevated blood sugars. Patients unlikely to need insulin coverage are those whose baseline blood sugars are normal or whose oral hyperglycemic agent therapy is small, such as less than 1000 mg of tolbutamide, 250 mg of chlorpropamide, 5 mg of glyburide, 10 mg of glipizide or 500 mg of tolazamide. Patients who are likely to need insulin are those who have elevated blood sugars despite taking maximum oral agent doses, e.g. glyburide 20 mg, glipizide 40 mg, tolbutamide 2000 mg, chlorpropamide 500 mg, or tolazamide 1000 to 1500 mg. Factors favoring the decision to change to insulin therapy would be surgical procedures expected to result in several days of nothing by mouth, intravenous feedings, and nasogastric suction.

## MANAGEMENT ON THE IMMEDIATE POSTOPERATIVE DAYS

Blood glucose should continue to be followed daily; that is, fasting, 11 A.M. and 4 P.M. after surgery. Insulin doses should be adjusted according to the blood glucose results as they return and according to blood sugar patterns from the previous days because recurring patterns may indicate the times of day when more or less insulin may be needed. Supplemental insulin may be needed to correct excessive elevations. The preoperative insulin regimen should also be kept in mind, because the stress associated with surgery and subsequent increased insulin requirements will diminish over several postoperative days. It should be expected that insulin requirements will return to preoperative baseline values if no complications develop. Overall nutritional consideration should be kept in mind and/or return to oral alimentation should be begun as promptly as possible to reduce nitrogen loss. If the period of time before oral intake can be instituted is prolonged, additional supplementation in the form of intravenous amino acids or total parental hyperalimentation should be considered.

## SUGGESTED READING LIST

### General

Alberti, K.G.M.M., and Thomas, D.J.B.: The management of diabetes during surgery. Br. J. Anaesth. 51:693, 1979.

Alberti, K. G. M. M., Gill, G. V., and Elliott, M. J.: Insulin delivery during surgery in the diabetic patient. Diabetes Care 5 (Suppl 1)65–77, 1982.

Cuthbertson, D.P.: Second Annual Jonathan E. Rhoads Lecture: The Metabolic Response to Injury and Its Nutritional Implications: Retrospect and Prospect. J. Parent. Extern. Nutr. 3:108, 1979.

Hardy, J.D. (ed.): Response to Surgery: Neuroendocrine and Metabolic Changes, Convalescence and Rehabilitation. Hardy Textbook of Surgery. Philadelphia, J.P. Lippincott Co., 1983.

Hirsch, I. B., and McGill, J. B.: Role of insulin in management of surgical patients with diabetes mellitus. Diabetes Care 13:980–991, 1990.

Schade, D. S.: Surgery and diabetes. Med. Clin. North Am. 72:1531–1543, 1988.

Stoner, H.B.: Carbohydrate metabolism after accidental injuries. Acta Chir. Scand. (Suppl.) 498:48, 1980.

Wilmore, D.W., Aulick, H.L., and Goodwin, C.W.: Glucose metabolism following severe injury. Acta Chir. Scand. (Suppl.) 498:43, 1980.

Watts, N. B., Gebhart, S. S. P., Clark, R. V., and Phillips, L. S.: Postoperative management of diabetes mellitus: Steady-state glucose control with bedside algorithm for insulin adjustment. Diabetes Care 10:722–728, 1987.

### ACTH, GH, Prolactin

Cooper, C.E., and Nelson, D.H.: ACTH levels in plasma in preoperative and surgically stressed patients. J. Clin. Invest. 4:1599, 1962.

Newsome, H.H. and Rose, J.C.: The response of adrenocorticotrophic hormone and growth hormone to surgical stress. J. Clin. Endocrinol. Metab. 33:481, 1971.

Noel, G.L., Suh, H.K., Stone, J.C., and Frantz, A.G.: Human prolactin and growth hormone release during surgery and other conditions of stress. J. Clin. Endocrinol. Metab. 35:840, 1972.

Russell, R. C. G., Ellis, B., Spargo, P., and Dudley, H. A. F.: The relationship between insulin and growth hormone before, during, and after minor surgery. B. J. Surg. 63:666–667, 1973.

Wright, P. D., and Johnston, I. D. A.: The effect of surgical operation on growth hormone levels in plasma. Surgery 77:479–486, 1975.

### ADH

Moran, W.H., Jr., Miltchberger, F.W., Shuayb, W.A., and Zimmermann, B.: The relationship of antidiuretic hormone secretion to surgical stress. Surgery 56:99, 1964.

### Thyroid

Burr, W.A., Black, E.G., Griffiths, R.S., and Hoffenberg, R.: Serum triiodothyronine and reverse triiodothyronine concentrations after surgical operation. Lancet 2:1277, 1975.

Brandt, M.R., Skovsted, L., Kehlet, H., and Hansen, J.M.: Rapid decrease in plasma triiodothyronine during surgery and epidural analgesia independent of afferent neurogenic stimuli and cortisol. Lancet 2:1333, 1976.

Adami, H.-O., Johansson, H., Thoren, L., et al.: Serum levels of TSH, $T_3$, $rT_3$, $T_4$ and $T_3$-resin uptake in surgical trauma. Acta Endocrinol. 88:482, 1978.

Tegler, L., Gillquist, J., Lindvall, R., and Almqvist, S.: Secretion rates of thyroxine, triiodothyronine and reverse triiodothyronine in man during surgery. Acta Endocrinol. 101:193, 1982.

### Catecholamines

Hafter, J.B., Pflug, A.E., and Porte, D., Jr.: Mechanisms of plasma catecholamine increase during surgical stress in man. J. Clin. Endocrinol. Metab. 45:936, 1977.

Mannelli, M., Gheri, R.G., Selli, C., et al.: A study on human adrenal secretion. Measurement of epinephrine, norepinephrine, dopamine and cortisol in peripheral and adrenal venous blood under surgical stress. J. Endocrinol. Invest. 5:91, 1982.

### Insulin and Glucagon

Mequid, M.M., Brennan, M.F., Aoki, T., et al.: Hormone-substrate interrelationships following surgery. Arch. Surg. 109:776, 1974.

Göschke, H., Bär, E., Girard, J., et al.: Glucagon, insulin, cortisol, and growth hormone levels following major surgery: Their relationship to glucose and free fatty acid elevations. Horm. Metab. Res. 10:465, 1978.

### FSH, LH, Testosterone

Charters, A.C., Odell, W.D., and Thompson, J.C.: Anterior pituitary function during surgical stress and convalescence. Radioimmunoassay measurements of blood TSH, LH, FSH, and Growth Hormone. J. Clin. Endocrinol. Metab. 29:63, 1969.

Aono, T., Kurachi, K., Miyata, M., et al.: Influence of surgical stress under general anesthesia on serum gonadotrophin levels in male and female patients. Levels in male and female patients. J. Clin. Endocrinol. Metab. 42:144, 1976.

# Chapter 18

# ANESTHESIA IN DIABETIC PATIENTS

ISTRATI A. KUPELI, M.D., DONALD W. FOSTER, M.D., and ELLISON C. PIERCE, Jr., M.D.

Nearly 50 per cent of diabetics will require surgery at some point during their lifetime, and undiagnosed diabetes often becomes manifest during the perioperative period. Although diabetes appears to hinder wound healing and immune response, new data suggest that in properly managed cases diabetics may not suffer increased risk of morbidity and mortality during anesthesia and surgery. The anesthesiologist now possesses a wide variety of anesthetic agents and monitoring techniques that can be tailored to fit the needs of the individual diabetic patient.

A careful preanesthetic assessment is an important factor with regard to the anesthetic plan. Newly discovered hyperglycemia requires further evaluation; the diagnosis of diabetes mellitus should be made as rapidly as the surgical condition allows. In patients with established diagnoses, diabetes should be evaluated with reference to glycemic control and the presence of end-organ pathology. A thorough review of medications and concurrent illness, as well as patient response to previous anesthetics, should be performed.

End-organ complications strongly influence the choice of anesthetic agents, techniques, and monitoring requirements. In long-standing diabetes, the presence of asymptomatic and subtle dysfunction without clear clinical signs should be expected. Chronic diabetes significantly increases the likelihood of intraoperative problems associated with the cardiovascular, genitourinary, alimentary, and autonomic nervous systems.

Cardiac disease is twice as common in the diabetic patient as in the general population. The increased risk of coronary artery disease, combined with severe diabetic autonomic neuropathy, may produce ischemia and silent myocardial infarction. The anesthesiologist preparing such a patient for a major surgical procedure may need to plan for pulmonary arterial catheter placement and arterial blood pressure monitoring and have a variety of vasoactive medications readily available to prevent myocardial compromise. Other considerations, such as impaired renal clearance of drugs and metabolites (as is seen in diabetic nephropathy) and gastroparesis (a manifestation of vagal autonomic dysfunction), will affect the choice of anesthetic agents and techniques. Anesthetic and analgesic drugs may, apart from any surgical influence, affect blood glucose levels; a basic understanding of these factors is necessary prior to the rational selection of anesthetic drugs.

## METABOLIC EFFECTS OF ANESTHESIA

Surgical stimulus is the principal factor causing hyperglycemia during the intraoperative period. The release of stress hormones (cortisol, glucagon, catecholamines, and growth hormone) causes hyperglycemia at the tissue level; glucagon and epinephrine suppress insulin release. The catabolic effects of stress hormones are insufficiently countered by the anabolic effects of insulin release, especially in the diabetic patient. The exaggerated response to stress hormones may result in hyperglycemia, dehydration, electrolyte imbalance, osmolar disturbances, and ketogenesis, leading to acidemia.

**177**

The inhalational anesthetics, halothane, enflurane, isoflurane, and desflurane, will cause stress hormone release and subsequent hyperglycemia in the absence of surgical stimulation. This response appears to be most prominent when the agents are utilized for face-mask induction of anesthesia. This effect can be attenuated by inducing anesthesia with a variety of intravenous agents or adding synthetic narcotics (i.e., fentanyl) to the anesthetic regimen. Sevoflurane, a newer inhalation anesthetic, appears to maintain plasma glucose levels at preanesthetic levels better than the other potent inhalational agents. It is unclear whether this property of sevoflurane will make it suitable for use in diabetics.

High-dose narcotic anesthetic techniques, as currently employed in cardiac anesthesia, have been shown to attenuate the stress response to anesthesia and surgery. This may be due to direct central nervous system effects or to superior analgesia. Hypothermia during cardiopulmonary bypass is probably responsible for an increase in circulating catecholamines despite adequate plasma narcotic levels. Hyperglycemia is often seen during this period; the effect is certainly more pronounced in diabetic patients.

Epidural, spinal, and other forms of regional anesthesia have no effects on carbohydrate metabolism and indeed may completely ablate the stress hormonal response to surgery. Epidural anesthesia, and some other forms of nerve blockade, may be carried on into the postoperative period (often for several days), thus allowing for smoother glycemic control as well as pain relief. Many diabetic patients, especially those with autonomic dysfunction and cardiac disease, may not easily tolerate the sympathectomy some of these techniques generate, however. Invasive monitoring, in combination with aggressive control of blood pressure and heart rate, provides a highly effective compensatory mechanism to deal safely with these problems.

## ANESTHETIC CONSIDERATIONS

Metabolic derangements and significant end-organ dysfunction resulting from diabetes mellitus complicate anesthetic management of diabetic patients. These often subtle systemic changes may alter the diabetic's response to anesthesia; an enhanced understanding of the processes involved has led to substantial reductions in morbidity and mortality.

In the past, diethyl ether was utilized as a complete anesthetic, alone, for induction and maintenance of general anesthesia. Today, few circumstances dictate use of general anesthesia by means of a single drug; balanced anesthetic techniques commonly employ five or more agents used in sequence or combination. Adjuncts to anesthesia such as neuromuscular blocking agents, intravenous antibiotics prepared in dextrose-containing solutions, and intraoperative steroids are but a few factors that may adversely affect the intraoperative and postoperative management of the diabetic patient. These influences, combined with the various stresses of laryngoscopy, anesthesia, and surgery, demand close coordination among the endocrinologist, anesthesiologist, and surgeon.

## PERIOPERATIVE METABOLIC CONTROL

For a variety of reasons, there is no consensus concerning the ideal perioperative insulin regimen for diabetics. Varying recommendations are dependent upon patient characteristics, surgical procedure, and institutional resources. Ambulatory surgery and surgical admissions on the same day as surgery present special challenges in the care of diabetic patients. In general, diabetics should be scheduled for early-morning surgical procedures to minimize problems related to fasting and diabetic control.

A primary concern is the diabetic's medical regimen. Since relative euglycemia is the preoperative goal, the adequacy of the regimen toward that end should be evaluated. The patient with wide swings in preoperative glucose levels is considered to be in poor glycemic control; hemoglobin $A_{1c}$ measurement may be a helpful indicator of patient compliance with diabetic medications. A past history of diabetic ketoacidosis (DKA) or hyperglycemic hyperosmolar state should be carefully evaluated, as should the patient's previous anesthetic encounters. Valuable predictive information can be gained in this manner and specific concerns underscored.

Diet-controlled diabetic patients essentially require nothing more than baseline fasting blood glucose determination prior to surgery, with intraoperative glucose measurement each one to two hours during major procedures. A postoperative glucose level can be obtained in the postanesthesia care unit. Other preoperative intervention is usually not required unless the fasting glucose level is 250 to 300 mg per dl or more. For elective procedures, especially in the ambulatory setting, a diet-controlled diabetic with hyperglycemia in this range should have surgery rescheduled after further work-up, with possible institution of oral hypoglycemic or insulin therapy in the interim.

Patients taking sulfonylurea compounds for control of diabetes mellitus are managed in a manner similar to that for diet-controlled diabetics. They are advised not to take short-acting oral hypoglycemic agents on the morning of surgery. Fasting blood glucose levels are obtained and intravenous dextrose-containing solutions are administered to prevent hypoglycemia. Postoperative glucose measurement is performed; sliding-scale insulin coverage each four to six hours can be instituted until the resumption of oral intake. Since the sulfonylurea preparation chlorpropamide has a one- to three-day duration of effect, it may cause hypoglycemia long after discontinuation in the fasted patient. It may be desirable to convert chlorpropamide to a short-acting agent preoperatively under the supervision of the patient's endocrinologist. Otherwise, it should be discontinued 48 to 72 hours prior to surgery.

Insulin-dependent (as well as non–insulin-dependent diabetics) can usually be safely fasted after midnight prior to surgery. In the morning, NPH insulin may be injected subcutaneously at 30 to 50 per cent of the normal NPH dose. Before insulin administration, baseline glucose levels are determined, and intravenous dextrose-containing solutions are begun at a rate of 3.5 to 5 gm of dextrose per hour.

Intraoperative glucose measurements should be performed on an hourly basis and regular human insulin administered as needed. Sliding-scale insulin coverage can be carried into the postoperative period via subcutaneous injection each four to six hours as needed. It should be noted that the subcutaneous deposition of insulin during the surgical procedure may result in incomplete or delayed absorption because of fluid shifts or changes in perfusion pressure. Subcutaneous

injection of insulin is therefore discouraged intraoperatively; intravenous insulin administration is the surest route.

More precise control of blood glucose levels can be achieved with continuous low-dose intravenous insulin infusion. This approach is certainly more appropriate physiologically than bolus techniques; it is standard therapy in the treatment of DKA and during pregnancy for labor and delivery complicated by diabetes. Treatment of hyperglycemia via intermittent intravenous insulin bolus poses the danger of high initial plasma insulin concentrations, which may result in hypoglycemia. Wide fluctuations in blood glucose levels that may then occur can exacerbate lipolysis and ketogenesis. In addition, intermittent intravenous bolus therapy can predispose the patient to cardiac dysrhythmias as a result of alterations in the plasma electrolytes magnesium, potassium, and phosphate.

One preferred method of continuous low-dose insulin infusion consists of the addition of regular insulin to normal saline (usually 50 units of regular insulin in 500 ml normal saline). The concern that insulin readily adheres to containers and intravenous administration sets is not a problem as long as the set is thoroughly flushed with infusate prior to use.

Continuous insulin therapy may then be administered as 10 units of regular insulin for each 50 gm of dextrose infused; (1 liter of 5 per cent dextrose, for instance, contains 50 gm of dextrose). A more exact dosing scheme calls for 0.3 to 0.4 units of regular insulin for each gram of dextrose infused per hour. Higher infusion rates, necessary for the treatment of severe insulin resistance seen in sepsis, liver disease, and obesity, could incorporate 0.4 to 0.8 units of regular insulin for each gram of dextrose administered per hour. Profound hypothermia, as is seen during cardiopulmonary bypass, may call for further increases to 0.8 to 1.2 units of regular insulin per gram of dextrose per hour.

Insulin infusion is subsequently adjusted, dependent upon the actual blood glucose levels. In addition to the above dosing schemes, obese or severely insulin resistant individuals may require 2 to 6 units of regular insulin per hour. Slender patients may require approximately one-half that amount.

Hyperglycemia in diabetics during emergency preparation for surgery is common and may be due to multiple factors such as sepsis, trauma, or resuscitation. Continuous intraoperative infusion of regular insulin, as outlined, may be desirable in this setting, with frequent intraoperative blood glucose determinations. Supplementary insulin may also be administered as necessary, but strict attention to the prevention of hypoglycemia is mandatory.

It is probably not necessary, nor is it considered advantageous, to attain strict euglycemia during the intraoperative and postoperative periods. The long-term sequelae of hyperglycemia are unlikely to develop during this period; tight glycemic control can once again be established in the late convalescent period. Hypoglycemia is a hazard under general anesthesia; its diagnosis can only be confirmed by obtaining blood glucose levels. Any sign or symptom of hypoglycemia may be masked by anesthesia during the intraoperative period, and brain damage, leading to coma or death, is certainly possible.

The awake diabetic may experience symptoms referable to hypoglycemia when blood glucose levels fall to 50 to 60 mg per dl, but these levels are highly variable. Tachycardia, diaphoresis, confusion, muscle weakness, and incoordination due to hypoglycemia may be mistaken for prolonged emergence from anesthesia or inadequate reversal of neuromuscular blockade. In the operating room, hypoglycemia must be rapidly treated with dextrose infusion; postoperative ventilatory support may also be required.

As discussed, mild hyperglycemia is acceptable during anesthesia and surgery. One must remember that an increase in urine output due to glycemic osmotic diuresis is expected, dependent upon the individual's renal glucose threshold. Frequent intraoperative blood glucose measurements are necessary—at least hourly—during extended surgical procedures. Portable glucometers, when properly calibrated, are ideal for this purpose, but acid-base status and electrolyte determinations may be required as well. Some patients (approximately 17 per cent of cases) will develop DKA with plasma glucose levels less than 300 mg per dl; DKA has been reported in patients with values less than 100 mg per dl. It is obvious that blood glucose determination, coupled with tests to detect enhanced ketogenesis and widened anion gap acidosis, will be necessary in this setting. Nonketotic hyperglycemic hyperosmolar phenomena may develop in greater than 90

per cent of the non-insulin-dependent diabetic population. This complication would be more commonly encountered than DKA perioperatively because of the greater number of susceptible patients. Both conditions can delay emergence from anesthesia and must be suspected in cases of altered anesthetic recovery.

Urinary glucose measurement provides an inaccurate reflection of plasma glucose levels and should not be utilized intraoperatively. Diabetic patients may have altered renal glucose thresholds; severe hyperglycemia may be present long before urinary detection is possible. Since diabetic patients are profoundly susceptible to urinary tract infection, the placement of urinary catheters should be considered only for long surgical procedures but never solely for glucose monitoring.

Metabolic homeostasis and significant diabetic co-morbidity are important aspects of diabetes mellitus that warrant careful preanesthetic evaluation. End-organ pathology associated with diabetes affects morbidity and mortality in the perioperative period; it is pertinent here to examine those aspects of the disease that can influence the anesthetic plan and intraoperative management.

The anesthesiologist must prepare for airway control regardless of chosen anesthetic technique. Since diabetic patients are prone to aspirate stomach contents when anesthetized, endotracheal intubation is required for all general anesthetic techniques. Unplanned tracheal intubation and mechanical ventilation may become necessary at any time during the operative course of a conscious, sedated patient. In many diabetics it is difficult to intubate the trachea because of limited atlanto-occipital extension. "Stiff joint syndrome," which appears to affect patients with juvenile-onset insulin-dependent diabetes with high frequency, is a cause of difficult laryngoscopy in up to one third of cases. Nonfamilial short stature, progressive microangiopathy, and small joint immobility are associated with the syndrome. Difficult laryngoscopy due to the obesity is also commonly noted in patients with adult-onset non-insulin-dependent diabetes; diabetics with renal failure may have friable, edematous tissues that obscure the laryngoscopist's view. These patients may commonly require awake fiberoptic tracheal intubation or other specialized techniques to safely secure the airway.

Cardiovascular disease is the most worrisome aspect of diabetic co-morbidity. Myocardial infarction is the leading cause of death in diabetes mellitus; hyperglycemia seems to be a prominent factor in the accelerated development of atherosclerotic coronary lesions. Although there appears to be no correlation between the duration of diabetic illness and the severity of coronary artery disease, diabetics are twice as likely to have cardiac disease as the general population. More than 50 per cent of diabetics have ST-segment abnormalities during stress electrocardiography, approximately double the expected frequency. At coronary arteriography, diabetics tend to have more vessel involvement, more collateralization, and more arteriosclerotic extension than the general population. Diabetics develop ventricular dysfunction early in the course of their disease; diastolic and systolic dysfunction commonly contribute to congestive heart failure, even in the absence of coronary artery disease.

Very often when diabetic myocardial ischemia and infarction are occult, electrocardiography provides the first evidence of the disease process. ECG evaluation is therefore essential even in the young diabetic patient presenting for surgery.

Diabetic neuropathy contributes to autonomic nervous system pathology, one cause of the "silent" cardiac disease process. As autonomic dysfunction progresses, cardiovascular instability can become more pronounced. In diabetic patients with the diagnosis of cardiac autonomic neuropathy the mortality rate within five years of diagnosis is 50 per cent, in comparison to diabetics with no autonomic dysfunction in whom the mortality is only 10 per cent for the same period. As a result of sympathetic nervous system decompensation, these patients have orthostatic hypotension, resting tachycardia, and a decrease or absence of heartbeat-to-heartbeat variability on voluntary deep breathing, and often they are resistant to beta blockade or atropine. During surgery and convalescence, they may be prone to severe bradycardia and even cardiac arrest. Reversal of neuromuscular blockade during anesthesia can lead to bradycardia as well.

Left ventricular hypertrophy due to hypertension (which is often renovascular in the diabetic patient) places the myocardium further at risk for ischemia during surgery. The anesthetic plan must incorporate measures to rapidly replenish fluid and blood loss during major procedures; hypotension will quickly develop under these conditions in the diabetic patient with decreased or absent sympathetic nervous system responses.

The severity of cardiac disease in diabetes mellitus is reflected in the observation that diabetics require five times more aortic counterpulsation and inotropic support during surgery for coronary revascularization. Additionally, in diabetics the perioperative mortality rate is 5 per cent, in comparison to 1.5 per cent for nondiabetics during these procedures.

It is evident, therefore, that the extent of cardiac and vascular disease is often underestimated in diabetic patients. The need and level of invasive monitoring are determined by the preanesthetic assessment and a high index of suspicion concerning occult processes. Transduced arterial, central venous, and pulmonary artery pressure monitoring provides information not available through noninvasive means. These methods will frequently allow quick anesthetic adjustments to promote cardiovascular stability. Standard monitoring techniques, including noninvasive blood pressure measurement, capnography, pulse oximetry, temperature measurement, and electrocardiography, are basic requirements and hence not considered optional. Urine output determination via Foley catherterization is not an adequate monitor of volume status due to the possibility of glycemic osmotic diuresis, which can occur even in the face of hypovolemia.

Computerized multilead ST-segment analysis is a valuable feature of newer-generation cardiac monitors; it has proven to be more accurate in the detection of myocardial ischemia than simple visual determination of ST trends. Sophisticated monitoring techniques such as intraoperative transesophageal echocardiography and continuous mixed venous oximetry are usually reserved for those with extraordinary cardiovascular compromise.

Diabetics suffer from the manifestations of vascular disease two times more frequently than the general population. Ischemic stroke is common; hyperglycemia may contribute to the severity of ischemic insult, thereby adversely affecting long-term outcome in these patients. Close attention to blood glucose levels during major vascular procedures (such as carotid endarterectomy) will be particularly advantageous; careful glycemic control in this setting may lower perioperative morbidity and mortality from neurological events.

Lower-extremity revascularization procedures are commonly performed on diabetic patients. Controversy has existed in recent years as to whether regional (i.e., spinal or epidural) anesthesia is superior to general anesthesia for this type of surgery. Some authorities believe that general anesthesia is associated with more major cardiac morbidity and graft thrombosis in the convalescent period. However, a recent major study at the New England Deaconess Hospital demonstrated that neither regional nor general anesthesia conferred an advantage in this regard. When patients were monitored with arterial lines and pulmonary artery catheters, and graft anastomotic integrity assessed with angioscopy, arteriography, and Doppler flow studies, no difference in outcome was observed with either general or regional anesthesia. It is conceivable that intensive monitoring is the key to maintaining low perioperative morbidity and mortality in these cases; the anesthesiologist needs to take these considerations into account when planning anesthesia for peripheral vascular procedures.

Diabetes mellitus leads to nephropathy in 30 to 60 per cent of cases. The severity of renal involvement in diabetes is directly related to the duration of diabetic disease and must often be suspected despite normal serum creatinine levels. Proteinuria is likely to precede changes in creatinine clearance; it provides a reliable indicator of the presence of nephropathy.

When renal disease is suspected, the anesthesiologist should choose agents that do not rely heavily on renal clearance; moreover, the nephrotoxicity of multiple drugs and antibiotics must be considered. All commonly used inhalational anesthetic agents are safe for use in this regard, although fluoride toxicity is a theoretical concern with the agent enflurane.

Neuromuscular blocking drugs preferentially metabolized and excreted by hepatobiliary processes are good choices when renal elimination is compromised. When renal failure is evident, neuromuscular blockers that are spontaneously degraded (atracurium) or metabolized by plasma cholinesterase (mivacurium) may be chosen.

The choice of analgesics is also affected by the preoperative assessment of renal function. Normeperidine, the demethylated byproduct of the narcotic meperidine, will accumulate in the nephropathic patient. It exerts a central nervous system excitatory effect, which may result in hyperreflexia, muscle twitching, and seizures. Since ketorolac, a parenteral nonsteroidal anti-inflammatory agent, can cause renal failure due to prostaglandin effects at the kidney, its sustained use should be avoided in diabetics with suspected renal compromise.

Neurogenic bladder, seen frequently in diabetics, is a manifestation of autonomic dysfunction. Ascending urinary tract infection due to urinary retention is common. Anesthesia may complicate this picture by delaying recovery of remaining autonomic and somatic nerve function in the immediate postanesthetic period. Epidural anesthetic techniques, when carried into the convalescent phase, often necessitate the use of indwelling urinary catheters; the benefits of epidural anesthesia and analgesia must be weighed against the increased risk of urinary tract morbidity in this population.

Diabetic patients are highly susceptible to the aspiration of gastric contents because of the gastrointestinal manifestations of autonomic neuropathy. Esophageal and gastric atony leads to increased residual gastric volume; passive regurgitation and aspiration (especially in the obese diabetic patient) during anesthetic induction is a significant hazard. Gastric volumes appear to be universally increased in diabetics. Even those without symptoms of delayed gastric emptying appear to be at significant risk. Pretreatment with an $H_2$ antagonist and metoclopramide can reduce residual gastric volume and may decrease the possibility of aspiration.

Diabetic peripheral neuropathy and vascular insufficiency require close attention to the proper positioning of anesthetized patients. Care must be taken to pad pressure points and assure that no peripheral nerves or vessels become compromised. The presence of peripheral neuropathy often allows debridement of foot ulcers and other minor procedures to be undertaken with a minimum of anesthesia. Peripheral nerve blocks, i.e., ankle blocks, are especially effective in these patients and are good options when spinal or epidural techniques are disallowed because of other concerns.

The anesthetic plan for the diabetic patient about to undergo surgery is strongly influenced by specific knowledge of the diabetic disease state as well as an understanding of diabetic co-morbidity. The diabetic's end-organ dysfunction can profoundly affect anesthetic and surgical outcome. Careful characterization of the diabetic patient's coexisting disease, combined with sophisticated monitoring and anesthetic techniques, can certainly improve outcome in this demanding patient population.

## SUGGESTED READING LIST

Berlauk, J. F., Abrams, J. H., Gilmour, I. J., et al.: Preoperative optimization of cardiovascular hemodynamics improves outcome in peripheral vascular surgery. Ann. Surg. 214:289, 1991.

Bode, R. H., Lewis, K. P., Zarich, S. W., et al.: Anesthesia does not alter cardiac outcome of peripheral vascular surgery [abstract]. In Moore, Roger A. (ed.): Society of Cardiovascular Anesthesiologists; 1993, San Diego. Richmond, 1993, p 244.

Bode, R. H., Lewis, K. P., Pierce, E. T., et al.: Graft occlusion after peripheral vascular surgery, general vs. regional anesthesia [abstract]. In Moore, Roger A. (ed.): Society of Cardiovascular Anesthesiologists; 1993, San Diego. Richmond, 1993, p 245.

Clarke, B. F., Ewing, D. J., and Campbell, I. W.; Diabetic autonomic neuropathy. Diabetologia 17:195, 1979.

Ewing, D. J., Campbell, I. W., and Clarke, B. F.: Assessment of cardiovascular effects in diabetic neuropathy and prognostic implications. Ann. Intern. Med. 92:308, 1980.

Gavin, L. A.: Perioperative management of the diabetic patient. Endocrinol. Metab. Clin. North Am. 21:457, 1992.

Hirsch, I. B., McGill, J. B., Cryer, P. E., and White, P. F.: Perioperative management of surgical patients with diabetes mellitus. Anesthesiology 74:346, 1991.

Page, M. M., and Watkins, P. J.: Cardiorespiratory arrest with diabetic autonomic neuropathy. Lancet 1:14, 1978.

Schade, D. S.: Surgery and diabetes. Med. Clin. North Am. 72:1531, 1988.

# Chapter 19

# AORTOILIAC RECONSTRUCTION

DAVID R. CAMPBELL, M.D.,
and DOROTHY V. FREEMAN, M.D.

Premature atherosclerosis is a major problem for the long-standing diabetic and has been discussed in detail in other chapters. The actual process is no different from that occurring in nondiabetics, but it does differ in relative distribution. Thus, "inflow" disease involving obstruction of the aortoiliac segment is more common in the nondiabetic, while "outflow" disease involving the femoral, popliteal, and tibial segments is much more frequent in the diabetic. Other risk factors, particularly smoking and hypercholesterolemia, may affect the distribution pattern of atherosclerosis. It is not uncommon to see young diabetic women who are heavy smokers with severe aortoiliac disease and who have a relatively normal outflow system. The high prevalence of outflow disease in the diabetic can be appreciated from the number of outflow and inflow operations performed in 1990 at the Deaconess Hospital on diabetic patients: There were 286 femoral-popliteal-tibial operations and 27 aorto-iliac-femoral operations. With the advent of increasingly distal procedures to the dorsalis pedis and plantar arteries in the last few years the preponderance of outflow procedures has increased significantly. Furthermore, the increasing utilization of transluminal angioplasty for isolated iliac disease has reduced the number of inflow procedures performed.

While calcification of an atherosclerotic plaque is seen in both diabetics and nondiabetics, diabetics develop calcification of the media that is unrelated to their atherosclerosis. This is particularly prominent in insulin-dependent diabetics and is most closely related to the development of neuropathy. The major significance of this calcification, whether in the plaque or in the media,

is the technical difficulty it may present with arterial reconstruction. Sometimes the aorta or iliac vessels are too calcified to tolerate clamping, and an alternative approach has to be devised. Clamping such a calcified aorta may result in uncontrollable hemorrhage with unfortunate consequences for the patient.

There are a number of other factors that make the diabetic patient with aortoiliac disease different from the nondiabetic. Hypertension and neuropathy are common as complications of diabetes. However, the renal arteries should still be evaluated in patients with severe hypertension and abnormal renal function to detect potentially correctable renal artery stenosis. Impotence is a common complication of diabetes, secondary to neuropathy, and is much less likely to be due to obstruction of the internal iliac arteries.

## EVALUATION OF PATIENT'S CONDITION

The diagnosis of aortoiliac disease can usually be inferred after a careful history and physical examination. It is also important to detect any other problems that affect the treatment plan for the patient. Risk factors such as a history of smoking, hypertension, and hyperlipidemia need to be carefully evaluated. The majority of diabetic patients with aortoiliac disease are non-insulin dependent and also have a history of smoking. The most common presenting symptom is claudication, which may be in the calf muscles, the thigh muscles, or the buttocks. Claudication usually occurs in the calf in both inflow and outflow disease, and it is assessed by determining the distance the patient can walk on the level. When the patient exercises there is an increased demand for blood. Because of the arterial obstruction, this demand cannot be met, and the most distal muscle groups become ischemic and the patient complains of a cramping pain. As soon as the patient stops exercising, the pain goes away and the patient can then walk the same distance again. If the patient has severe neuropathy, then, instead of pain, he may complain of fatigue in the legs that immediately resolves with rest. With inflow disease, the patient may initially develop pain in the calves that extends to the thighs and buttocks as he continues to walk. Isolated buttock claudication implies severe disease of the internal iliac arteries, which supply the blood to the gluteal muscles. Iliac disease may also cause vasculogenic impotence. Characteristically the patient can attain erection but cannot maintain it once sexual activity has started. The diabetic often also has neurogenic impotence caused by neuropathy, and this may mask a history of vasculogenic impotence.

After claudication develops, the patient's symptoms may progress so that he complains of pain in his toes at night, relieved by getting up. This is because, without the help of gravity, not enough blood reaches the feet to maintain tissue viability. Further progression may result in gangrene of one or more toes or a nonhealing ulcer. Ischemic lesions are usually exquisitely painful. However, in the diabetic with severe neuropathy with loss of sensation, they may be painless. The most difficult differential diagnosis is between aortoiliac disease and the cauda equina syndrome. The cauda equina syndrome is due to pressure in the nerve roots from either a prolapsed disc or degenerative arthritis. This produces pain that runs down the back of the leg that is often worse with exercise. Severe cardiac disease associated with reduced cardiac output may worsen the symptoms of arterial insufficiency, and the patient may note significant improvement when the cardiac disease is treated. The use of beta-adrenergic blocking agents has been said on occasion to result in deterioration of the patient's symptoms, although this must be uncommon, as so many of these patients are receiving beta blockers.

In the physical examination, careful evaluation of the pulses is essential. The diagnosis can be made by noting absence or reduction of femoral pulses. Sometimes this is difficult because of the patient's obesity, which not uncommon is seen in older non–insulin-dependent diabetics. Many patients with symptoms of aortoiliac disease have normal pulses at rest that disappear with exercise. A pocket Doppler is useful in the office to measure the ankle-brachial ratio, and this can be rechecked after the patient has exercised. A value below 0.75 is consistent with significant peripheral vascular disease. It should be remembered, however, that, because of calcification in vessel walls seen in the diabetic, these values may be artifactually high. More complete evaluation in the vascular laboratory is usually indicated and may be essential to distinguish between aortoiliac disease and the cauda equina syndrome. The vascular laboratory may also be helpful in evaluation of the complaint of impotence.

## INDICATIONS FOR INTERVENTION

The indications for arteriography and surgery or balloon angioplasty are the same as for outflow disease and can be divided into absolute indications and relative indications. Classically the absolute indications for intervention include ischemic rest pain and gangrene or a nonhealing ulcer of the foot. When neuropathy is not present the situation is relatively straightforward. However, a neuropathic ulcer may fail to heal because there is inadequate circulation or conservative treatment is inadequate or the patient is noncompliant. Sometimes a neuropathic lesion may heal with total non-weight bearing, but it recurs whenever the patient tries to walk on it despite adequate shoeing. In this situation revascularization may be necessary to allow the patient to walk and stay healed, even though he has no lesion at the time of surgery. This situation is, however, relatively rare, and it requires experience to determine the best approach for an individual patient.

Disabling claudication is a much more common indication for intervention in diabetics with inflow disease than in those with outflow disease who more usually have a foot lesion. Before any intervention is done, it is important to have the patient stop smoking and start on an exercise program and, perhaps, try a three-month course of pentoxifylline (Trental). The decision as to when clau-

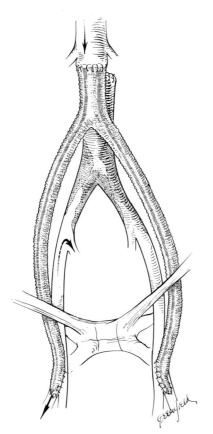

**Figure 19–3** Aortofemoral bypass graft with end-to-side anastomosis to aorta.

bleeding and, as they have less give than Dacron grafts, need to be more accurately sized. There are now some coated knitted Dacron grafts that handle well and yet are nonporous, and these may prove to be very useful. Most commonly, the graft is sewn proximally in an end-to-end manner. This involves transecting the aorta below the renals and oversewing the distal aorta above the inferior mesenteric, which is preserved. The graft is usually sewn in using a running monofilament nonabsorbable suture such as 2–0 Prolene. The end-to-end anastomosis results in the graft lying better so that it can be more easily covered with retroperitoneum at the end of the procedure. It should be noted, however, that in a number of large series no improvement in patency or reduction in complications has been detected in comparison to the end-to-side anastomoses. The end-to-side anastomosis is usually performed above the inferior mesenteric artery and below the renals (Fig. 19–4). If the graft does

very difficult, particularly in heavy men with a narrow pelvis. As the risk of infection has diminished, the femoral has become the preferred site for the distal anastomosis. One advantage of proximal placement of the graft is that the aortic bifurcation does not need to be extensively dissected, and the function of the autonomic nerves is less likely to be affected.

There are numerous grafts available for performing an aortofemoral bypass. These are made of either Dacron or polytetrafluoroethylene (PTFE). The Dacron grafts are either knitted or woven. The knitted grafts handle well, but require preclotting with blood, as they are relatively porous. The woven grafts are stiffer and tend to fray when cut to size for the distal anastomoses. They, however, do not require preclotting and, therefore, are particularly useful when the graft cannot be preclotted. The PTFE grafts are nonporous and simple to use. However, they may be associated with some suture line

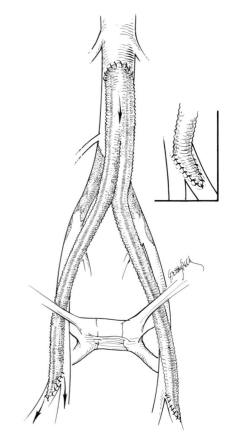

**Figure 19–4** Aortoiliac bypass graft with end-to-end anastomosis to aorta.

become infected, it is easier to remove, but it tends to stick out of the retroperitoneum and is more difficult to cover. When both external iliacs are occluded but the aorta and internal iliacs are open, then it would seem to make sense to perform an end-to-side anastomosis, as this allows for continued perfusion of the viscera via the internal iliacs and, it is hoped, reduces the likelihood of postoperative colonic ischemia.

The preoperative arteriogram allows for evaluation of the mesenteric and renal arteries, which may need to be addressed at the time the aortoiliac segment is bypassed. The inferior mesenteric artery is frequently occluded and can be ignored. Occasionally the superior mesenteric is diseased, and the inferior mesenteric becomes the only supply to the lower bowel and therefore may need to be anastomosed to the bypass graft to prevent postoperative colonic ischemia. Concomitant renal artery stenosis is quite common, and the decision when to add a renal artery revascularization can be controversial. It has been shown that adding a renal artery procedure to an aortofemoral bypass significantly increases the operative morbidity and mortality. We therefore restrict it to those patients with severe bilateral stenoses or with unilateral stenosis and uncontrolled hypertension. With bilateral diseases, endarterectomy of the renal arteries is frequently performed at the time of the bypass. With unilateral disease, a bypass from the renal artery to the graft is performed using either autogenous saphenous vein or a prosthetic graft. Occasionally in high-risk patients, it may be prudent to perform the renal artery bypass extra-anatomically at a separate operation.

Once the proximal anastomosis has been accomplished, the graft is tunneled in a retroperitoneal fashion into the groins, and the distal anastomoses are performed to the common femoral arteries in an end-to-side fashion using 5–0 monofilament suture. This allows retrograde perfusion of the iliacs if they are open. When the common femoral arteries are severely diseased or the superficial femoral arteries are occluded, it may be necessary to anastomose the graft to the profunda femoris artery. Occasionally endarterectomy of the femoral vessels has to be performed prior to the distal anastomosis, though this is avoided whenever possible.

## Iliofemoral Bypass

This bypass from the common iliac to the femoral artery has become increasingly popular in the last few years in the management of patients with external iliac and femoral artery occlusion. The proximal anastomosis to the common iliac is carried out via a retroperitoneal "renal transplant" incision. This is well tolerated in high-risk patients and gives good exposure. If the iliac artery turns out to be more calcified than anticipated and unusable, then exposure of the distal aorta can also be obtained. The graft material most commonly used is PTFE, and after the iliac anastomosis, the graft is tunneled anatomically into the groin and the distal anastomosis effected to the common, superficial, or profunda femoris artery. Though usually performed as a unilateral procedure, a bifurcated graft can be used to run to both groins. This graft is often preferred to a femoral-femoral graft, as it avoids operating on the other femoral artery, which may well be required for a later outflow procedure.

## COMBINED DISEASE

The presence of combined disease may result in a difficult problem in the patient with an ischemic foot. The most common situation in the diabetic is to have a localized lesion in the iliac combined with severe outflow disease. Clearly, fixing the iliac lesion alone would do nothing for the patient's ischemia, and yet the inflow is too poor to allow an outflow procedure alone. In the past, this was handled by doing a combined inflow-outflow procedure using a two-team approach. This was tolerated fairly well, given the magnitude of the procedure, and acceptable results were obtained. However, the advent of transluminal angioplasty has certainly facilitated the situation. We started doing intraoperative angioplasty, but soon found that things went much smoother if the angioplasty was done first in the radiology suite and the result assessed by pressure measurements and postprocedure noninvasive studies. If the preoperative arteriogram reveals an external iliac lesion not amenable to angioplasty, then a combined iliofemoral outflow procedure can be performed. This is well tolerated and does not take too long if a two-team approach is used. The autogenous-vein-proximal-anastomosis can be done directly into the hood of the distal PTFE anastomosis or, alternatively, to the native femoral vessel in tandem with the PTFE graft. The situation in which there is extensive aortoiliac disease combined with bilateral superficial femoral artery occlusion is also commonly seen in the nondiabetic, and the decision has to be made whether to combine an aortobifemoral bypass with an outflow procedure or to stage them. There have been many attempts to use data derived from the noninvasive laboratory to assist in this decision, though none have been generally adopted. In most cases the aortofemoral bypass can be safely performed first. Often an outflow procedure is not necessary after a successful inflow procedure, but if it is, it can easily be performed within a few days of the inflow procedure.

## DISTAL EMBOLIZATION ("TRASH FOOT")

The sudden appearance of painful ischemic lesions of the extremities in the presence of good distal pulses is not an uncommon condition of either diabetics or nondiabetics. Whether this is more common in diabetics has never been defined. If these patients are treated only with anticoagulation, many will end up with amputation as further embolization takes place. The work-up includes echocardiography to rule out a cardiac source and abdominal ultrasound to rule out an abdominal aortic aneurysm. If these are normal, then an aortography and a bilateral femoral follow-through procedure are indicated. The most common source of embolization is atheroma of the aortoiliac segment, which is often seen as a ground-glass appearance to the aorta. It is important to note that digital subtraction films do not give enough definition to allow this to be ruled out. When the aorta is transected at surgery, it is found to be full of material with the consistency of toothpaste. Obviously, aortobifemoral bypass for embolization demands an end-to-end proximal anastomosis.

## EXTRA-ANATOMICAL BYPASS

The aortobifemoral and iliofemoral bypasses are described as anatomical bypasses

as they are laid alongside the native vessel. On occasion, this cannot be done because of infection, previous operation, or the patient's general condition, and an extra-anatomical bypass has to be used. The most commonly used extra-anatomical bypass is the femoral-femoral bypass, which was first described in the early 60's. This involves bypassing an occluded iliac artery by running a graft from the opposite side to the femoral artery (Fig. 19–5A and B). A successful graft can be performed as long as there is less than 50 per cent stenosis of the donor iliac artery and no significant outflow disease in the recipient femoral. The graft material is not critical, and good results have been obtained with

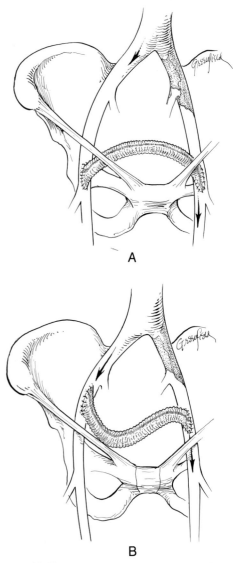

**A**

**B**

**Figure 19–5** Femorofemoral bypass graft. *A,* C-shaped graft. *B,* S-shaped graft.

both Dacron and PTFE. We routinely use an 8-mm PTFE graft and run the graft subcutaneously. The operation is simple and can be carried out under local anesthesia; patency rates of over 70 per cent at five years have been reported. The femoral-femoral bypass has been accomplished with increasing frequency as an adjunct to open heart surgery in critically ill patients. These patients need an intra-aortic balloon so the pump can be removed and to get them through the first couple of days. If placement of this device via the femoral artery results in ischemia in that leg, then a femoral-femoral bypass can be performed to maintain the viability of the leg until the balloon is removed.

When both iliac arteries are obstructed and an anatomical bypass cannot be achieved, then the axillobifemoral bypass is the procedure of choice. A PTFE or Dacron graft is run subcutaneously from the axillary artery to the femoral artery, and then a second graft is run from this to the opposite femoral (Fig. 19–6). It has been shown that an axillobifemoral bypass stays open better than an axillounifemoral graft, and so even if

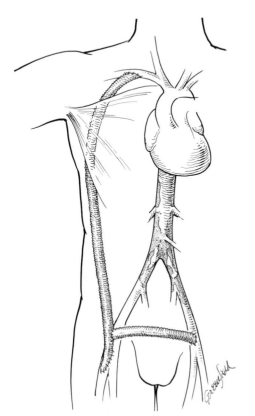

**Figure 19–6** Axillobifemoral bypass graft.

one leg is asymptomatic, a crossover limb is inserted. It does not matter which axillary artery is used, provided that it is not obstructed, as evidenced by reduced blood pressure in the corresponding arm. It is important to position the graft sufficiently laterally so that it is not kinked by the rib margin when the patient sits up. Some authors have claimed that externally supported PTFE reduces the likelihood of occlusion by compression, though this has not been proved. It is certainly true that most grafts occlude at night, but this may well be related to the reduced flow associated with inactivity. We do encourage the patient not to sleep on the side of the axillary graft, and we have been prescribing Coumadin for all patients postoperatively, as it has been claimed that this reduces the incidence of postoperative occlusion. Early graft thrombosis is not uncommon, but it can often be corrected by thrombectomy.

With improvements in anesthesia and perioperative management, we now perform fewer axillofemoral grafts than in the past, as we prefer the aortobifemoral bypass if the patient can tolerate the procedure. However, it would appear to be a durable procedure as a number of recent reports have described a five-year patency rate of greater than 70 per cent. Our preference is for the anatomical route, since few of our extra-anatomical bypasses have survived 5 years.

## INFECTION

One of the most feared complications of bypass with prosthetic materials is the development of infection. Fortunately the diabetic does not seem to be particularly more predisposed to developing this than the nondiabetic. Superficial wound infections in the groin are not uncommon and can usually be handled by adequate debridement, packing, and antibiotic therapy. Deep-seated infection, however, requires removal of the graft and revascularization via an extra-anatomical pathway that stays out of the infected area. For an aortofemoral graft infection, the graft has to be removed, the aorta oversewn, and the legs revascularized by means of an axillobifemoral bypass. Better results are obtained if the axillobifemoral bypass is in place prior to removal of the old graft. For infections isolated to the groin, the obturator bypass can be used. The abdominal aorta or either iliac artery may be used as the proximal inflow vessel and may be approached retroperitoneally or transperitoneally. The graft is tunneled through the upper medial portion of the obturator foramen and along the adductor muscle to the adductor canal. This is demonstrated in Figure 19–7. With the increasing frequency of "redo surgery" and multiple re-explorations of the groin, this is a useful way of staying out of the difficult groin even when there is no infection.

## LUMBAR SYMPATHECTOMY

Lumbar sympathectomy used to be common as an isolated procedure or in conjunction with aortofemoral bypass grafting. While it was effective in producing a warm foot, it did so by shunting blood to the skin at the expense of the nutrient vessels and therefore

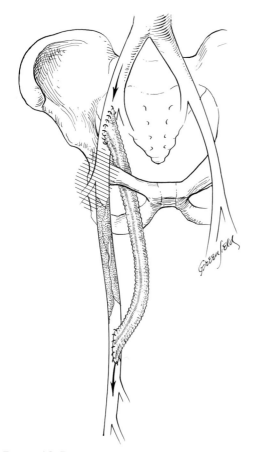

**Figure 19–7** Obturator bypass from external iliac to distal superficial femoral artery. Shaded area shows infected groin.

did nothing to reduce the ischemia. Diabetics with significant neuropathy also have an autosympathectomy, and so there is a theoretical reason why sympathectomy would be ineffective. Currently, sympathectomy is not regarded as helpful and is never performed at the Deaconess Hospital except for occasional cases of reflex sympathetic dystrophy.

## PERIOPERATIVE MANAGEMENT

The most important feature of the perioperative management of the diabetic is the special cardiovascular monitoring required. Many of the patients have some degree of renal dysfunction that may worsen following the arteriography despite liberal use of fluids and Lasix prior to and after the study. As mentioned earlier, 80 per cent of all diabetics have a positive thallium-dipyridamole scan, and that is poor correlation with clinical history. For this reason, we now employ Swan-Ganz catheter monitoring and intravenous nitroglycerin for all patients undergoing vascular surgery. We have developed a step-down unit on the vascular floor so we can continue to monitor the patient closely until the preoperative weight has been obtained. In the past it was noted that the most dangerous time for the patient was 48 hours after surgery, when diuresis would start to affect the perioperative fluid gain. With a Swan-Ganz catheter in place, the patient can be given diuretics as soon as the filling pressures start to rise and before clinical congestive heart failure with its attendant hypoxia develop. By looking at how the patient's filling pressures respond to fluids given perioperatively, it is possible to predict which patients are at risk of having problems. Antibiotics are given preoperatively to all patients undergoing vascular surgery and generally are continued until all the lines are out. The patients are aggressively mobilized as soon as their condition allows. Anticoagulation is prescribed on a case-by-case basis. We are increasingly using Coumadin in patients with long PTFE grafts, as this has been shown to improve patency.

## COMPLICATIONS

In looking at any large experience, including ours, cardiac complications represent the

**TABLE 19–1.  CONSECUTIVE AORTOILIAC RECONSTRUCTION RESULTS IN DIABETICS***

| PATIENTS | FOLLOW-UP MONTHS (MEAN) | GRAFT FAILURE | SEPSIS | REOPERATION (yr) Inflow | Outflow |
|---|---|---|---|---|---|
| 57 | 48 | 6 | 0 | 5 | 6 |
| Disabling claudication | | 18 patients (31.6%) | | | |
| Threatened limb loss | | 51 limbs, 39 patients (68%) | | | |

*New England Deaconess Hospital.
Compiled by Wheelock and Gibbons.

major source of morbidity and mortality. With the increased monitoring already described, these are being kept to a minimum. Early complications include distal embolization, bleeding, and early graft failure. Pulmonary, urinary, or local wound infection may also occur. For intra-abdominal procedures, bowel obstruction or ischemia and ureteric injury or obstruction are rare but significant problems. Late complications include false aneurysm formation, graft failure, and infection. Infection of an aortofemoral bypass is the most feared complication, particularly if associated with an aortoenteric fistula. Detailed management of these problems is beyond the scope of this chapter, but it can certainly be said that inflow reconstruction, even in the diabetic, has become safer and more effective over the last few years. Table 19–1 shows the results of a study of aortoiliac reconstruction in diabetic patients at the Deaconess Hospital and reported in 1984.

## SUGGESTED READING LIST

Bartlett, F. F., Gibbons, G. W., Wheelock, F. C., Jr.: Aortic reconstruction for occlusive disease: Comparable results in diabetics. Arch Surg. 121:1150, 1986.

Blaisdell, F. W., Holcroft, J. W., Ward, R. E., et al.: Axillofemoral and femoro-femoral bypass: History and evaluation of technique. In Greenhalgh, R. M. (ed.): Extra-anatomic and Secondary Arterial Reconstruction. Bath, Pitman, 1982, p. 84.

Brewster, D. C., and Darling, R. C.: Optimal methods of aorto-iliac reconstruction. Surgery 84:739, 1978.

Couch, N. P., Clowes, A. W., Whittemore, A. D., et al.: The iliac origin arterial graft: A useful alternative for iliac occlusive disease. Surgery 97:83, 1985.

Crawford, E. S., Bomberger, R. A., Glaeser, D. H., et al.: Aorto-iliac occlusive disease: Factors influencing survival and function following reconstructive operation over a twenty-five year period. Surgery 90:1555, 1981.

Lane, S. E., Lewis, S. M., Lane, S. E., et al.: Predictive value of quantitative dipyridamole-thallium scintigraphy in assessing cardiovascular risk after vascular surgery in diabetes mellitus. Am. J. Cardiol. 64:1275, 1989.

LoGerso, F. W., Johnson, W. C., Carson, J. D., et al.: A comparison of the late patency rates of axillobilateral femoral and axillounilateral femoral grafts. Surgery 81:33, 1977.

Szilasyi, D. E., Elliott, J. P., Jr., Smith, R. T., et al.: A thirty year survey of the reconstructive surgical treatment of aorto-iliac occlusive disease. J. Vasc. Surg. 3:421, 1986.

VanDet, R. J., and Brand, L. C.: The obturator foramen bypass: An alternative procedure in ilio-femoral artery revascularization. Surgery 89:543, 1981.

# Chapter 20

# ARTERIAL RECONSTRUCTION: FEMORAL TO POPLITEAL, TIBIAL, PERONEAL, AND PEDAL

GARY W. GIBBONS, M.D., FRANK B. POMPOSELLI, M.D.,
and FRANK W. LoGERFO, M.D.

The advances in vascular surgery since the first edition of this book are astonishing and probably best summarized by the fact that our major lower-extremity amputation rate for purely ischemic problems has been reduced from 28 per cent in 1984 to the current rate of less than 5 per cent. This is important because the incidence of type II diabetes is increasing, and peripheral vascular disease is 20 times more common in the diabetic than in the nondiabetic. While the severity of diabetes is not crucial to the development of atherosclerosis, the relationship between the two exceeds the commonly recognized risk factors for macrovascular disease in both men and women. These include hypertension, hyperlipidemia, obesity, cigarette smoking, hypercoagulability, and genetics.

While diabetic patients have a 17-fold increased risk of developing gangrene over nondiabetic patients, it must not be assumed that this is totally the result of macrovascular atherosclerosis. It is the triopathy of neuropathy, vascular insufficiency, and inability to handle infections normally that—either singularly or, more commonly, in combination—makes the diabetic patient uniquely susceptible to the development of any foot problem. In two of our studies of diabetic patients with limb-threatening foot infections, neuropathy was present in more than 98 per cent, and significant ischemia was identified in 50 per cent.

## PREVENTION OF PROBLEMS

Lower-extremity ischemia is only one component of diabetic foot problems, and prevention and effective treatment must always be directed at the three primary pathological situations. Many diabetic patients remain free of foot problems yet have diminished pulses or even absence of pulses at the femoral, popliteal, pedal, or all of these levels. The role of patient and physician education—especially in proper foot care—cannot be overemphasized. Daily foot inspection, proper hygiene, and appropriate shoeing are essential to protect the ischemic foot. Periodic vascular examinations help to identify patients at high risk and to observe them.

Controlling the other risk factors is also essential. While good control of hyperglycemia will not prevent macrovascular complications, it may reduce the genesis of thrombotic complications frequently seen in the diabetic state. Hyperglycemia significantly increases platelet aggregation, increases thromboxane production by platelets, and inhibits vessel wall prostacyclin production, all of which have important consequences.

# PATHOLOGY OF ATHEROSCLEROSIS

The pathophysiology of diabetic atherosclerosis is detailed in Chapter 5; key points are summarized here to illustrate the need for modern concepts of management. Diabetic macrovascular disease fundamentally involves the arterial wall in two ways. Medial calcinosis involves calcification in and around the smooth muscle cells of the media; it may be of neuropathic origin, and, since there is usually no significant intimal injury, it does not occlude the actual lumen but does affect the ability of the artery to pulsate. Medial calcinosis results in a rigid noncompressible artery and is responsible for the frequent erroneous noninvasive segmental pressure results; it also makes surgical or laser manipulation difficult.

The actual pathology of atherosclerosis is similar for diabetic and nondiabetic patients, but several distinguishing features are characteristic of the diabetic patient. Most important, while all arteries are at risk, there is a predilection for diabetic macrovascular occlusive disease to involve the more distal outflow vessels (tibial/peroneal), especially between the knee and foot. This is evidenced by the fact that 40 per cent of diabetic patients with gangrene or ulceration have a palpable popliteal pulse, a finding not characteristic of the nondiabetic. When this pulse is found, diabetes should be suspected in the future of such patients. Crucial is the fact that the foot arteries are usually spared in diabetic atherosclerosis. The continued misconception that diabetic patients have occlusive disease involving the foot arteries that impairs perfusion and causes ulceration leads to an attitude of hopelessness on the part of many health care professionals treating diabetic foot problems. It is responsible for inappropriate care extended to many. Simply put, there is no "macrovascular lesion or small vessel disease" uniquely affecting the diabetic foot, even in patients with gangrene and palpable foot pulses.

The other two characteristic features of diabetic atherosclerosis are the more frequent involvement of the distal profunda femoris artery and infrageniculars and the diminished ability to develop collateral circulation when major vessel occlusion occurs. The intimal and medial complex plaque also tends to have more calcium. The diffuse pattern of atherosclerotic disease with tibial/peroneal involvement and limited collateralization produces more serious limb-threatening symptoms and complications in the distal aspect of the leg and foot than occlusive disease in the nondiabetic patient. Again, this situation does not arise from any involvement of the foot arteries, and tissue perfusion in these ischemic diabetic feet can be restored by appropriate revascularization procedures.

# CLINICAL PRESENTATIONS AND CONSERVATIVE MANAGEMENT

This chapter discusses macrovascular disease below the inguinal ligament when significant symptoms are manifested by stenosis or occlusions of the common femoral, superficial femoral, deep femoral, popliteal, and/or tibial-peroneal arteries. It must be remembered that hemodynamically significant disease can involve the infrainguinal arterial tree yet the patient exhibits minimal or no symptoms. The adequacy of collateral pathways, the patient's activity level, and the degree of neuropathy affect clinical presentation.

Below-the-knee claudication is the earliest symptom of infrainguinal macrovascular disease, but for the diabetic may not always take the form of pain, the patient instead describing a numb or dead feeling in the leg or foot on walking a given distance that is made worse by going up an incline or by hurrying. It is always alleviated by a short period of rest and never occurs immediately on standing.

As the disease progresses the next symptom is rest pain, usually an aching in the foot muscles, most likely to occur at night when the patient is in bed and gravity no longer aids circulation to the foot. This symptom often is relieved when the patient sits up and hangs the legs over the side of the bed. Elevating the head of the bed 4 to 6 inches often helps.

Claudication and rest pain must be distinguished from symptoms of nerve root irritation caused by intervertebral disc herniation, spinal stenosis, arthritis, or other nerve compression syndromes. Neuropathy originating from diabetes or other causes most frequently confuses the clinical presentation. Night leg cramps are rarely related to ischemia and most frequently are associated with electrolyte imbalances or strain and respond to correction of the disturbance or administration of quinine sulfate at bedtime.

The third symptom represents further progression of macrovascular disease and is the development of ischemic ulcerations or gangrene (a term we avoid using within the patient's hearing). Starting as small cracks in the skin of the distal aspect of the toes, heel, or other areas, these areas may go unrecognized if neuropathy leaves the patient insensate to claudication or rest pain. Ischemic gangrene is usually dry, but the presence of infection compounds the issue. Confusing the picture is the presence of gangrene and palpable distal pulses, but one has to remember that gangrene has other causes, e.g., it may be secondary to pressure necrosis and/ or uncontrolled infection.

The significance of the patient's presenting symptoms and the examination help determine the appropriate course of treatment. It must be remembered that intermittent claudication is not a precursor of limb loss, especially in its early stages, since only 10 to 15 per cent of cases progress to limb-threatening symptoms. Claudication, however, may be more progressive in diabetic patients, especially those who continue to smoke.

Conservative management is the first line of treatment, with good control of diabetes, cessation of smoking, reduction to or maintenance of ideal weight, control of hypertension, correction of lipid abnormalities, reduction or discontinuance of beta blockers, and tailored exercise. While the use of Trental (pentoxifylline) is somewhat controversial, it may improve the walking distance in up to one third of diabetic patients with claudication. It is the only medication available for this particular use, so patients know that more aggressive treatment is ahead if symptoms worsen. Use of low-dose aspirin to reduce thromboembolic complications has not been proved, but it has not been associated with worsening of any associated eye problems and is relatively safe.

Rest pain and ischemic ulcerations represent limb-salvaging situations, as these extremities are immediately threatened. Depending on the patient's associated risk factors and well-being, more aggressive intervention is recommended.

## EXAMINATION

The diagnosis of diabetic peripheral vascular disease is confirmed by a detailed physical examination. While exact assessment is detailed in Chapter 3, key points deserve emphasis again. Clinical evaluation, judgment, and experience are still the essential means for assessing vascular insufficiency and are only complemented, not replaced, by noninvasive testing, even with all of the technological advances (Ch. 14). We still have not found any noninvasive test that uniformly predicts primary healing with or without surgery or that can be used in follow-up of patients after the procedure.

Most diabetics who have had their diabetes for an extended period have autonomic neuropathy, which creates the same effect as surgical sympathectomy. (This is the reason that this procedure has no value in treating critical lower-extremity ischemia.) Sweating is eliminated, leaving the skin dry and quite susceptible to cracking and fissuring. Blood is shunted from the deeper nutrient vessels to the skin so that the skin is warm and capillary filling appears good. The resulting false impression of vascular integrity often entices the inexperienced health care provider into local procedures doomed to failure.

Again, the palpation of a popliteal pulse does not ensure vascular integrity, since 40 per cent of ischemic diabetic feet have this finding. Like Andros et al., we have found a small number of patients who have palpable pedal pulses at rest and yet have nonhealing foot ulcers and severe foot ischemia. An excellent rule of thumb is to proceed with arteriography whenever there is a question of ischemia associated with an unresolving diabetic foot problem.

## OPTIMAL MANAGEMENT

There are four essential components for optimal management of the diabetic patient with critical lower-extremity ischemia: (1) understanding the specific pattern of diabetic atherosclerotic vascular disease, especially its predilection for tibial/peroneal vessels; (2) recognizing the nonexistence of occlusive macrovascular disease of the diabetic foot; (3) utilizing precise, up-to-date techniques of arteriography; and (4) adopting modern approaches to arterial revascularization.

Since 1984, when this chapter was originally written, several medical and technological advances not only have made optimal management of diabetic lower-extremity ischemia a reality, but also they have made it routine. Components one and two have been discussed. Arteriography is discussed in Chapter 15: key points deserve emphasis. Precise and up-to-date arteriography is mandatory for successful vascular reconstruction, and the vascular surgeon should accept nothing less. This includes visualization of the foot vessels whenever possible. The arterial digital subtraction technique has been a major advance in accomplishing this, but the vascular surgeon must understand that the clinical pathology and severity of the involved vessels at the time of reconstruction is worse than depicted by the arteriogram. Much less contrast dye is needed—important for the diabetic patient in whom there is a definite increased risk of dye-induced renal failure. Avoidance of major vascular reconstruction immediately following arteriography is recommended, except in emergency situations.

## MODERN APPROACH TO ARTERIAL RECONSTRUCTION

A modern approach to arterial reconstruction (the final component of optimal management) is best exemplified by the proud and rich history of the New England Deaconess Hospital and the Joslin Diabetes Center. The changes and refinements in the principles and techniques of our approach to the diabetic are best understood by reviewing this experience, because so much has changed.

The vision of a modern team approach to diabetic foot problems dates back to Dr. Leland McKittrick, who first set up a "foot room" at the New England Deaconess Hospital in the 1930's at the request of Dr. Elliot Joslin of the Joslin Clinic. At that time there was no vascular surgery and antibiotics were yet to come. Treatment options were local debridement and minor or major amputation, depending on the adequacy of the circulation. A weekly foot conference was held in which patients and their problems were presented; it included all members of the subspecialties interested in the diabetic foot. It is tradition that continues. Dr. McKittrick popularized the transmetatarsal amputation (TMA) and published the first reported series of TMA's in 1949.

The specialty of vascular surgery was developed in the early 1950's once Dos Santos had introduced the concept of arteriography.

While Kunlin of France was the first to popularize the long venous bypass graft, Robert Linton's success in this country with the reversed saphenous vein bypass established this method as the procedure of choice for arterial reconstruction below the inguinal ligament. One of Linton's students, Dr. Frank Wheelock, was brought to the New England Deaconess Hospital by Dr. McKittrick to develop vascular surgery techniques and principles for the ischemic diabetic patient. In 1969, Wheelock reported the first large experience of 104 reversed saphenous vein bypasses in diabetic patients at the New England Deaconess Hospital and Joslin Clinic; 86 of these graft procedures were performed for critical limb ischemia. Initial success was 98 per cent with one death and one early graft failure. These incredible results demonstrated the success of a team approach. Of interest was the fact that in 69 of the 103 successful bypasses, no pedal pulse was palpable postoperatively, the pedal pulses being absent because of blocks in the tibial arteries of the calves, according to Dr. Wheelock in his discussion. The Doppler and other forms of noninvasive testing were yet to be invented. Sixty per cent of the patients had gangrene, and post bypass only 4 toe amputations and 23 TMA's (quite different from our experience today) were performed to achieve limb salvage. Only one of these procedures failed, and it was in a limb with a functioning bypass graft. Long-term patency was 91 per cent at two years and 72 per cent at five years. The only major difference noted in this diabetic population was that one third of the patients were dead at five years, in sharp contrast to series reporting nondiabetic patients.

This important paper was presented before the International Cardiovascular Society in 1969, and in the discussion following Wheelock noted that only about 20 per cent of diabetic patients with advanced ischemia were bypass candidates. Of the diabetic patients at risk, 40 per cent already had a palpable popliteal pulse that he did not think he could improve upon. At that time, artery grafts performed were about equal in number per year to major amputations at our institution, and routine distal bypass grafting in the diabetic patient was yet to come. As experience was gained, it became obvious that autogenous vein was the conduit of choice to provide satisfactory long-term patency. When

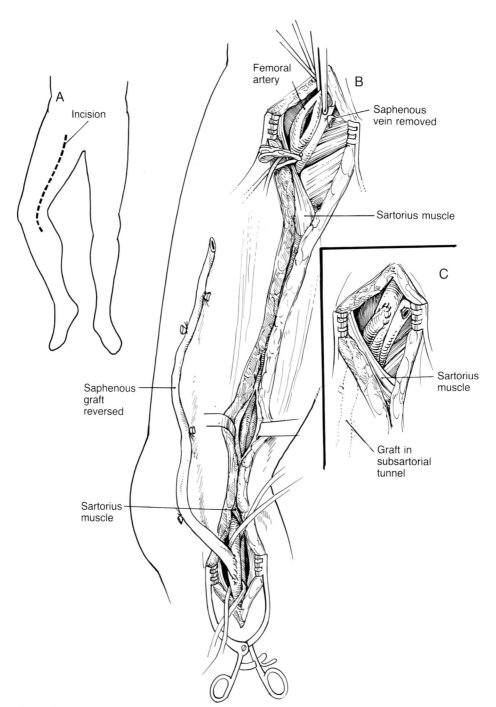

**Figure 20–2** Standard femoral-to-popliteal artery reversed saphenous vein bypass. *A,* Continuous incision along the course of the greater saphenous vein. *B,* Distal anastomosis is completed, and the graft is ready for tunneling through the subsartorial plane to the common femoral artery. *C,* Completed femoral anastomosis.

foot vessels challenged our skills to bypass to these vessels when restoration of pulsatile flow was needed to achieve limb salvage. Because we were encouraged by the reports of others and our own early results, pedal artery bypass grafting became our standard approach to achieve limb salvage in cases in which restoration of pulsatile flow to the foot

## TABLE 20–1.  CLINICAL DATA AND INDICATIONS FOR SURGERY

| CLINICAL DATA | NO. OF PATIENTS (n = 96) | % |
|---|---|---|
| Males | 64 | 67 |
| Females | 32 | 33 |
| Diabetes | 90 | 94 |
| Myocardial infarction/ angina | 33 | 34 |
| Previous peripheral vascular surgery | 28 | 29 |
| Previous amputation | 41 | 43 |
| Previous transmetatarsal amputation | 6 | 6 |
| Indications* | | |
|   Ischemic ulcer | 51 | 49 |
|   Rest pain | 36 | 35 |
|   Failed amputation | 6 | 6 |
|   Gangrene | 31 | 30 |
|   Secondary infection | 44 | 42 |

From Pomposelli, F. B., Jepson, S. J., Gibbons, S. W., et al.: Efficacy of the dorsal pedal bypass for limb salvage in diabetic patients. J. Vasc. Surg. 11:745, 1990.
*Some patients had more than one indication.

would not be possible by grafting to the tibial or peroneal vessels.

Our combined experience at the New England Deaconess Hospital between August 1986 and May 1989 included 104 pedal artery bypasses attempted in 96 patients. The patient profile is presented in Table 20–1. All bypass procedures were performed for limb salvage; 42 per cent of patients had associated infection of the extremity requiring initial surgical debridement and intravenous administration of antibiotics prior to revascularization. Misleading noninvasive vascular laboratory testing was evident by the fact that the mean preoperative ankle brachial index was .64, but all patients had fewer than five boxes on pulse volume forefoot recordings.

Arterial digital subtraction angiography was performed in all patients. The most common finding was occlusion of all three tibial vessels, either proximally or distally, and no demonstrable continuity with a reconstituted pedal or posterior tibial artery below the ankle. Angiography successfully visualized the dorsalis pedis artery in 92 patients, but in 12 patients that artery was not visualized despite an audible Doppler signal.

In the 92 cases in which the dorsalis pedis artery was visualized, 91 pedal artery bypasses were successfully performed. In the 12 cases in which the pedal artery was explored because of an audible Doppler signal but failed visualization by arteriography, six successful bypasses were performed (five of the other six patients underwent below-knee amputation), making 97 cases available for analysis.

All bypasses were performed with vein, the type of bypass varying with the adequacy of the inflow source and the size and adequacy of the vein (Table 20–2). The technique of pedal artery bypass grafting will not be discussed here. It is important to note, however, the need to keep the pedal artery incision away from the vein harvest incision and tunnel the vein superiorly and not through the skin bridge between the two incisions, to avoid the occurrence of necrosis in this area. During the tunneling any sharp angulation should be avoided, and the distal incisions are best closed with a running skin plus subcutaneous single layer monofilament closure, avoiding double-layer closure or clips that gather up too much tissue and can result in necrosis of the skin edges. Routine intraoperative angioscopy has become an important adjunct to intraoperative angiography in performing these bypasses to ascertain vein size, quality, and adequacy of valve lysis and to evaluate the anastomoses. Routine valve lysis under direct angioscopic visualization has reduced the incidence of complications associated with this procedure.

Two patients died within 30 days of surgery (1.92 per cent), and six bypasses failed within

## TABLE 20–2.  TYPES OF CONDUIT AND SOURCE OF ARTERIAL INFLOW

| CONDUIT/SOURCE OF ARTERIAL INFLOW | NO. OF BYPASSES (n = 97) |
|---|---|
| Type of conduit | |
|   ISV | 48 |
|   RSV | 21 |
|   NRSV | 16 |
|   AV | 6 |
|   COM | 6 |
| Inflow source | |
|   FEM | 48 |
|   POP | 45 |
|   TIB | 2 |
|   FEM-TIB | 2 |

From Pomposelli, F. B., Jepson, S. J., Gibbons, G. W. et al.: Efficacy of the dorsal pedal bypass for limb salvage in diabetic patients. J. Vasc. Surg. 11:745, 1990.
ISV = In situ saphenous vein; RSV = reversed saphenous vein; NRSV = nonreversed saphenous vein; AV = arm vein; COM = composite vein; POP = popliteal; FEM = femoral artery; POP = popliteal artery; TIB = tibial artery; FEM-TIB = femoral-tibial bypass graft.

this period (16.1 per cent). Further bypass reconstructive foot surgery was required in 33 patients, and the limbs of all patients who were discharged with patent grafts were saved. Actuarial life table analysis of graft patency, limb salvage, and patient survival was 82 per cent, 87 per cent, and 80 per cent, respectively, at 18 months.

Several reports in the literature note comparable patency rates for reversed saphenous vein grafts to distal tibial or pedal vessels and question the superiority of the in situ technique. It has become obvious to us that a rigid commitment to one technique or another is inappropriate. From October 1985 to August 1989 we performed 156 dorsalis pedis artery bypass grafts in 146 patients. All bypasses were performed for limb salvage. The patient profile is outlined in Table 20–3. A variety of surgical techniques were utilized as well as inflow sources, as detailed in Table 20–4. The 30-day mortality rate was 2.6 per cent with seven grafts failing (4.5 per cent) in this period. Actuarial patency and limb salvage in the 6- to 60-month follow-up were 87 per cent and 92 per cent, respectively. Most important, however, was the fact that there was no significant difference in patency between in situ and ex situ vein grafts (93 per cent versus 90 per cent) or on the basis of inflow site (common femoral 89 per cent versus distal superficial femoral artery or popliteal 88 per cent). It is clear that excellent results can be obtained by adapting

### TABLE 20–4. DORSALIS PEDIS BYPASS GRAFTS (10/16/85–8/28/89)

| CONDUIT/INFLOW SOURCE | NO. (156) |
|---|---|
| Conduit | |
| In situ | 75 |
| Ex situ* | 62 |
| Arm | 9 |
| Composite† | 9 |
| PTFE | 1 |
| Inflow source | |
| Common femoral | 58 |
| Distal SFA/popliteal | 88 |
| Tibial artery | 3 |
| Previous bypass graft | 7 |

*Includes reversed and nonreversed translocated saphenous veins.
†All were totally autogenous, including saphenous- and arm-vein segments.
PTFE = polytetrafluoroethylene; SFA = superficial femoral artery.

all modern vascular surgical techniques to the specific circumstances involved with each individual patient: a flexible approach. In the operating room, patience, excellent lighting, routine magnification, meticulous technique, and gentle preparation and handling of the vein graft are most important (Table 20–5).

Certain principles remain basic to any lower-extremity revascularization in a diabetic. First, it must be realized that current laser recanalization techniques (including balloon angioplasty) have an extremely limited application to the diabetic with critical lower-extremity ischemia. Preoperative preparation includes control of any foot infection with intravenous broad-spectrum antibiotics combined with incision and drainage of abscesses and debridement or open partial forefoot amputation prior to any major vascular

### TABLE 20–3. DORSALIS PEDIS BYPASS GRAFTS (10/16/85–8/28/89)

| CLINICAL CHARACTERISTICS/ INDICATIONS | NO. PATIENTS (156) |
|---|---|
| Characteristics | |
| Male | 105 |
| Female | 51 |
| Age (mean) | 65.6 |
| Diabetes mellitus | 148 |
| Mean ankle/brachial ratio | .67 |
| Mean PVR forefoot trace | 4 mm |
| Indications* | |
| Ischemic ulcer | 82 |
| Gangrene | 44 |
| Rest pain | 53 |
| Failed amputation | 9 |
| Secondary infection | 79 |
| Osteomyelitis | 12 |

*All procedures were performed for limb salvage.
Some patients had more than one indication.

### TABLE 20–5. ARTERIAL VASCULAR SURGERY PROCEDURES AT NEW ENGLAND DEACONESS HOSPITAL*

| | |
|---|---|
| **INFLOW** | |
| Aorto-iliac-femoral bypass | 201 |
| Axillo-femoral bypass | 10 |
| Femoral-femoral | 19 |
| **OUTFLOW** | |
| Femoral-popliteal bypass | 168 |
| Femoral-popliteal to tibial | 186 |
| Femoral-popliteal to peroneal | 66 |
| Femoral-popliteal to dorsalis pedis | 154 |
| Local endarterectomy | 23 |

*Oct 1990–Oct 1992.
Compiled by D. R. Campbell, M.D., and F. LoGerfo, M.D.

reconstruction. Aggressive evaluation and management of concurrent cardiovascular disease and control of diabetes are essential. While all anesthetic choices have been found to be equally safe, these procedures are best performed with Swan-Ganz catheter and arterial monitoring.

Once it has been determined that a bypass is needed to restore circulation to a clearly threatened limb, there are several clear-cut requirements to ensure patency and success. Obviously, patients with severe dementia or mental deterioration who do not ambulate certainly are not candidates for bypass grafting. In patients with extensive tissue destruction in whom there would be a question of limb salvage even if circulation were restored, evaluation must be carefully carried out to determine whether a primary below-knee amputation may better suit their needs. Bedridden patients with long-standing flexion contractures are not good candidates for reconstruction.

The ideal situation for successful lower-extremity bypass grafting is occlusion of the superficial femoral artery with an open popliteal artery distally and good runoff via the three distal vessels onto the foot. From the previous discussion it can be noted that this situation is rare for the diabetic patient. Specifically, the type of bypass performed usually will depend on the outflow vessels visualized during arteriography and the reason for which the bypass is being performed. One would prefer a femoral to popliteal artery bypass graft in patients whose only symptom is disabling claudication or early rest pain. We would not recommend a femoral to distal tibial, peroneal, or pedal artery bypass for patients with claudication. These grafts should be limited to those patients with limb-threatening ischemia. Because of limited collateralization, very distal tibial or pedal bypass grafting may not eliminate claudication in the calf.

Diabetic patients with extensive tissue loss or gangrene of the foot probably need restoration of pulsatile flow to the foot whenever possible. Blind popliteal segments or tibial reconstructions without vessel continuity to the foot may be successful and remain patent but many fail to achieve limb salvage. Pedal artery bypass grafting is a less demanding procedure technically than bypassing to the distal peroneal artery, at which there is continuity only via collateral flow to the dorsalis pedis or distal posterior tibial artery onto the foot. One must also consider the outcome if the bypass graft should fail. There may be fewer consequences to healing a below-knee amputation when a more distal bypass is performed than when a below-knee amputation is preceded by a deep dissection of the lower leg.

When an audible Doppler signal is present but visualization by arteriography fails, blind exploration of the pedal artery and grafting are successful 50 per cent of the time and should be carefully considered before proceeding with a major amputation, particularly in patients who already have had a major amputation of the other extremity. The same can be said for a distal posterior tibial artery, especially when the primary problem is located in the heel or proximal plantar aspect of the foot.

The present reduction in our major amputation rate for severe diabetic lower-limb ischemia to under 5 per cent is a result of tremendous team commitment to these patients and a modern flexible approach to vascular reconstruction applied to the diabetic. Our post-bypass local forefoot amputation requirements have also changed dramatically since the Wheelock/Hoar era. In our efforts to preserve as much of the walking foot as possible to achieve maximum function, the number of TMA's performed after distal tibial or pedal artery bypass has dramatically declined in favor of more localized procedures. This even has been applied to the toes (especially the first toe and metatarsal), in which local resection of osteomyelitis and involved tissue is preferred over amputation when possible. The restoration of pulsatile forefoot flow makes this possible.

Because of all of the technical complexities involved, distal diabetic vascular reconstruction may not be preferable for the vascular surgeon who is called upon to perform it only occasionally. Distal diabetic arteries are frequently extensively calcified, and distal tibial and pedal arteries often are only 1 mm in internal diameter. A team approach addressing all associated diabetic risk factors is essential for success.

## COST VERSUS BENEFIT

Caring for diabetic patients with lower-extremity problems is not inexpensive. Diagnosis-related groups (DRG's) and health care cost constraints have placed additional burden on caring for these patients. The alternative of major amputation as opposed to an aggressive approach to limb salvage must be considered at all levels. It must be remembered that in 30 to 50 per cent diabetics a contralateral limb-threatening problem will develop in the next several years. While life expectancy for the diabetic with critical limb ischemia is reduced, subjective factors such as quality of life and the ability to live and function independently are foremost in the minds of these patients. While an aggressive revascularization and limb salvage program involves an initial and often lengthy period of hospitalization and higher cost, its success far outweighs the total financial and emotional cost of primary amputation as a procedure of choice. The diabetic's greatest fear is amputation, and our responsibility to the patient and society is best served by an aggressive team approach to saving diabetic lower extremities.

## SUGGESTED READING LIST

Andros G., Harris, R. W., Dulawa, L. B., et al.: The need for arteriography in diabetic patients with gangrene and palpable foot pulses. Arch. Surg. 119:1984.

Gibbons, G. W.: Vascular surgery of the diabetic lower extremity. In Frykberg, R. G. (ed.): The High Risk Foot in Diabetes Mellitus. New York, Churchill Livingstone, 1991, pp. 273–296.

Gloviczki P., Morris, S. M., Bower, T. C., et al.: Microvascular pedal bypass for salvage of the severely ischemic limb. Mayo Clin. Proc. 66:243–253, 1991.

Leather, R. P., Shah, D. M., Buchbinder, D., et al.: Further experience with the saphenous vein used in situ for arterial bypass. Am. J. Surg. 142:506, 1981.

LoGerfo F. W., and Coffman, J. D.: Vascular and microvascular disease of the foot in diabetics: Implications in foot care. N. Engl. J. Med. 311:1615, 1984.

LoGerfo, F. W., and Gibbons, G. W.: Ischemia in the diabetic foot: Modern concepts and management of clinical diabetes. Clin. Diabetes 7:72, 1989.

Pomposelli, F. B., Jepson, S. J., Gibbons, G. W., et al.: A flexible approach to infra-popliteal vein grafts in patients with diabetes mellitus. 17th Annual Meeting of the New England Society for Vascular Surgery, Newport, R. I., September 1990.

Pomposelli, F. B., Jepson, S. J., Gibbons, G. W., et al.: Efficacy of the dorsal pedal bypass for limb salvage in diabetic patients. J. Vasc. Surg. 11:745, 1990.

Reichle, F. A., Rankin, K. P., Tyson, R. R., et al.: Long-term results of femoroinfrapopliteal bypass in diabetic patients with severe ischemia of the lower extremities. Am. J. Surg. 137:653, 1979.

Veith, F. J., and Gupta, S. K.: Femoral-distal artery bypasses. In Bergan, J. J., and Yao, J. S. T. (eds.): Operative Techniques in Vascular Surgery. New York, Grune & Stratton, 1980, pp. 141–150.

Wheelock, F. C., Jr., and Filtzer, H. S.: Femoral grafts in diabetics. Arch. Surg. 99:776, 1969.

Wheelock, F. C., Jr., and Gibbons, G. W.: Arterial reconstruction—femoral-popliteal-tibial. In Kozak, G. P., Hoar, C. S., Jr., Rowbotham, J. L., et al. (eds.): Management of Diabetic Foot Problems. Philadelphia, W. B. Saunders Co., 1984, pp. 173–187.

# Chapter 21

# TRANSLUMINAL ANGIOPLASTY AND LASER TREATMENT

KENNETH R. STOKES, M.D., FRANK B. POMPOSELLI, M.D.,
and H. ESTERBROOK LONGMAID, III, M.D.

## PERCUTANEOUS TRANSLUMINAL ANGIOPLASTY

Since the first arterial dilatation by Dotter and Judkins in 1963 and development of the double-lumen angioplasty balloon by Gruntzig in 1974, percutaneous transluminal angioplasty has firmly established its role as either primary or adjunctive treatment of lower extremity atherosclerotic disease. The mechanism of dilatation has been understood only more recently. Dilatation fractures the endothelial plaque, causing intimal and medial dehiscence, and then stretches the media and adventitia, resulting in a dilated lumen. This plaque separation and underlying dissection create an intimal flap that can be seen on 70 per cent of postdilatation arteriograms. Within a period of days, the dissection is remodeled by thrombus deposition and organization. By one month, this remodeling results in a smooth luminal surface within the dilated segment.

Whether a patient is a candidate for angioplasty or surgical bypass is determined by history, physical examination, noninvasive examination, and arteriography. In general, a clinical assessment is made of either the degree of disability from claudication or the threat to further limb viability by the presence of ischemic rest pain, ulceration, and gangrene.

Although controversial, angioplasty may be used for claudication that is severe enough to affect the individual's life-style, but not severe enough for surgical revascularization.

These patients are ideal in that usually the stenoses are short, readily crossed, and easily dilated. Both the patient and other physicians involved should understand, however, that complications, although unusual, do occur. Although long-term patency rates are much reduced, angioplasty should also be considered for patients with diffuse or multisegmental disease who are too ill for surgical revascularization.

Performing diagnostic arteriography, and, if needed, angioplasty at the same time, is efficient and spares the patient the potential risks of subsequent contrast studies—an especially important consideration in those diabetic patients with underlying renal insufficiency. Communication and cooperation between the arteriographer and vascular surgeon greatly facilitate the arteriographer's task of making treatment decisions while the patient is being studied. The greater expense and morbidity of surgery must be weighed against the generally lower patency rates of angioplasty. A cooperative relationship is essential in tailoring the best treatment for the individual's clinical situation.

Techniques for angioplasty are the same in diabetic patients as in nondiabetic patients and are well described elsewhere. Once the lesion has been crossed with the angiographic guide wire, the balloon catheter can easily be exchanged for the existing diagnostic catheter and then angioplasty performed (Fig. 21–1). Our patients routinely receive heparin 3000 units intravenously at the time of the angioplasty and aspirin 80 mg/day for maintenance after the procedure. For infra-

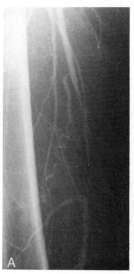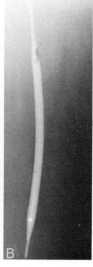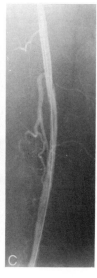

**Figure 21–1** Superficial femoral angioplasty. *A,* Severe stenosis of the mid superficial femoral artery. *B,* Expanded 5-mm-diameter angioplasty balloon. *C,* Postangioplasty arteriogram reveals adequate dilatation with luminal irregularity typical of arterial dissection.

popliteal arteries, patients are fully heparinized for 24 hours following the procedure.

For 10- and 12-mm iliac arteries, we prefer the Olbert balloon catheter. Its design eliminates the large "wings" found on other deflated balloons, resulting in a smaller, less irregular arterial puncture site after removal. For small arteries, we presently use a variety of the 5 F catheter thin-wall high-pressure balloons now available. These balloon catheters will tolerate inflation pressures up to 10 atmospheres, which is often necessary with densely calcified atherosclerotic plaques. These high-pressure balloons are also less likely to be damaged by calcified lesions than previous 5 F catheter balloons, and the thin balloon wall and small catheter size result in a smaller and less traumatized puncture site on removal. For arteries less than 3 mm, we use coronary angioplasty catheters.

Complication rates vary, but are generally decreasing with improved techniques and catheter designs. One review of almost 2000 procedures identified an overall complication rate of 5.1 per cent with 0.67 per cent requiring surgical repair. Specific complications were as follows (with the rate of surgical intervention given in parentheses): hematoma, 2.5 per cent (0.12 per cent); thrombosis, 1.3 per cent (0.2 per cent); distal embolization, 0.8 per cent (0.15 per cent); false aneurysm, 0.25 per cent (0.15 per cent); and perforation, 0.25 per cent (0.05 per cent).

As a general rule, the larger the artery and shorter the stenosis, the better the long-term patency rates, the short iliac artery stenosis

being an ideal lesion for angioplasty. Long stenoses or multiple stenoses greater than 8 cm in total length have a lower long-term patency rate. Chronic occlusions have a lower patency rate than stenoses, although short occlusions have similar results to stenoses of similar length. Acute embolic or thrombotic occlusions and occlusions of unknown age should not be treated solely by angioplasty because recently formed thrombus can embolize distally. If the patient's limb can tolerate continuing ischemia and there are no contraindications, a trial of lytic therapy can be used to eliminate any fresh thrombus and the underlying stenosis can then be treated with angioplasty.

Long-term angioplasty results in diabetic patients are not readily available. Our review of 122 angioplasties evaluated by life table analysis revealed results comparable to those in nondiabetic patients with similar severity of vascular disease, findings supported by others. Better results were obtained in both iliac and femoral angioplasties when the patients had patent, although possibly diseased, two- or three-vessel runoff ("good runoff") rather than more severe diffuse disease with no runoff or one-vessel runoff ("poor runoff"). Among these patients, 76 per cent were insulin dependent and 71 per cent had rest pain, ulceration, or gangrene.

Of 66 successful iliac angioplasties, the overall patency rate was 85 per cent at one year, 67 per cent at three and four years, and 34 per cent at five years (Fig. 21–2). Among all patients, 49 per cent had good runoff at

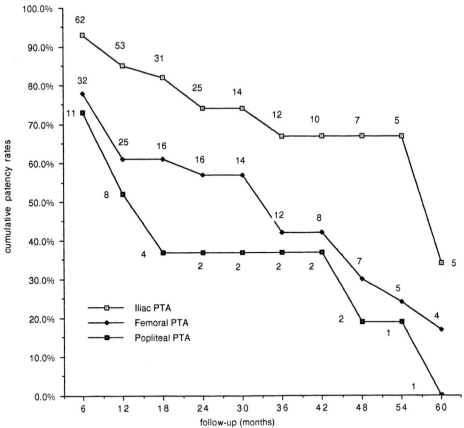

**Figure 21–2** Life table analysis of iliac, femoral, and popliteal angioplasty patency rates. *PTA* = percutaneous transluminal angioplasty.

presentation, whereas 51 per cent had poor runoff. The three- and five-year patency rates of iliac angioplasties with good runoff were 76 per cent as opposed to 60 per cent three-year and 20 per cent five-year patency rates with poor runoff (Fig. 21–3).

Our review of 40 superficial femoral angioplasties revealed overall patency rates of 61 per cent at one year, 42 per cent at three years, and 17 per cent at five years. Patients with good runoff had patency of 82 per cent at one year, 46 per cent at three years, and 46 per cent at five years, whereas patients with poor runoff had 48 per cent one year, 40 per cent three-year and 8 per cent five-year patency (Fig. 21–4).

All 16 popliteal angioplasties were performed for limb salvage in the presence of poor runoff (see Fig. 21–2). Patency rates were 52 per cent at one year and 37 per cent at three years. None was patent at five years.

Frequently diabetic patients with limb-threatening ischemia have multiple segments of atherosclerotic disease involving the aortoiliac segment, superficial femoral artery, and proximal infrapopliteal vessels (so-called *inflow/outflow disease*). When ischemic tissue loss or gangrene is present in the foot, bypass of the aortoiliac segment (inflow disease) without bypass of the more distal occlusions (outflow disease) may not allow healing. In these circumstances the vascular surgeon is faced with two unappealing options: either to perform a lengthy combined procedure involving simultaneous correction of both inflow and outflow disease or to sequentially perform the inflow procedure first and the outflow procedure several days later. This latter option exposes the patient to the morbidity and mortality associated with two separate surgical procedures. When iliac angioplasty is possible, the potential morbidity to the pa-

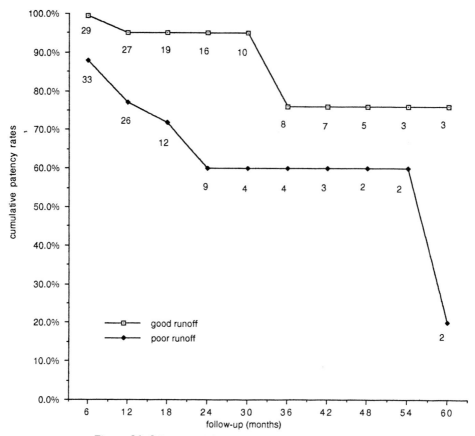

**Figure 21–3** Patency of iliac angioplasty with respect to runoff.

tient can be significantly reduced by removing the need for the inflow surgical procedure.

Atherosclerotic lesions occurring below the inguinal ligament are also amenable to percutaneous transluminal angioplasty. Occasionally a patient may require distal tibial reconstruction, but will not have an adequate length of venous conduit for bypass. When angioplasty of the superficial femoral artery is possible, the length of vein necessary for bypass can be reduced by performing the proximal anastomosis with the popliteal artery instead of with the usual common femoral artery. Although the durability of percutaneous transluminal angioplasty below the inguinal ligament is significantly less than surgical bypass, it still may be the appropriate primary procedure in patients with isolated superficial femoral artery stenosis and disabling claudication when the risks of surgery are great or when venous conduit is not available.

## THROMBOLYSIS

Thrombolytic agents have been used to treat arterial thrombosis since 1955, but only recently has the technique of regional intra-arterial thrombolysis been used extensively. Early studies involved streptokinase administered in low doses directly into the thrombosed artery. We presently use urokinase, which is more expensive but is more effective and safer with fewer systemic thrombolytic side effects than streptokinase.

Urokinase (UK) is a nonantigenic thrombolytic agent derived from human fetal renal cell cultures. The drug lyses thrombus by directly activating plasminogen. Its half-life is approximately 20 minutes, but its anticoagulant effects persist for hours because of depletion of clotting factors and fibrinogen. Currently an additional thrombolytic agent, tissue plasminogen activator (t-PA), is under investigation. This endogenous agent activates plasminogen only in the presence of

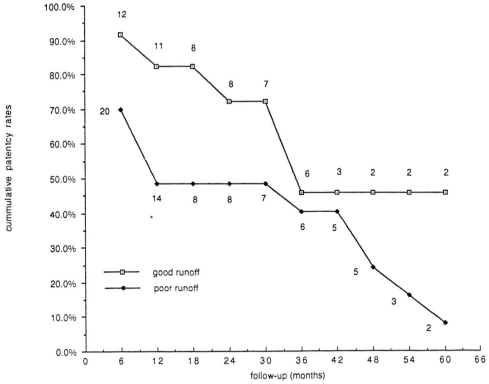

**Figure 21-4** Patency of femoral angioplasty with respect to runoff.

fibrin. Initial results suggest t-PA is as effective as urokinase and may require shorter infusion times.

Local intra-arterial thrombolysis involves selective placement of an arteriographic infusion catheter into the thrombosed artery and, if possible, into the thrombus itself. This placement allows direct infusion of relatively low doses of urokinase into the thrombus, resulting in improved thrombolysis without the bleeding complications associated with high-dose systemic therapy. Dosage regimens for urokinase vary, the most popular being continuous infusion of 60,000 to 80,000 units per hour, or infusion of 240,000 units per hour for two hours followed by 60,000 units per hour. We routinely administer heparin, 500 to 1000 units per hour, into the urokinase arterial catheter.

During infusion, the patient's status is monitored closely in an intensive care unit. Repeat angiography is performed periodically to determine the extent of lysis and to reposition the catheter into the residual thrombus if necessary. The infusion is continued until no further lysis is detected for 12 to 24 hours or until complications such as he-

morrhage necessitate premature termination of the infusion. Generally the longer the length of infusion, the more likely that systemic bleeding complications will occur. When infusion is completed, the underlying cause of the thrombosis, such as atherosclerotic narrowing, should be treated immediately either by surgery or angioplasty. Since lytic therapy may be prolonged, it should be performed only when the limb is in no immediate danger of loss. The average infusion time varies between 18 and 26 hours, depending upon the length and the age of thrombosis.

Intra-arterial thrombolytic therapy can be successfully used for occluded native arteries and occluded bypass grafts. Our principal use of thrombolytic therapy is in the salvage of thrombosed saphenous vein grafts to the tibial or pedal arteries (Fig. 21-5). The length of the graft often eliminates the use of arm veins as adequate conduit, and ischemia of the other leg prevents the use of the opposite saphenous vein. It is also useful for postarteriographic or postangioplastic arterial thrombosis and in many cases of arterial embolus (Fig. 21-6).

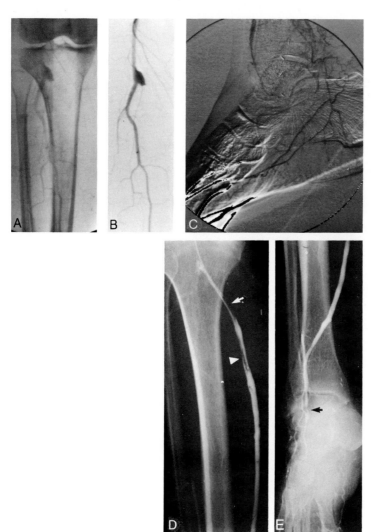

**Figure 21-5** Nonsubtracted *(A)* and subtracted *(B)* DSA of distal popliteal artery revealed a thrombosed popliteal-to-dorsalis pedis graft. Lateral foot view *(C)* failed to show the dorsalis pedis artery. *D,* After 12 hours of intra-arterial urokinase infusion through a catheter placed into the graft *(arrow),* partial lysis is noted with residual thrombus proximally *(arrowhead).* *E,* after 20 hours of urokinase infusion, complete lysis has occurred with flow into the previously nonvisualized dorsalis pedis artery. The distal anastomosis was severely narrowed by intimal hyperplasia *(arrow)* and was repaired surgically.

The more recent the thrombosis, the higher the success rate of thrombolytic therapy, with lysis of acute thromboses in up to 90 per cent of cases. In general, thrombolytic therapy is successful in approximately 80 per cent of all cases. At the present time, little information exists on the long-term patency of thrombolysed vein grafts.

Complication rates vary from 15 to 23 per cent, the most common being mild to marked bleeding. For this reason, contraindications to thrombolytic therapy involve those conditions in which bleeding is likely to occur (such as recent surgery or trauma, pregnancy, recent stroke, central nervous system tumor or other disease, or active internal bleeding). In diabetic patients, the possibility of retinal hemorrhage should be considered.

Other complications include pericatheter thrombosis and distal embolization, both of which generally can be treated with continued thrombolytic therapy, and complications of arteriography such as contrast-medium–induced renal failure.

## INTERVENTIONAL DEVICES

### Atherectomy Devices

The atherectomy devices rather recently developed offer an additional potential method for percutaneous treatment of atherosclerotic disease. As opposed to angioplasty, which disrupts the plaque and stretches the arterial wall, atherectomy de-

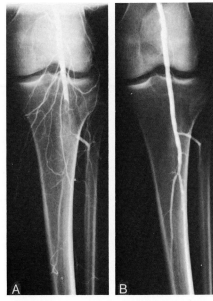

**Figure 21-6** Acute thrombosis of distal popliteal artery and peroneal-tibial trunk probably due to embolism *(A)*. Complete lysis after 16 hours of intra-arterial urokinase therapy into thrombus *(B)*. Distal posterior tibial and peroneal arteries are now patent.

vices mechanically remove atheromatous material. At this time only three devices have been approved for clinical use: the Simpson atherectomy catheter, the transluminal endarterectomy catheter, and the Kensey dynamic angioplasty catheter.

Only the Simpson catheter is designed to remove the bulk of the plaque, restoring patency without angioplasty. This approach is useful in relatively short stenoses or occlusions, but it is not used for diffuse disease. In theory, removal of atheromatous material results in a smooth surface with less turbulence and a lower incidence of dissection, improving long-term patency rates compared with angioplasty. Using this device, Althaus et al. reported a one-year patency rate of 92.5 per cent, which compares favorably to most angioplasty series.

The two other devices bore a small hole through the occluded artery to allow passage of an angiographic guide wire. Both require adjunctive angioplasty to open the artery completely. Neither of these devices has been studied in diabetic patients, and no long-term results are yet available. Wholey et al. reported 14 per cent recurrence with stenoses and 24 per cent recurrence with occlusions treated with the transluminal endarterectomy catheter.

The limited experience with the Kensey catheter prevents adequate evaluation at this time. Snyder et al. successfully recanalized 14 of 23 superficial femoral arteries using open surgical techniques, but only four of these were totally occluded arteries. Wholey et al. recanalized seven of eight totally occluded femoral arteries; of these, four reoccluded early, and one suffered distal embolization with only three arteries patent at 18 months.

## Laser Angioplasty

Initial enthusiasm for lasers in recanalizing femoral and popliteal arteries has waned as the technique has been found to have limited usefulness. Limited data on long-term patency are available in the nondiabetic patient but none specifically in the diabetic patient. In the hands of an experienced angiographer, most severe stenoses and short occlusions can easily be crossed with standard catheter and guide-wire techniques. The laser can be used successfully, however, to cross femoral and popliteal occlusions not treatable with other techniques. Like some atherectomy devices, the laser, whether argon or neodymium:yttrium-aluminum-garnet and whether a hot tip, sapphire tip, or direct-fiber design, forms only a 2- to 3-mm path through the occlusion to permit passage of a guide wire for subsequent angioplasty. In this respect, it has been a successful technique with up to 90 per cent of total occlusions being recanalized. The long-term patency rates, however, have not been shown to be appreciably better than those for angioplasty alone.

Cost of the laser unit exceeds $100,000 in some cases, in addition to the cost of installation and operation. Thus it is difficult to recommend it over mechanical atherectomy catheters that have similar success rates. Additional laser systems are being investigated, the most notable of which are the excimer laser and the directed laser. Their efficacy is not yet determined.

A radiofrequency thermal angioplasty system is also under investigation. A radiofrequency generator heats a hot-tip probe that is then used in the same fashion as the hot-tip laser. The uses and shortcomings are the same as those of the laser, although this system will be appreciably less expensive. At this time, few clinical data are available.

## SUGGESTED READING LIST

Althaus, S.J., Maynar, M., et al.: Clinical-pathologic-angiographic correlation following transluminal atherectomy. Presented at the Annual Meeting of the RSNA, Chicago, IL, 1989.

Becker, C.J., Rabe, F.E., Richmond, B.D., et al.: Low-dose fibrinolytic therapy: Results and new concepts. Radiology 148:663, 1983.

Belkin, M., Belkin, B., Bucknam, C.A., et al.: Intraarterial fibrinolytic therapy; efficacy of streptokinase versus urokinase. Arch. Surg. 121:769, 1986.

Casteneda-Zuniga, W.R., Formanek, A., Tadavarthy, M., et al.: The mechanism of balloon angioplasty. Radiology 135:565, 1980.

Dotter, C.T., and Judkins, M.P.: Transluminal treatment of arteriosclerotic obstruction: Description of a new technique and a preliminary report of its application. Circulation 30:654, 1964.

Gardiner, G.A., Meyerovitz, M.F., Stokes, K.R., et al.: Complications of transluminal angioplasty. Radiology 159:201, 1986.

Gardiner, G.A., Koltum, W., Kandarpa, L., et al.: Thrombolysis of occluded femoropopliteal grafts. AJR 147:621, 1986.

Grapr, R.A., Risius, B., Yound, J.R., et al.: Peripheral artery and bypass graft thrombolysis with recombinant human tissue type plasminogen activator. Circulation 72:III–XV(58), 1985.

Gruntzig, A., and Hopff, H.: Perkutane recakanalisation chronischer arterieller vershlusse mit newen. Dilatation skatheter. Dtsch. Med. Wochenschr. 99:2502, 1974.

Hewes, R.C., White, R.I., Murray, R.R., et al.: Long-term results of superficial artery angioplasty. AJR 146:1025, 1986.

Johnson, K.W., Rae, M., Hogg-Johnston, S.A., et al.: Five-year results of a prospective study of percutaneous transluminal angiography. Ann. Surg. 403, 1987.

Katzen, B., and van Breda, A.: Transluminal angioplasty of the iliac arteries. Semin. Intervent. Radiol. Suppl. 2:196, 1985.

Kensey, K.R., Nash, J.E., Abrahams, C., et al.: Recanalization of obstructed arteries with a flexible, rotating tip catheter. Radiology 165:387, 1987.

Lally, M.E., Johnston, K.W., and Andres, D.: Percutaneous transluminal dilatation of peripheral arteries: An analysis of factors predicting early success. J. Vasc. Surg. 1:704, 1984.

Lammer, J., Pilger, E., Neumayer, K., and Schreyer, H.: Intra-arterial fibrinolysis: Long-term results. Radiology 161:159, 1986.

Litvack, F., Grundfect, W.S., Adler, L., et al.: Percutaneous excimer-laser and excimer-laser-angioplasty of the lower extremities: Results of initial clinical trial. Radiology 172:331, 1989.

Lyon, R.T., Zarins, C.K., Lu, C-T, et al.: Vessel, plaque and lumen morphology after transluminal balloon angioplasty: Quantitative study in distended human arteries. Arteriosclerosis 3:306, 1987.

Maynar, M., Reyes, R., Cabreara, V., et al.: Percutaneous atherectomy with Simpson atherectomy device in the management of arterial stenosis. Semin. Intervent. Radiol. 5:247, 1988.

McNamara, T.O., and Fischer, R.: Thrombolysis of peripheral arterial and graft occlusions: Improved results using high dose urokinase. AJR 144:769, 1985.

Meyerovitz, M.F., Goldhaber, S.Z., Reagan, K. et al.: Tissue plasminogen activator versus urokinase: Randomized controlled trial in peripheral arterial occlusion. Presented at Annual Meeting of RSNA, Chicago, December, 1988.

Mok, W.Y.: Construction of the MCM smart laser. In Moore, W.S., and Ahn, S.S. (eds.): Endovascular Surgery. Philadelphia, W. B. Saunders Co., 1989, p. 453.

Nordstrom, L.A., and Young, E.G.: Direct laser recanalization of occluded superficial femoral and iliac arteries: Primary success and low complication rates. Semin. Intervent. Radiol. 5:277, 1988.

Sanborn, T.A., Cumberland, D.C., Greenfield, A.S., et al.: Percutaneous laser thermal angioplasty: Initial results and one-year follow-up in 129 femoropopliteal lesions. Radiology 168:121, 1988.

Simpson, J.B., Johnson, D.E., Thapliyal, H.V., et al.: Transluminal atherectomy: A new approach to the treatment of atherosclerotic vascular disease. Circulation 72(Suppl. 2):111, 1985.

Snyder, S.O., Wheeler, J.R., Gregory, R.T., et al.: Kensey catheter—early results with a transluminal atherectomy tool. J. Vasc. Surg. 8:541, 1988.

Stokes, K.R., Strunk, H.M., Campbell, D.R., et al.: Five-year results of iliac and femoropopliteal angioplasty in diabetic patients. Radiology 174:977, 1990.

van Breda, A., and Katzen, B.: Femoral angioplasty. Semin. Intervent. Radiol. Suppl. 1:251, 1984.

van Breda, A., Katzen, B.T., Picus, D., and Steinberg, D.L.: Intra-arterial urokinase infusion for treatment of acute and chronic arterial occlusions. Radiology 116:104, 1986.

van Breda, A., Robinson, J.C., and Feldman, L.: Local thrombolysis in the treatment of graft occlusions. J. Vasc. Surg. 1:103, 1984.

Walden, R., Siegel, Y., Rubinstein, Z.J., et al.: Percutaneous transluminal angioplasty. J. Vasc. Surg. 3:583, 1986.

Wholey, M.H., Jarmolowski, C.R., Rein, D. et al.: Multicenter trial with the transluminal endarterectomy catheter in 200 patients with peripheral vascular occlusive disease. Presented at the Annual Meeting of the RSNA, Chicago, 1989.

Wholey, M.H., Smith, J.A.M., and Godlewski, P.: Recanalization of total arterial occlusions with the Kensey dynamic angioplasty catheter. Radiology 172:95, 1989.

Zarins, C.K., and Glagov, S.: Histopathology of plaque dilatation and remodeling following balloon angioplasty. In Moore, W.S., and Ahn, S.S. (eds): Endovascular Surgery. Philadelphia, W. B. Saunders Co., 1989, p. 141.

Zarins, C.K., Lu, C-T, Gewertz, B.L., et al.: Arterial disruption and remodeling following balloon dilatation. Surgery 92:1086, 1982.

# Chapter 22

# RECONSTRUCTIVE FOOT SURGERY FOR THE DIABETIC PATIENT

GEOFFREY HABERSHAW, D.P.M.,
JAMES CHRZAN, D.P.M., and JOHN GIURINI, D.P.M.

Reconstructive foot surgery is designed to preserve as much viable tissue in the foot as possible. It is done when surgery becomes the conservative thing to do. The avoidance of even minor amputation is the major objective. We have shown with pedobarographic studies that force is distributed through distally preserved structures. To indiscriminately remove this tissue deprives the patient of more functional mechanical dissipation of forces. Amputation having been avoided with anatomical preservation keeps hope alive in these patients that they will not be a victim of limb loss, one of the greatest fears of the diabetic patient.

## INDICATIONS FOR SURGERY

1. Presence of nonhealing, chronic neuropathic ulceration with or without osteomyelitis after reasonable nonsurgical techniques have failed
2. Presence of a nonhealing, chronic ischemic ulceration with or without osteomyelitis after bypass surgery has been performed
3. Chronically recurring ulceration that will not remain healed with nonsurgical care

The guidelines for consideration of surgery must take into account certain factors. Acute sepsis must be absent. Incision and drainage with debridement of all necrotic tissue must be completed before a definitive procedure. Antibiotics are continued throughout the perioperative period. Cultures and sensitivities are used to adjust antibiotic coverage throughout. Vascular disease must be fully evaluated. Palpable dorsalis pedis and posterior tibial pulses are preferable when surgery is being considered. If they are absent, noninvasive vascular studies are recommended. Arteriography is necessary if it is apparent that adequate healing is not taking place despite bed rest, intravenous antibiotics, dressing changes, and good metabolic control of the diabetes mellitus. If bypass surgery is necessary, reconstructive surgery can be delayed until the patient's condition is stable and performed during the same admission.

Patients undergoing hemodialysis or peritoneal dialysis are particularly at risk for complications. Preoperatively, the diabetes should be under good control. Surgery should be planned for the day after hemodialysis because of the heparinization on the day of dialysis. Nephropathic patients should be admitted earlier and kept longer after surgery than non-nephropathic patients. Meticulous attention to non-weight bearing is very important. Physical therapy is of great help in getting these patients mobile enough to leave the hospital. Preoperative physical therapy consultation is recommended if possible. Post-transplant patients are at risk for complications due to immunosuppression. Peripheral neuropathy tends to be dense in these patients. Protection from decubitus heel ulcers is imperative.

## GOALS OF FOOT SURGERY

Goals of foot surgery in the *sensate* foot are to (1) decrease pain, (2) correct deformity, (3) improve function, and (4) improve ap-

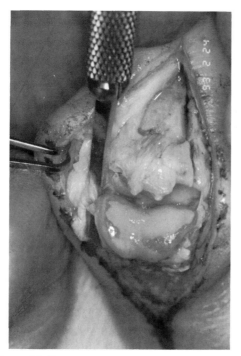

**Figure 22-3** Although no deep abscess or necrotic tissue was encountered, there is obvious destruction of the cartilage surface of the proximal phalangeal head. It will be removed, along with the base of the middle phalanx. There is no deep closure; only the skin is closed.

mal phalangeal head of the fifth toe and the proximal phalangeal base of the fourth toe pinch the skin in the web space. Chronic ulceration at this location can quickly lead to severe cellulitis and deep space infection.

Arthroplasty with hemiphalangectomy is the usual method of treatment. It is done whether or not osteomyelitis is present. The approach is usually a dorsolinear incision. We do not advise closed techniques or exostosectomy. A complete hemiphalangectomy or joint excision appears to work the best.

## LESSER METATARSAL ULCERATION—2, 3, 4, AND 5

After infection has been brought under control and peripheral vascular status is deemed adequate, consideration for lesser metatarsal osteotomy should take into account a few major factors. The location of the ulcer should be correlated as closely as possible with the offending metatarsal head. Clinical inspection alone may be all that is necessary to determine which metatarsal

head is implicated. Lead-marked anterior/posterior radiographs taken at 90 degrees to the foot and compared with physical examination are best. The depth of ulceration is very important when one is considering the surgical approach to the involved metatarsal.

If the ulceration can be probed to joint capsule but not into it and there is no synovial drainage, dorsal approach is preferred for metatarsal osteotomy (Fig. 22–5). If the joint may be entered with a sterile probe and/or synovial fluid is present where there is palpable bone, a plantar approach with excision of the ulcer and removal of the joint should be considered. This excision must include the metatarsal head, base of the proximal phalanx, and certainly all necrotic or avascular tissue, including flexor tendon when necessary.

It is true that isolated metatarsal osteotomy will upset the vertical force and shear distribution across the forefoot during gait. Central-column metatarsals 2, 3, and 4 function as a unit during gait. Whatever is done to one metatarsal will have profound effects on the forces that are transmitted to the skin by the remaining metatarsal. This may stimulate the development of transfer lesions. Orthotics and shoeing should be used to manage transfer lesions if they develop as hyperkeratoses. Chronically recurrent transfer ulcerations should be managed with additional metatarsal surgery.

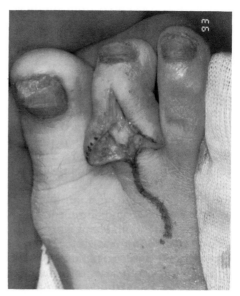

**Figure 22-4** The bone has been resected; the redundancy of the skin will allow for adequate closure.

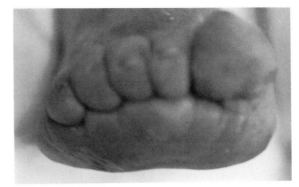

**Figure 22-5** Chronically recurrent neuropathic ulcer below the 4th metatarsal head. The ulcer is shallow with no evidence of joint involvement. Dorsal approach for osteotomy is the procedure of choice.

Multiple osteotomies should be delayed as an initial procedure if possible. It is reasonable, however, to proceed with multiple metatarsal osteotomies if transfer ulceration is a likely possibility. Previous lesser-metatarsal head resection of 2, 3, or 4 may justify the osteotomy of the remaining two metatarsals. Two long central-column metatarsals may also support multiple osteotomies. Osteotomy of all three mid-column metatarsals is occasionally done if the area of ulceration is widely spread below the mid-metatarsal heads. The ulceration does not have to be healed before surgery is carried out. Walling off the area with a preferred drape is all that is necessary. It prevents handling of the ulcer during surgery and helps avoid spread of infection from the ulcer to the surgical site.

Osteoclasis with a double-action bone cutter is the preferred procedure of choice (Fig. 22–6, 22–7). Through a dorsal incision the bone is cut just proximal to the plantar condyles. The long extensor tendon may be lengthened, but it is not necessary if the toe is straight with weight bearing. The long flexor tendon may be left alone. With fixed, rigid contracture of the distal toe, hemiphalangectomy should be done at the same time. This will lessen retrograde forces of the newly osteotomized metatarsal.

Digital dislocation, when it occurs, is invariably dorsal. The toe must be relocated. Preservation of the metatarsal heads should be foremost. Relocation can be achieved only by shortening the metatarsal. This is done by removing a section of the metatarsal shaft, approximately 0.5 to 1.0 cm. The base of the

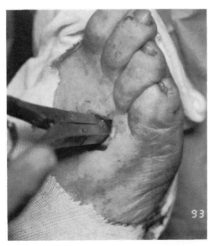

**Figure 22-6** A double-action bone cutting forceps is used to fracture the metatarsal at the surgical neck. The bone is cut with the forceps at 90 degrees to the long axis of the metatarsal. Crepitus at the osteotomy site should be palpated before closure.

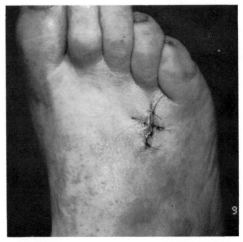

**Figure 22-7** Only the skin is closed after metatarsal osteotomy. The patient may use a postoperative surgical shoe to get to the bathroom and meal table only over the 1st week. The shoe should be worn for at least 4 weeks. Regular activity should not be resumed for 6 weeks.

phalanx should be preserved, if possible. Internal fixation is usually not done in these cases. Fixation with an 0.45 K wire exiting the end of the toe may be considered with normal peripheral vascular status in a cooperative patient. Concentration on non-weight bearing is the mainstay of postoperative care. Patients are usually kept in a postoperative shoe for three to four weeks. They are encouraged to remain off the foot, especially if there is still a plantar ulceration.

Ulceration below the fifth metatarsal head is treated quite nicely with isolated metatarsal osteotomy. The same rules apply for preoperative care as to bone infection or deep space involvement. Osteoclasis is just as effective as oblique osteotomy with power equipment. Postoperative and follow-up care is the same as with central-column osteotomy.

## FIRST RAY SURGERY

The most common location for plantar ulcerations in the neuropathic foot is the region of the first ray. Typical location for ulceration includes: (1) distal tip of the hallux, (2) plantar medial aspect of the interphalangeal joint, (3) direct plantar interphalangeal joint, (4) medial base of the proximal phalanx, or (5) directly below the first metatarsal phalangeal joint.

The etiology of ulceration in this region includes limited motion at the first metatarsal phalangeal joint, i.e. structural or functional hallux rigidus and hallux valgus. This can lead to heavy callous formation and blistering leading to ulceration. Arthritic changes seen in the first metatarsal phalangeal joint will structurally limit joint motion, increasing the risk of ulceration.

Ulcerations at the plantar medial aspect of the first metatarsal head and proximal phalangeal base may also be seen in the excessively pronated foot causing functional hallux limitus, usually in association with hallux abducto valgus. Morton divided the forefoot into sixths and estimated that two sixths of the forefoot pressure was borne by the first metatarsal. The lesser metatarsals bear one sixth of the body weight each. Studies performed by Cavanagh support these early observations.

## Interphalangeal Joint Arthroplasty

Ulcerations directly plantar to or medial to the interphalangeal joint or at the distal tip of the hallux respond quite nicely to interphalangeal joint arthroplasty. This procedure is typically done in the absence of hallux valgus. Bunionectomy would be considered in these cases.

A rigidly contracted digit, hallux hammer toe results in shoe irritation and ulceration dorsally or distally. Hyperextension of the joint typically results from hallux limitus, either functional or structural, resulting in a direct plantar or medial ulcer at the level of the interphalangeal joint. Excessive pronation loads the medial aspect of the hallux and the first ray such that the patient pivots on the medial condyle of the proximal phalanx. Both these situations can lead to ulceration. The arthroplasty relieves the intrinsic pressure from within the toe, allowing the ulceration to heal.

A curved incision is made over the interphalangeal joint. This allows excellent exposure of this wide joint, with minimal traction on the skin. The extensor mechanism is transversely incised, and the collateral ligaments are cut. The head of the proximal phalanx is exposed and transected. The cartilage is then rongeured off the base of the distal phalanx. This will most times lead to a rigid fibrous union between the proximal and distal phalanges. No form of external or internal fixation is required. The extensor mechanism is reapproximated with absorbable sutures and shortened if necessary. The long flexor tendon should not be disturbed if the toe is straight upon reapproximation of the distal phalanx. The dressing should be changed daily if there is open ulceration. If there is no ulceration, dressings may be changed at the third or fourth postoperative day. A postoperative shoe is used until the sutures are removed in two to three weeks. Weight-bearing status is determined by the condition of the ulcer. The ulcer should be fully healed before total weight bearing resumes. Complications may be masked by the peripheral neuropathy and further aggravated by excess activity. Condylectomy and exostosectomy have proven to be inadequate and should be avoided. These procedures can lead to joint instability and neuropathic fracture. It is best to proceed directly to complete arthroplasty.

## Keller Arthroplasty

Hallux limitus or rigidus, whether due to functional or structural changes, can lead to ulceration. These generally result from arthritic changes within the joint due to degenerative joint disease, trauma, or neuropathic fracture. Because there is lack of dorsiflexion at the first metatarsal phalangeal joint during propulsion, the leg will externally rotate and the toe may ulcerate at the head or base of the proximal phalanx. There may be some degree of hallux valgus. This procedure may also be applied to interphalangeal joint ulcers instead of arthroplasty when there is extensive degenerative joint disease at the first metatarsal phalangeal joint. We, however, have found that interphalangeal joint arthroplasty is simpler and avoids the greater degree of dissection required by the Keller arthroplasty when there is minimal degenerative joint disease.

The incision over the joint is made to bone. The skin is not undermined. The capsule is incised linearly. The base of the proximal phalanx is cut free from collateral ligament attachments and removed with a power saw. Sesamoids are removed only if there is any ulcer or preulcerative lesion below the first metatarsal head.

Hematoma can complicate this procedure. Close inspection of the wound for bleeding is imperative before closure. Closing all dead space is also important. The extensor hallucis longus tendon may be lengthened when necessary if it is contracted. After a Keller arthroplasty in neuropathic patients, seven to ten days of total non-weight bearing are preferred. No casting is necessary.

## Sesamoidectomy

The factors that predispose diabetic patients to the development of ulcerations directly below the first metatarsal head are increased weight bearing and shear forces that are significant through this area and progressive motor and sensory neuropathy. Early work and subsequent study by Cavanagh indicating greater forces below the first metatarsal phalangeal joint has already been cited. The intrinsic musculature is subject to progressive denervation. This leads to instability at the level of the metatarsophalangeal joints resulting in progressive plantarflexion defor-

mities of the metatarsals. Tibial and fibular sesamoid bones, normally located plantar to the first metatarsal head, play an important role in the normal function of the joints. As the first ray becomes progressively more plantarflexed, sesamoid bones become more prominent and contribute to the development of sub first metatarsal head ulceration. Planing procedures of the sesamoids for ulcer treatment have been ineffective in our hands. First metatarsal osteotomy carries increased morbidity and potential for complications. We have found sesamoidectomy to be extremely successful, with little morbidity for the patient, and to be highly effective in solving the problem of recurrent ulceration.

This procedure is not recommended if the ulceration probes into the joint or if osteomyelitis is present. Sesamoidectomy is preferred as an initial procedure, even in the presence of a rigidly plantarflexed first ray. Recurrence of the ulceration after sesamoidectomy will then lead us to perform condylectomy of the first metatarsal head. This is preferred over first metatarsal osteotomy at the head or the base.

Surgical approach for sesamoidectomy is through a plantar medial incision at the level of the first metatarsal phalangeal joint. This allows for excellent exposure of the tibial sesamoid and adequate exposure of the fibular sesamoid, should it be necessary to resect at the same time. Following a linear capsulotomy, further dissection and excision are facilitated by a No. 64 Beaver blade and sesamoid clamp. It is always necessary to excise the tibial sesamoid. The decision whether to proceed and excise the fibular sesamoid is based on intraoperative evaluation. Once the tibial sesamoid has been excised, if a plantar prominence remains directly under the first metatarsal head with the foot loaded to a weight-bearing position, it is recommended that the fibular sesamoid be excised as well. Care should be taken not to cut the flexor hallucis longus tendon when removing the fibular sesamoid. This is often necessary when the first metatarsal phalangeal joint is in rectus alignment. In the presence of a severe hallux abducto valgus deformity, the fibular sesamoid is often rotated dorsally into the first interspace and therefore does not contribute to the etiology of ulceration. The fibular sesamoid can be left alone in this case, with little risk of recurrent ulcer.

Two potential complications of this procedure are development of hallux hammer toe and hallux valgus. While we have not seen an increased incidence of hallux valgus in these patients, we have seen cases of hallux hammer toe develop when both sesamoids are removed in a rectus toe. We have elected not to attempt fusion of the interphalangeal joint in the primary procedure. One important modification that we believe reduces the risk of hallux hammer toe is lengthening of both the extensor and flexor hallucis longus tendons. This is done if there is flexible hammer toe of the digit preoperatively. Since incorporating this modification into our procedure, we have noted a significant reduction in the development of hallux hammer toe. As with any plantar incision, weight bearing should be restricted for three to four weeks. Ambulation should not be allowed while the ulcer remains opened.

If osteomyelitis of the sesamoid is present, it may be necessary to proceed with excision of the first metatarsophalangeal joint. Occasionally the osteomyelitis is not extensive, and an attempt is made to preserve the joint. In this case both sesamoids are removed through a plantar approach. The joint is copiously flushed and the wound is 90 per cent closed and left opened proximally. If drainage stops and cultures are negative, non-weight bearing is continued for four weeks. If drainage persists and cultures continue to grow pathogens from the osteomyelitis, then the joint is excised. It is also left partially opened proximally (Fig. 22–8, 22–9).

## PANMETATARSAL HEAD RESECTION

It is advisable to preserve the forefoot to distribute forces during gait and to allow continued use of conventional shoeing. Panmetatarsal head resection should be considered as an alternative to transmetatarsal amputation. When multiple osteotomies or metatarsal head resections have failed to alleviate the ulcerative process, panmetatarsal head resection should be used. It is done when acute sepsis is controlled. It is done through three or four dorsal linear incisions, or a plantar transverse incision for metatarsals 2 through 5 and medial incision for the first joint. The long extensor and long flexor tendons are left alone, unless they are infected. The metatarsal heads are degloved with the use of

McGlamry elevators. The osteotomies are done at the anatomical neck of the metatarsals. A Keller arthroplasty is done in conjunction with the first metatarsal head resection. The sesamoids should also be removed. Wounds are closed primarily when possible. When osteomyelitis is excised from a specific metatarsal, appropriate dependent drainage should be used from this site. Postoperative compression dressing along with posterior splint is commonly used after this procedure.

Conventional, extra-depth, and athletic shoes along with soft, molded orthotics are commonly used after this procedure. It is usually not necessary for the patient to obtain molded shoes or any other external bracing. Continued close follow-up of these patients is a must because of the propensity for heterotopic bone to develop at the cut bone surfaces. If specific ulcers begin to recur, suspicion of heterotopic bone should be entertained and metatarsal revision should be considered.

## SURGERY FOR THE CHARCOT FOOT

The vast majority of patients with Charcot foot should be able to be protected by the use of appropriate shoeing, orthoses, and altered habits. Regular follow-up is an absolute necessity for continued protection. It is not necessary to surgically restore an arch in every Charcot foot. Treating the acute Charcot deformity with total non-weight bearing until it consolidates assures a foot that can be shoed. The resulting deformity can be accommodated accordingly. Failure of the skin to remain closed in spite of attempts to treat nonsurgically should then require a more aggressive approach.

Surgery for the Charcot deformity can be done only in the absence of acute spreading sepsis. Incision and drainage, antibiotics, metabolic control of diabetes, and bed rest are imperative before further surgery is planned. All infected tissues should be radically excised. Only when acute sepsis is under control can elective surgery be planned. As stated earlier, the patient and the patient's family should understand that these procedures are being attempted to avoid the necessity of amputation.

There are two basic categories of surgery for the Charcot foot, exostosectomy—with

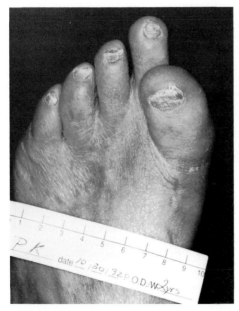 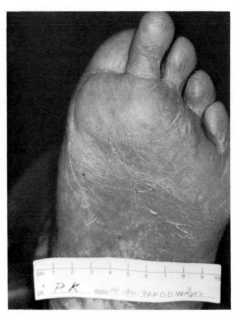

**Figures 22–8 and 22–9** A diabetic patient who had excision of the 1st metatarsophalangeal joint 2 years previously. He walks with extra-depth shoes and molded plastazote orthotics. There have been no recurrences and no transfer ulcers.

primary closure, split-thickness skin grafting, fasciocutaneous flaps or free flaps—and reconstruction of the mid foot, rear foot, and/or ankle.

Exostosectomy and planing procedures are done to remove a bony prominence that has surfaced as a result of adjacent bone destruction by the Charcot process. These procedures will not change the overall shape of the foot. Most common locations are plantar to the first metatarsal cuneiform joint and beneath the tarsal cuboid. The presence of an ulceration does not preclude surgery.

## First Metatarsal Cuneiform Joint

A medial approach to this ulceration gives the best exposure to the first metatarsal cuneiform joint (Fig. 22–10). The ulceration is walled off with the drape of choice so that the ulcer is not manipulated during surgery. If the ulcer probes to bone, it may be excised or left open to granulate and skin grafted at a later time. The incision is made to bone and the distal expansion of the tibialis anterior tendon is elevated along with the periosteum. A generous portion of bone is removed with an osteotome and mallet from the area of the first metatarsal cuneiform

joint plantarly. A drain is usually not necessary. A mild compression dressing is applied to thwart hematoma. A posterior splint is commonly used to limit motion and inhibit weight bearing.

The medial aspect of the foot tends to be straight (rectus) when this ulceration occurs. It is reasonable to expect that these patients should then return to extra-depth shoes with molded inserts alternating during the day with athletic shoes. It is an exception that they should require molded shoes.

The expected outcome of this procedure is nonrecurrence of ulceration and ambulation. It does not seem to matter whether the first metatarsal cuneiform joint is fused and fixated with staples or planed at the plantar aspect of the joint. Both groups of patients appeared to do equally as well inasmuch as they returned to ambulation without recurrence of ulceration. Arthrodesis is reasonable to consider if there is an excessive degree of motion at the joint. Care must be taken to ensure complete healing of the arthrodesis with eight weeks of strict non-weight bearing in a splint or removable cast.

## Cuboid Exostosectomy

This common location of ulceration in the Charcot foot will eventually deteriorate to

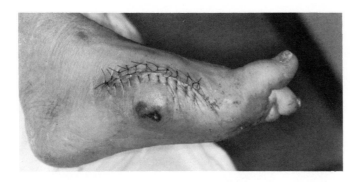

**Figure 22–10** Surgical approach to first metatarsal cuneiform exostosectomy. The ulcer is covered during the surgery. The surgical debridement is done through the ulcer if there is osteomyelitis or deep sepsis.

sepsis and loss of the foot if steps are not taken to alleviate them. The best treatment is to prevent ulceration by following the guidelines for management of Charcot fracture, i.e. total non-weight bearing until bony consolidation, then advancement to appropriate molded shoeing and thick padded soft orthotics.

When the midfoot collapses, including the metatarsal bases and the cuneiforms, the cuboid is usually spared. The forefoot abducts and dorsiflexes, transferring weight bearing from the ball of the foot to the midfoot. Talar declination increases, and the calcaneal inclination decreases. This places additional stress over the dorsum of the cuboid, driving it against the plantar skin where pressure and shear are intensified, leading to blistering and ulceration.

When nonsurgical measures fail to allow the ulcer to close, exostosectomy should be considered. As long as there is no abscess, peripheral vascular disease, or distal bypass graft, an ankle tourniquet is usually used during this procedure. The patient is best positioned prone or in the right decubitus position for right foot ulcer or left decubitus position for left foot ulcer. This gives a good view of the plantar surface of the foot and will expedite protection of vital plantar structures. An ulcer less than 2.0 cm in size can usually be excised and closed primarily. If the ulcer is larger than this, grafting can be considered after exostosectomy. Grafting should not be attempted without exostosectomy because of the importance of removing the plantar bony prominence. A full-thickness fasciocutaneous flap based on the posterior tibial blood supply, with split-thickness skin graft over the harvest area, is usually the coverage of choice (Fig. 22–11). This allows almost complete removal of scarred tissue at the ulcer site. Usually a large amount of ad-

ventitious bursal tissue is encountered at the level of the plantar fascia. This can be left in place if it was not exposed through the ulcer. Exposure of this tissue through the ulcer site requires its complete removal. This bursal tissue has poor blood supply and may remain as a source of sepsis if left behind.

Sharp and blunt dissection should then continue to the peroneal ridge of the cuboid. Just medial to the ridge is a large branch of the lateral plantar artery that usually must be ligated. The peroneus longus tendon distal to the ridge is then sacrificed to expose the

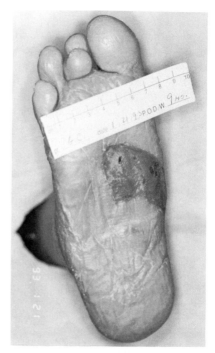

**Figure 22–11** Fasciocutaneous flap after exostosectomy and removal of the ulcer below the cuboid. This is 9 months after operation. The split-thickness skin graft is holding up nicely, despite its plantar location. A molded shoe with plastazote insert is the shoe of choice.

plantar surface of the cuboid. A large plantar section of the cuboid is then saucerized with an osteotome and mallet. Copious flushing ensues. The tourniquet is released, and all active bleeding must be controlled before closure.

Hematoma is a common complication of this procedure. A drain may be used if active bleeding cannot be stopped or capillary oozing persists. The peroneus longus tendon may be reopposed; however, no difference in outcome has been observed when this has not been done. Closure is done in layers. Total non-weight bearing must be prescribed for one month or longer if the ulceration fails to heal. It is common to encounter superficial dehiscence, especially if the ulcer has been ellipsed out. A repeat of the procedure should be considered if the ulcer fails to heal, especially if it continues to probe deeply. Walking should not be resumed until all healing has occurred. Reconstruction is usually reserved until exostosectomy, grafting, and flaps have failed.

## Reconstructive Foot Surgery of the Midfoot

The goal of reconstructive foot surgery is to stabilize the foot. The failed union of a

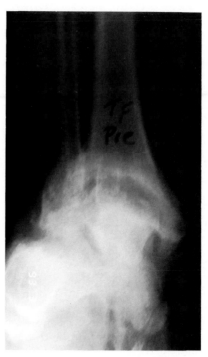

**Figure 22–13** Anteroposterior radiograph of a 59-year-old diabetic with neuropathic fracture of the os calcis and talus, depression fracture of the tibial plafond, and lateral malleolar fracture. Lateral deviation of the foot is seen. Ulceration over the lateral malleolus was a chronic problem.

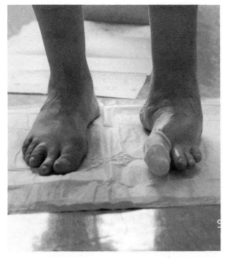

**Figure 22–12** This post-transplant diabetic patient continually develops ulceration in the area of the fifth metatarsal base. He lost the peroneus longus and peroneus brevis tendons to infection. The tibialis posterior has inverted the foot. There is no neuropathic fracture. Triple arthrodesis is the preferred procedure.

Charcot fracture may allow motion through fibrous and/or nonunion fracture sites. Correction of deformity in the transverse plane, with rectus medial and lateral columns, should be attempted. Sagittal plane correction, or restoration of an arch, is not necessary. These procedures are usually accompanied by Achilles tendon lengthening. This significantly shortens stride length, thereby diminishing deforming forces through the midfoot during gait. The use of a rigid, padded, ankle-foot orthosis is also recommended after these procedures. Ankle-foot orthoses minimize the chance of additional Charcot fracture at the ankle when walking resumes.

The midfoot is approached with a long medial and lateral incision made directly to bone. The dissection is carried across the dorsum and plantar aspects of the midfoot at the level of the periosteum. Perforating arteries can be avoided if the dissection is kept proximal to the metatarsal bases. An appropriate section of bone is removed, including fibrous tissue and nonunion fracture fragments. Grafting is not necessary as long as bleeding bone surfaces are opposed. Fixation should be rigid with desired technique, for example, pins, staples, screws. A drain should be used because of the extensive dissection. A posterior splint is left in place for several days, then a below-knee non-weight-bearing cast is used. This is changed every two to three weeks for the next three to four months. X-rays are obtained monthly to follow progress of the fusion. The extended period of non-weight bearing may necessitate preoperative placement planning in a nursing or rehabilitation facility. The use of molded shoes with thick molded orthotics is usually necessary after these procedures.

## Triple Arthrodesis

Triple arthrodesis is selected as an isolated procedure when deformity at the subtalar joint and midtarsal joint is contributing to ulcerative changes that cannot be controlled with shoeing, orthosis, and bracing (Fig. 22–12). There is not necessarily a Charcot fracture. It is most common to use this procedure when there is isolated or combined uncompensated rear foot varus and forefoot varus and equinus deformity. The ankle joint is intact. The ulcer will usually be along the lateral aspect of the foot at the fifth metatarsal base. The fifth metatarsal base is planed at the same time the triple arthrodesis is accomplished. Talonavicular dislocation with severe calcaneal valgus and chronic medial ulceration should also cause triple arthrodesis to be considered. The ankle joint should be intact.

The procedure is done with medial and lateral incisions exposing the talonavicular, calcaneal cuboid, and subtalar joints. All cartilage is removed, along with subchondral bone, and fixated with staples, screws, or pins. Tendo Achillis lengthening is also done for reasons previously described. It is best to attempt to correct the varus and valgus deformities at the time of surgery. It is always best to leave the foot in a slight degree of valgus. Splints, casts, and extended non-weight bearing are similarly utilized as with midfoot fusion. Rigid, padded ankle-foot orthoses are used when ambulation begins.

## Pantalar Arthrodesis

Pantalar arthrodesis should be attempted when the foot has moved medially or laterally off the tibial plafond. This usually means the medial or lateral malleolus has fractured as part of the Charcot process. This type of fracture is not conducive to continual weight bearing because of the high probability of ulceration and infection. The objective of surgery is to stabilize the foot under the tibia so it will not move medially or laterally. Viability and integrity of the talus and calcaneus will lead to the greatest chance of successful fusion. The greater the talar and calcaneal involvement in the Charcot process, the less chance there will be of bony union and eventual stability (Fig. 22–13). Talectomy is necessary if the talar body and neck are comminuted. Calcaneotibial fusion has a low potential for success, but it is reasonable to attempt before amputation. The midtarsal joint and calcaneal cuboid joints are fused at

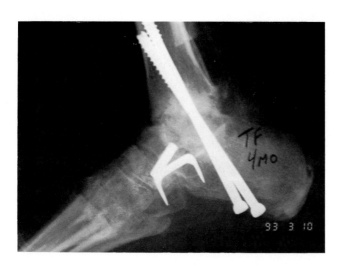

**Figure 22–14** Four months after pantalar arthrodesis. The distal fibula was resected and used for bone graft. The patient wears a padded ankle-foot orthosis. He began to ambulate at 4 months after operation with a walker and close supervision by physical therapists.

the same time, along with Achilles tendon lengthening. Although the efficacy of bone stimulation devices has not been definitively proven in this setting, we are in favor of using one. Implantable, intraoperative coil placement at the fusion site is preferred. Bone grafting of choice is an important part of the procedure for expected successful arthrodesis.

The procedure and the method of fixation must be individually selected by the clinical situation and surgeon's preference. Internal fixation with crossed cannulated screws is the preferred method. External fixation should be considered if there is sepsis at the ankle joint, especially if it must be left open. Nonweight bearing must continue for four or more months. Extensive physical therapy preoperatively and postoperatively and during the recuperative period is vitally important to try to maintain musculoskeletal flexibility and strength.

## SUGGESTED READING LIST

Cavanagh, P. R., Hennig, E. M., Rodgers, M. M., Sanderson, D. J.: The measurement of pressure distribution on the plantar surface of diabetic feet. In Whittle, M., Harris, D. (eds.): Biomechanical Measurement in Orthopedic Practice. Oxford, Clarendon Press, 1985, pp. 160–166.

Habershaw, G. M., Gibbons, G. W., Rosenblum, B. I.: A historical look at the transmetatarsal amputation and its changing indications. J. Am. Podiatry Assoc. 83:79–81, 1993.

Barry, D. C., Sabacinski, K. A., Habershaw, G. M., et al.: Tendo achilles procedures for chronic ulcerations in diabetic patients with transmetatarsal amputations. J. Am. Podiatry Assoc. 83:96–100, 1993.

Giurini, J. M., Basile, P., Chrzan, J. S., et al.: Panmetatarsal head resection: a viable alternative to the transmetatarsal amputation. J. Am. Podiatry Assoc. 83:101–107, 1993.

Giurini, J. M., Chrzan, J. C., Gibbons, G. W., Habershaw, G. W.: Sesamoidectomy for the treatment of chronic neuropathic ulcerations. J. Am. Podiatry Assoc. 81:167–173, 1991.

Giurini, J. M., Habershaw, G. M., Chrzan, J. S.: Panmetatarsal head resection in chronic neuropathic ulceration. J. Foot Surg. 26:249–252, 1987.

Tillo, T. H., Giurini, J. M., Habershaw, G. M., et al.: Review of metatarsal osteotomies for the treatment of neuropathic ulcerations. J. Am. Podiatry Assoc. 80:211–217, 1990.

McGlamry, E. D., Banks, A. S., Downey, M. S.: Comprehensive Textbook of Foot Surgery, Volumes I and II. Baltimore, Williams & Wilkins, 1992.

# Chapter 23

# AMPUTATIONS

FRANK C. WHEELOCK, Jr., M.D.,
GARY W. GIBBONS, M.D., and
DAVID R. CAMPBELL, M.D.

There may be 12 million diabetics in the United States at this time, counting both those with recognized disease and those whose disease is undiagnosed. Practically 25 per cent of these will sooner or later need to consult a physician or podiatrist for problems with a foot, and a certain number of these will eventually require an amputation of one type or another. In this chapter we will discuss simple toe amputations, toe plus metatarsal head amputations, transmetatarsal amputations (of all the toes and metatarsal heads), guillotine leg amputations, and below- and above-knee amputations of the leg. We will consider the pathological conditions leading to this type of operation, make a few comments about the prevention of amputations, and describe preoperative and postoperative care, and surgical principles and technique. Results to be expected from the various procedures will be outlined as well. One interesting observation that we have made through the years is that most diabetics, when informed of the need of some form of amputation, accept the fact with greater equanimity than do nondiabetics. The presumption is that ever since they have known of their disease, they have been made aware by way of reading and contact with others that the day might come when such a procedure would be indicated for them.

## HISTORICAL PERSPECTIVE

Fifty years ago Dr. Eliott Joslin asked Dr. Leland McKittrick to be the surgeon responsible for his diabetic patients. He set up the foot room where a foot nurse and a podiatrist were always available. He was the first to pub-

licize the transmetatarsal amputation as a useful procedure in limb salvage in the diabetic. The patients selected for this operation fell into two basic groups: The first was those with good circulation and severe neuropathy. Paralysis of the intrinsic foot muscles led to foot deformity and chronic toe and metatarsal head injury. Superficial lesions were treated with bed rest and antibiotics. Deep lesions involving the bone required toe, ray, and transmetatarsal amputation (TMA). The second group was basically ischemic; it was found that if there was no dependent rubor at the level of the amputation, a transmetatarsal amputation would heal with a good rate of success. This was particularly true of those patients who had isolated tibial disease. As this situation was peculiar to diabetics, the TMA became known as the "diabetic operation."

From the mid fifties through the seventies there was tremendous progress in vascular surgery. Drs. Wheelock and Hoar performed numerous femoral popliteal bypasses on diabetics with ischemic feet. They were able to produce results that were as good as reported series for nondiabetics. This significantly reduced the number of patients requiring below-knee or TMA's. However, there remained the large group of patients with isolated tibial disease who were not candidates for revascularization, and for them TMA offered an opportunity for limb salvage.

Since 1980 a number of advances have occurred to significantly reduce the number of patients requiring major leg or partial foot amputations. First, with improved understanding of the way in which neuropathy leads to tissue loss, our podiatric group is straightening toes and performing metatarsal

## TABLE 23–1.  CURRENT INDICATIONS FOR AMPUTATIONS

**MINOR AMPUTATIONS**
1. Open amputation as part of debridement in control of acute infection.
2. Chronic neuropathic ulcer: When too much tissue loss has occurred to save digit.
3. Ischemia: After infection is controlled and limbs revascularized to create functional walking foot.

**MAJOR AMPUTATIONS** (below knee and above knee)
1. Extensive tissue loss.
2. Unreconstructible ischemia.
3. Failed revascularization.
4. Charcot's disease of the ankle causing instability of the foot.

osteotomies to prevent the consequences of the claw foot. This has dramatically reduced the number of toe amputations that we now perform. Second, with chronic infection involving the metatarsal heads, it is now possible to remove the metatarsal heads and leave the toes. In the right situation this produces a better cosmetic and functional result than the TMA. Finally, the introduction of the in situ technique and arterial digital subtraction arteriography has allowed us to revascularize many patients with isolated tibial arterial occlusion who, in the past, would not even have been subjected to arteriography. It can certainly be said that the popliteal to dorsalis pedis artery bypass graft has displaced the TMA as the "diabetic operation." These changes are reflected in the decreased incidence of major and minor amputations at the Deaconess, and the current indications for amputation (Table 23–1).

## PREVENTION OF AMPUTATIONS

As in all fields of medicine and surgery, prevention is by far the better approach; therefore, a few words about it seemed appropriate. Dealing with the infection, it is important to realize that it usually will follow trauma to the foot by such mundane causes as improperly fitting shoes, lack of good care of the toenails, injury on walking barefoot, problems arising from epidermophytoses, and so on. If the portal of entry for the infection does not exist, infection is uncommon.

If a diabetic patient has neuropathy with a numb foot, this should be recognized as a dangerous situation. The foot needs to be inspected daily. If the patient cannot do this because of poor vision or any reason, someone else should look at the feet every night. If a build-up of callus is noted, podiatric care should be sought and perhaps the pressure in areas of the foot redistributed by appropriate appliances. Small injuries should also be noted and appropriate treatment provided. Since in many neuropathic feet circulation is excellent, it should be possible to avoid amputations secondary to neuropathic complications by simple preventive measures.

The most common pathological situation leading to an amputation is ischemia. Prevention would take two forms. An attempt should be made by the patient to prevent arteriosclerotic blockages of the artery by avoiding the presently recognized contributors to arteriosclerotic changes. Tobacco in any form should not be used, excess weight should be avoided, a tendency to hypertension should be carefully controlled, good diabetic control should be sought enthusiastically, elevated triglycerides or cholesterol levels should be lowered by appropriate means, and an exercise program should be instigated, tailored to the patient's situation.

When arterial occlusive disease has occurred and the foot is in an ischemic state, consideration should be given to arterial reconstruction as described in Chapters 19 and 20. In addition, once the state of ischemia has been recognized, great care should be taken to prevent injury to the foot by the simple means previously discussed. An extremely ischemic foot can continue to serve the patient in many instances if skin breakdown can be avoided. Therefore, any amount of effort to avoid the initial ulceration or necrosis of the skin is important because once it has occurred, the situation may be irreversible.

## PREOPERATIVE CARE

It is important that patients facing an amputation, however minor, be suitably prepared for it. We will not discuss the general situation in depth because it has been covered elsewhere. Diabetics who reach the state of needing any type of amputation probably have major cardiovascular and renal problems and therefore warrant a careful general evaluation before any operation is done.

The patient who enters the hospital in

need of a local amputation of the foot because of infection or neuropathy and who has good circulation would presumably be able to have amputation carried out relatively soon after admission. If a local abscess is present, this would be drained initially in some instances and a more definitive procedure done secondarily. In cases of life-threatening infection, it may be necessary to perform a guillotine amputation initially to allow the infection to be brought under control prior to definitive closed amputation and drainage. At other times when the infection might not be serious, control could be attained with antibiotics alone and then definitive surgery carried out. Patients with significant infection in the foot should be kept at absolute bed rest and their diabetes controlled effectively prior to operation.

The diabetic foot with ischemia and infection is a more complex problem. After infection is controlled with intravenous antibiotics and appropriate incision and drainage or open amputation, the leg must be revascularized, and then closed amputation as indicated can be performed to restore a walking foot. In the occasional patient with unreconstructible ischemia, infection must be controlled and a closed amputation performed because open amputations rarely heal in the presence of ischemia.

## ANESTHESIA AND PRINCIPLES OF TECHNIQUE

The anesthesiologist will decide on the type of anesthesia as a rule, whether general, spinal, regional, or local. In many neuropathic feet the procedure can be carried out without pain to the patient and without anesthesia. In several patients we have carried out amputations of toes or a transmetatarsal amputation in such circumstances with no anesthesia and no pain. On at least two occasions one of us has been able to do a below-knee amputation on a patient in a similar fashion.

Good general surgical principles and technique demand that tissues of diabetics, whether they have ischemic problems or neuropathic ones, be handled very delicately because they are easily injured. Gentleness in handling of tissues at the operating table is of paramount importance. Clean, carefully made incisions that are not undermined are

essential. Bleeding points are controlled by hemostats, with only the vessel or extremely small bites of tissue being taken when the instrument is applied. Usually each hemostat is tied after it has been placed so that it does not dangle from the incision and injure the tissue by its weight or by hands or instruments brushing against it. Very fine ties are used for the vessels in foot surgery.

It is important to achieve excellent hemostasis, since a small hematoma may further damage the blood supply or lead to sinus formation and result in an unsuccessful operation. No dead space should be left if an operation is to succeed in the face of ischemia, since serum will collect there and easily become infected. If a dead space must be left, as is the case when removing the second, third, or fourth toes and metatarsal heads, it is necessary to place a small, dependent gauze drain. Simple gauze drains work well. These are made by appropriately twisting a small $2 \times 2$ or similar piece of gauze into a tubular structure and placing it through a dependent skin opening into the area to be drained. Skin closure is usually made with small monofilament interrupted skin sutures of fine stainless steel wire or plastic material. In the foot, subcutaneous sutures are not used because it is thought that they produce more injury to the blood supply and accomplish little. As noted previously, one should aim for *primary wound closure in the ischemic foot* and not expect an open amputation to heal. Any retraction should be done with great care to avoid injury to these vulnerable tissues. For instance, in doing a transmetatarsal amputation of the forefoot, we never permit any retractor to be placed on the skin of the dorsum of the foot, lest it be pulled from the deeper tissues through which the blood supply is coming.

## SINGLE TOE AMPUTATION

### Indications

In its simplest form, which we will first discuss, amputation implies the removal of a single toe through the proximal phalanx. In a neuropathic foot such a procedure might be indicated because so much skin has been lost that healing cannot be accomplished in the presence of osteomyelitis or a septic interphalangeal joint, or because of recurring ulcers on the tip or the dorsum of the toe as in hammer toe. In an ischemic foot the procedure might be indicated to treat severe necrotic ulceration of the distal third or even the distal half of the toe. Osteomyelitis distally located would be another indication to remove such a toe.

## Requirements

It must be decided whether the amputation can be accomplished by a conservative operation such as transphalangeal removal of the digit. In the neuropathic foot with good circulation, this procedure could be accomplished if there were enough viable skin left to permit healing, either by primary or secondary intention. If enough uninfected, healthy skin were available, healing could be expected from such a procedure. The requirements are more difficult to meet in the ischemic foot. The lesion in this circumstance must be distally located so that the proximal skin will be healthy enough to heal. This means that the lesion would usually need to involve only the distal third of the toe or perhaps the distal half. If the necrosis and discolored skin are too close to the necessary skin incision line, healing will not occur. Circulation must be evaluated by means previously discussed including the venous filling time* and presence of dependent rubor.†

## Surgical Technique
(Figs. 23–1 to 23–3)

After a careful skin preparation of the operative field and draping, the adjacent toe or toes are gently retracted medially and laterally by gauze slings placed around them. The toe to be removed is grasped at the tip with a towel clip as a convenient means of holding it. Usually medial and lateral flaps are used because this is the area in which the digital

*Venous filling time is measured by first elevating the patient's feet while he lies supine on the examining table. The patient then sits up and hangs his feet over the side of the table. The first second that any vein is seen protruding above a tangent to the skin surface is taken as the venous filling time. Normally this might be around 10 seconds. A level higher than 20 to 25 seconds indicates severe ischemia.

†Dependent rubor is a dark red discoloration of the skin of the foot on dependency, a sign of severely impaired circulation at the level of redness. In general, amputations performed through such a red area will not heal.

arteries run. These flaps also give the added advantage of allowing dependent drainage onto the dorsum of the foot in case infection develops. Infrequently it is preferable to use anterior and posterior flaps, depending on the location of the skin lesions. These may be initiated with a first toe amputation because of the shape of the first phalanx. In creating the flaps, great care is taken not to undermine the skin so that all possible blood supply is preserved right up to the very cut edge of epidermis. The flexor and extensor tendons are divided in line with the skin incisions. We think it is poor practice to pull the tendons down, cut them, and allow them to retract up into the sheaths, because this leaves an empty cylinder in the tendon sheath to collect fluid, which may become infected. We believe it is preferable to have the cylindrical tendon sheaths filled with tendon right to the point of division but not protruding beyond. The proximal phalanx is then divided with a double-action bone cutter. The end of the bone is very carefully rongeured back as far as necessary for closure to be easily attained and so that the toe will not protrude more than a few millimeters below the level of the web spaces. It is dangerous to have the toe protrude 1 cm or more because it may then rub the adjacent

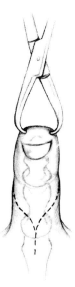

**Figure 23–1** This illustrates the lateral skin flaps, the proximal incision for drainage if necessary, and the level of cutting the proximal phalanx to leave a button of bone. (From Wheelock, F. C., Jr.: Surgical Techniques Illustrated. Little, Brown, Boston, Vol. 3, No. 3, 1978.)

incision directly down to the bone, saving all possible subcutaneous tissue in which blood is circulating. In separating the metatarsophalangeal joint of the involved toe from the next one, great care is taken to avoid entering into the joint that will be left behind since an incision would probably introduce infection and result in failure later. After removing the specimen by dividing the metatarsal shaft at an appropriate angle, the bone end is rongeured smooth to give a good contour to the foot. The skin flaps are approximated from time to time by hand and held while the contour of the foot is felt to be sure that there is no projecting shelf of metatarsal bone. Once this is accomplished and hemostasis is securely attained, the incision is irrigated very thoroughly with antibiotic solution and then closure of the distal portion is made with interrupted monofilament sutures. Flaps are trimmed so there is not an excess of skin but enough so that an easy closure with a minimum of dead space left behind may be achieved. A gauze wick drain is placed from the open, dependent portion of the incision and pushed up into the cavity. A suitable dressing is applied.

In the case of the second, third, or fourth toe and metatarsal heads, a similar procedure is carried out except that in this case the "handle" of the racquet incision runs down the sole of the foot. Again the incision is

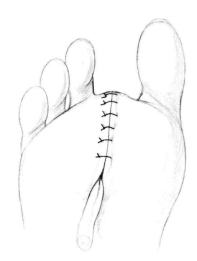

**Figure 23–9** The distal wound is closed (re-roofed) and a wick is placed in the proximal wound to drain the underlying dead space. (From Wheelock, F. C., Jr.: Surgical Techniques Illustrated. Little, Brown, Boston, Vol. 3, No. 3, 1978.)

carried sufficiently far so that dependent drainage will be achieved. At the proximal end of the incision, the skin is cut farther than the fat, which is cut farther than the fascia so that any fluid can run smoothly out of the cavity and not be dammed by a shelf-like end of the incision.

## Postoperative Care
(Figs. 23–7 to 23–9)

The healing of this type of operation will take longer than that of a simple toe amputation. Only when healing is complete and the defect firmly closed in should weight bearing be permitted. Usually, special shoes will not be required for a patient who has had a single-digit amputation, either through the phalanx or through the metatarsal shaft. Occasionally if there are problems with other portions of the foot, a special innersole and a special shoe are invaluable.

We have not mentioned a disarticulation procedure. This is because we consider it to be a very poor choice of operation. Cartilage has poor resistance to infection and has essentially no blood supply, so that healing can become a serious problem. Therefore it seems inappropriate to disarticulate a digit and expect a good result.

During the postoperative period, dressings are changed at frequent intervals and as soon

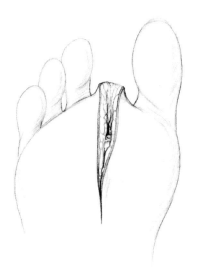

**Figure 23–8** The toe and its metatarsal head are removed, taking great care *not* to injure or enter the joint space of the adjacent toes. (From Wheelock, F. C., Jr.: Surgical Techniques Illustrated. Little, Brown, Boston, Vol. 3, No. 3, 1978.)

as the gauze wick loosens in the incision, it is changed daily, lest it act as a cork. Sutures are usually left in for several weeks.

## TRANSMETATARSAL AMPUTATION

### Indications

Transmetatarsal amputation is the removal of all five toes and all five metatarsal heads, producing a short foot. Coverage of the end of the foot is achieved by an appropriately long plantar flap brought up over the end of the foot much like a Turkish slipper. In a neuropathic foot, it is an appropriate operation when there has been destruction of several toes or several metatarsal heads. If the problem has previously involved two adjacent metatarsophalangeal joints, transmetatarsal amputation is needed because healing is difficult in a foot from which two adjacent metatarsals have been removed. Such a foot is also limited in function. Consequently, when the problem in a neuropathic foot has reached this stage, a more useful foot is produced by means of a transmetatarsal amputation.

In the case of the ischemic foot, a transmetatarsal amputation has the advantage over a more distal operation in that the blood supply is better proximally in the foot. In addition to this advantage is the fact that this operation is often needed because of the proximal location of ischemic ulceration on the foot. Thus it is frequently used when there is an area of gangrenous ulceration in the webbed space, over a metatarsal head, medially, laterally, or inferiorly, or in the proximal area of the toe itself. On some occasions even a distal toe lesion requires a transmetatarsal amputation because the blood supply at the proximal portion of the toe is too poor to permit healing. If an ulcer is present beneath a metatarsal head, it can frequently be excised by means of a V-shaped incision in the plantar flap with removal of the triangular area of skin containing the ulcer. The closure in such a case eventually is made in the form of a T.

Another indication for a transmetatarsal procedure is the presence of multiple toe lesions in an ischemic foot. In this case it may not be prudent to amputate individual toes lest the failure of any one amputation cost the patient the extremity.

### Requirements for Success

In the case of neuropathic feet, which account for less than one third of our transmetatarsal amputations, the only requirement is that there be enough skin somewhere to use for closure and that any seriously active or spreading infections be controlled preoperatively by antibiotics and appropriate drainages. Even if skin destruction has occurred to such an extent that complete closure cannot be made because of lack of skin on either the plantar or dorsal aspect, it still may be possible to carry out a transmetatarsal amputation with skin grafting either at the time of surgery or subsequently. In the case of the ischemic foot careful evaluation is made of the circulation before a decision is made to use this procedure. The requirement to be met is control of all active infections, because primary closure is made when there is ischemia. This may take from several days to three weeks to achieve. If it cannot be accomplished in three weeks, a higher amputation should be chosen. The venous filling time should be 20 to 25 seconds or less and dependent rubor should be minimal or absent at the area where incision is proposed. The forefoot tracing of the pulse volume recording is also helpful in determining whether the amputation is likely to heal.

### Technique (Figs. 23–10 to 23–16)

After suitable preparation and draping, the operator places a sponge around the toes and holds the toes in his nondominant hand until a specimen has been removed, following which he changes his glove. A slightly curving incision is made across the dorsum of the foot 1 cm or so proximal to the web spaces; it ends just proximal to the bones of the first and fifth metatarsal heads. It is carried straight down through all the tissues to the metatarsal shaft. No retractors are placed on the dorsal skin and bleeding vessels are secured with small hemostats. Each one is tied as it is placed, so that at no time does anything pull at the dorsal skin. Plantar incision is then made in a gentle sweep from the two corners of the dorsal incision, creating a plantar flap that comes down to within 1 cm of the web spaces. Again the incision is carried down to the subcutaneous tissues and through the tendons, which are kept on the

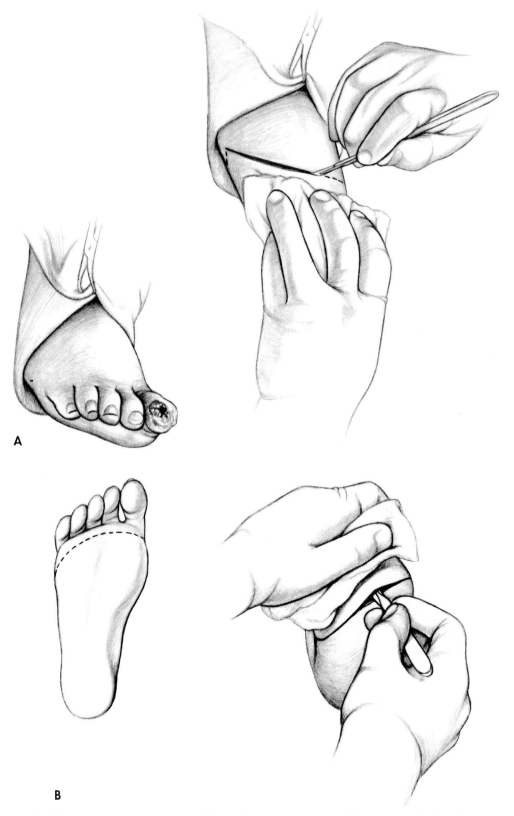

**A**

**B**

**Figure 23–10** *A,* The forefoot is grasped and held with a sponge or towel while the incisions are being made and until the specimen has been removed. The dorsal incision is made straight down to the metatarsals, leaving a full-thickness incision from skin to bones. *B,* The plantar incision is made easier if the toes are sharply dorsiflexed. (From Wheelock, F. C., Jr.: Surgical Techniques Illustrated. Little, Brown, Boston, Vol. 3, No. 3, 1978.)

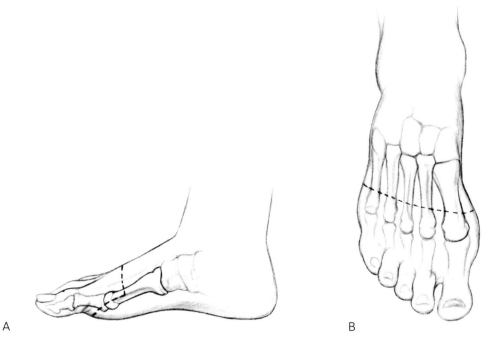

A                                                                                      B

**Figure 23-11** The transmetatarsal amputation is done with a short straight incision across the dorsum of the foot 1 cm proximal to the metatarsal heads. The plantar incision is long and curved and goes almost up to the base of each toe. (From Wheelock, F. C., Jr.: Surgical Techniques Illustrated. Little, Brown, Boston, Vol. 3, No. 3, 1978.)

flap. When the level of the metatarsophalangeal joint capsules is reached, the dissection of the plantar flap to the heel is carried out until the shafts of the metatarsals are exposed. It should be remembered that the metatarsal bones are not club-shaped but are L-shaped, with the short limb of the L pointing to the sole of the foot. Consequently as the plantar flap is elevated, probing must be done to find this space and follow the contour of the bone precisely. Failing to do this may destroy some of the blood supply to the plantar flap. The metatarsal shafts are then divided with double-action bone cutters, with care taken not to splinter the bone by avoiding any twisting motion in using this instrument. A specimen is then removed. The bone ends are rongeured back appropriately and contoured in a smooth arc from left to right and from top to bottom so that the foot will eventually have satisfactory shape. Hemostasis is carefully checked. Any protruding bits of tendon are removed, but the tendons are not pulled out of their sheaths to be divided and allowed to retract for reasons previously mentioned. The incision is then very thoroughly irrigated with antibiotic solution

and closed with a single layer of monofilament suture, usually 6-0 wire. The plantar flap is appropriately trimmed so that it meets without being too tight or too loose. There will be a certain amount of scalloping of the plantar flap because the plantar incision is considerably longer than the dorsal. This can be easily accomplished if the bites are taken farther apart in the plantar flap from the first suture to the last. If there is an excuse to take out a piece of skin from the plantar flap by reason of an ulcer, the closure is then obviously easier, because the T will come together smoothly. Following closure an appropriate dressing is placed.

## Postoperative Care

It is even more important in transmetatarsal amputations to keep the patient off that foot until it is completely healed. This varies from 3 to 6 weeks depending on the circulation. A short healing sandal is useful initially but usually a special shoe is not required. Lamb's wool is utilized to fill up space in the end of the shoe.

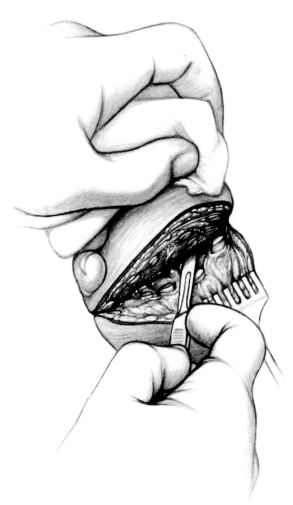

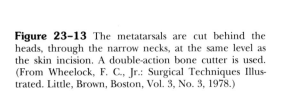

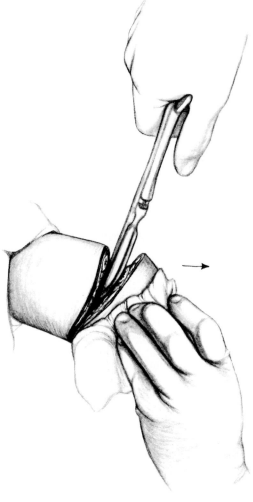

Figure 23–12 The plantar flap is long, curved, and full thickness. The flexor tendons are left in the flap. Care is taken to cut up behind the metatarsal heads in order to preserve the plantar flap circulation. (From Wheelock, F. C., Jr.: Surgical Techniques Illustrated. Little, Brown, Boston, Vol. 3, No. 3, 1978.)

Figure 23–13 The metatarsals are cut behind the heads, through the narrow necks, at the same level as the skin incision. A double-action bone cutter is used. (From Wheelock, F. C., Jr.: Surgical Techniques Illustrated. Little, Brown, Boston, Vol. 3, No. 3, 1978.)

## Results

As expected in the neuropathic group, the success rate was found to be higher than in the ischemic group (Table 23–2).

## BELOW-KNEE AMPUTATIONS

### Indications

The indication for a major amputation is the presence of tissue destruction or uncontrollable infection in the foot, so severe that salvage of the foot by a lesser procedure is impossible.

### Requirements

The considerations in choosing a below-knee amputation rather than an above-knee amputation fall into three main categories. The first is whether the patient's condition will allow use of a prosthesis if a below-knee amputation is done. If the answer to this is *no*, by reason of severe cardiac disease or pre-

**TABLE 23–2. RESULTS OF LARGE SERIES OF TMA's FROM PRE IN SITU REVASCULARIZATION ERA**

| | |
|---|---|
| 1. Neuropathic patients | |
| Early success 97% | Three years 93.5% |
| 2. Ischemic patients (not revascularized) | |
| Early success 85% | Three years 61% |

vious stroke, an above-knee amputation is simpler and more likely to heal; this should be carried out. Secondary consideration must be given to circulation. Is the circulation sufficiently good to permit healing of a below-knee amputation? Many elaborate ways of evaluating circulation have been described and used, including methods involving use of radioactive isotopes. We have found that clinical judgment is sufficient in this area. No particular pulse must be present for below-knee amputation because some of these have healed successfully in the absence of even a femoral pulse. The important consideration is whether there is an area of gangrene or ischemic ulceration above the ankle, and

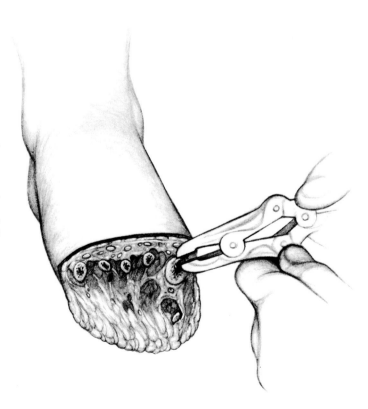

**Figure 23–14** The rough ends of the metatarsals are cut away with the rongeur, and the lateral edges of the first and fifth metatarsals are beveled away and rongeured smooth to prevent bone protrusion through the corners of the wound. (From Wheelock, F. C., Jr.: Surgical Techniques Illustrated. Little, Brown, Boston, Vol. 3, No. 3, 1978.)

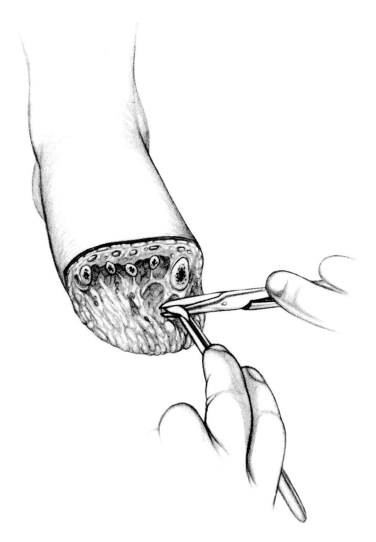

**Figure 23-15** Exposed tendon in the plantar flap is cut away. It is *not* pulled out and cut. (From Wheelock, F. C., Jr.: Surgical Techniques Illustrated. Little, Brown, Boston, Vol. 3, No. 3, 1978.)

whether there is a line of temperature demarcation between reasonable and cold above the ankle. If either of these circumstances is present, probably a below-knee amputation will not heal. If not, the below-knee amputation should heal.

A third consideration is whether infection has been appropriately controlled to permit a below-knee amputation at a level not too far above a septic foot. If the foot sepsis is out of control and it is feared that bacteria are passing into the lymphatics, it is probably not wise to do a below-knee amputation as a primary procedure. A guillotine amputation should be done first, and then, a few days later, it will be safe to do a definitive closed, below-knee amputation a few inches higher up.

## Technical Considerations

### Guillotine Amputations

A guillotine amputation is exactly what the word implies, a single cut through all layers with no formation of flaps and no attempt at closure. This operation should be done for uncontrolled sepsis in the foot; the incision is located just barely above the ankle. Any large muscle groups are thus avoided, and the procedure is made simple. No effort should be made to go above the cellulitis or lymphangitis, of course. If an abscess or necrotic muscle is found extending upward from this incision, it should be drained by appropriate longitudinal incisions up the leg, but not by a higher amputation if there is

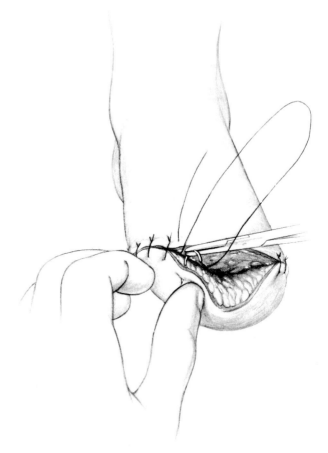

**Figure 23–16** The plantar flap is sutured loosely to the dorsal incision line. No subcutaneous sutures are used. Each corner is sutured first. Scalloping may occur, but is corrected with Steri-strips. Excessive skin on the plantar flap may have to be excised, leaving a T incision. (From Wheelock, F. C., Jr.: Surgical Techniques Illustrated. Little, Brown, Boston, Vol. 3, No. 3, 1978.)

hope to eventually save the knee joint. Hemostasis is obtained. A petroleum jelly gauze dressing is applied and a splint to prevent knee contracture. A closed, below-knee amputation is done four to seven days later. A small dressing is put on the guillotined area and careful walling off is obtained by use of appropriate adhesive drapes. The final formal closed below-knee amputation is done a few inches proximal in the usual location.

### Below-Knee Amputations
(Figs. 23–17 to 23–25)

Following a careful preparation and draping, the skin incisions are made in one of several ways. The technique that we prefer is that of creating equal, very short anterior and posterior flaps at such a level that the tibia will ultimately be about 12 cm in length from the anterior tibial tubercle. The measurements are made so that the skin incisions are approximately equal in length and thereby

set up for easy skin closure later. The fascia and muscles are divided in line with the skin. The three major vascular bundles are carefully identified and the vessels secured with 2–0 chromic catgut ties. The two major nerves are similarly treated. The anterior flap is then elevated for a distance of 5 cm from the original line of incision. This will almost always be far enough to permit a satisfactory closure. Next the muscle attachments to the fibula are dissected free and the fibula is divided at a level approximately 3 cm higher than the proposed line of division of the tibia. This is accomplished with a double-action angled bone cutter. A little rongeuring is then carried out to smooth the end and care must be taken that no bone chips are left in place. The tibia is then beveled with a straight saw at about 45 degrees and cut square across from there. At this point in time, the surgeon should become a sculptor for a few minutes and appropriately shape the end of the tibia in order that the stump will have a satisfactory contour when the skin is closed. This can be done with a double-

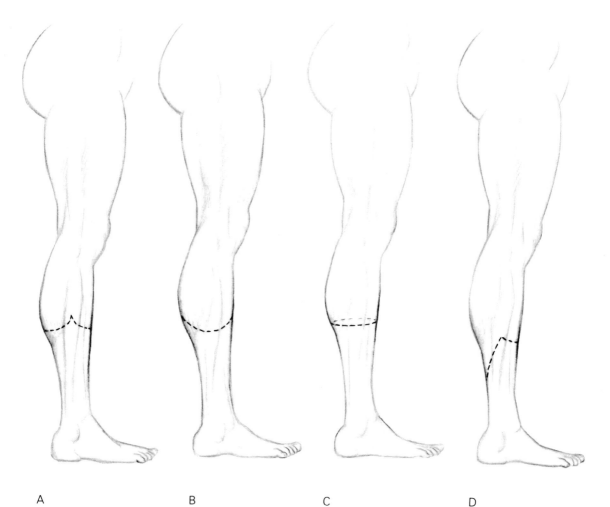

A                    B                    C                    D

**Figure 23–17** This illustrates the *level* for a below-knee amputation, and *types* of incisions commonly used. We usually use the type A. (From Wheelock, F. C., Jr.: Surgical Techniques Illustrated. Little, Brown, Boston, Vol. 3, No. 3, 1978.)

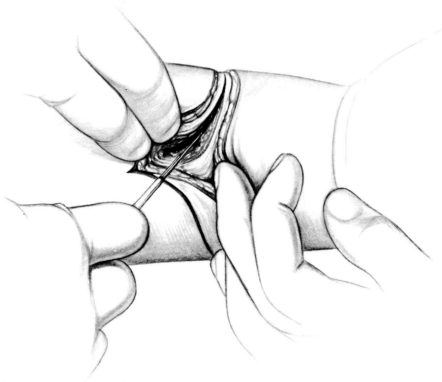

Lateral view

**Figure 23-18** The fascia, muscles, and tendons are divided at the level where the skin and subcutaneous layer have retracted. All bleeding vessels are clamped and tied when encountered. (From Wheelock, F. C., Jr.: Surgical Techniques Illustrated. Little, Brown, Boston, Vol. 3, No. 3, 1978.)

action, fairly narrow rongeur if one has a strong hand. After the area is irrigated carefully with diluted antibiotic solution, a closure is made with 3–0 fascial sutures with the knots buried. Great care is taken to be sure that these fairly closely spaced sutures are in the fascia that surrounds the calf and not simply in the muscle fascia. This suture line is very important because if it gives way, there will be so much stress on the skin that probably a dehiscence of the incision will occur. Next the skin is closed with a layer of monofilament sutures. An appropriate dressing, using Kling, is applied, with great pains taken to contour it to the stump. Not many circular turns are made lest they act like a tourniquet proximal to the end of the stump; rather, a more diagonal bandaging is carried out with oblique turns around the stump to avoid a tourniquet effect and so that the corners of the stump are turned in, giving it a round shape. This portion of the dressing is very important. A knee immobilizer is then applied to prevent flexion contracture.

## Postoperative Care

There have been major changes in our postoperative management of major limb amputations since the introduction of disease related groups (DRG's). The initial dressing is taken down on the second postoperative day. The wound is examined and the limb measured for a temporary prosthesis. The prosthesis, a Boston leg, arrives three days later, and if the stump is ready the patient tries it on and is then transferred to a rehabilitation facility for intensive gait training. We do not use stump shrinkers, preferring to allow the postoperative swelling to resolve spontaneously. Further shrinkage due to muscle atrophy occurs over the next four months, and the prosthesis can be tightened to accommodate this. After the stump has reached its final size, a permanent prosthesis can be ordered. The adjustable temporary prosthesis remains in the patient's closet and can be used as a backup if edema prevents the permanent prosthesis from being worn.

*Text continued on page 247*

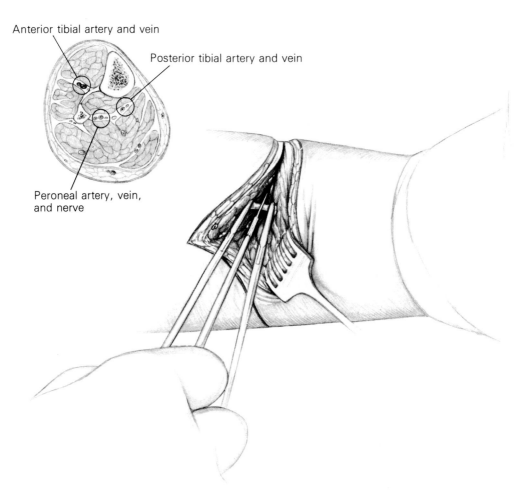

**Figure 23–19** The three vascular bundles are found as illustrated. The posterior tibial and peroneal arteries are in the same plane. The anterior tibial artery is in the anterior compartment. All vessels are carefully tied. The rake retractor is used only on the part that will be removed. (From Wheelock, F. C., Jr.: Surgical Techniques Illustrated. Little, Brown, Boston, Vol. 3, No. 3, 1978.)

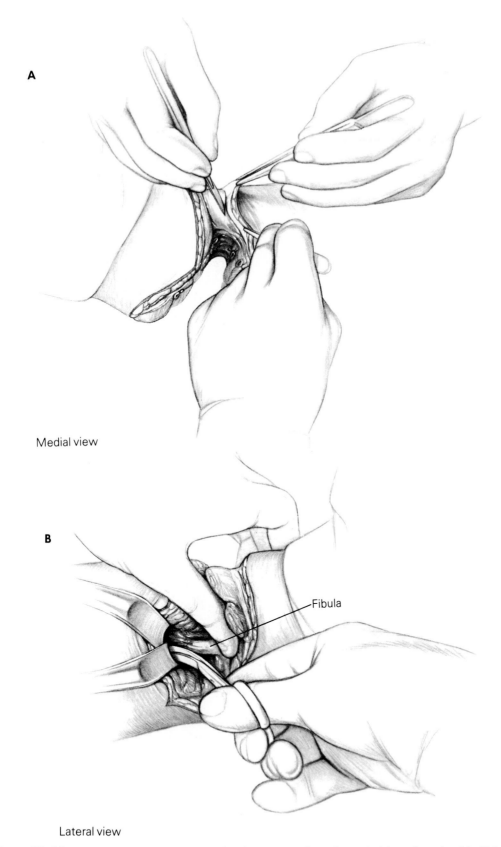

A

Medial view

B

Fibula

Lateral view

**Figure 23–20** *A,* The skin, subcutaneous fat, and periosteum are elevated as a *single* layer from the tibia. This must be done to preserve a viable anterior flap. *B,* The muscles are stripped off the fibula with a periosteal elevator or scissors. (From Wheelock, F. C., Jr.: Surgical Techniques Illustrated. Little, Brown, Boston, Vol. 3, No. 3, 1978.)

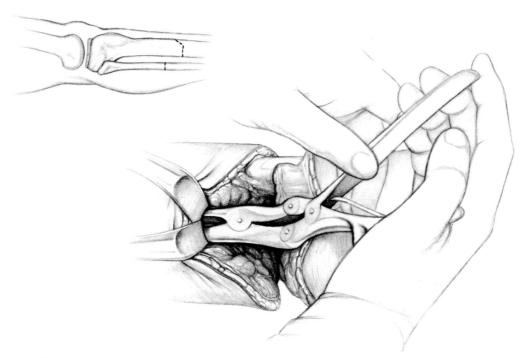

**Figure 23–21** The fibula is divided 2 to 3 cm above the level of the tibia. It is cut with a Gigli saw or a double-action bone cutter. A rough end is nipped smooth with a rongeur. (From Wheelock, F. C., Jr.: Surgical Techniques Illustrated. Little, Brown, Boston, Vol. 3, No. 3, 1978.)

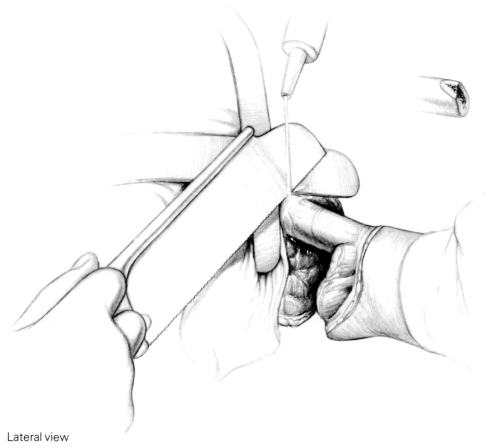

Lateral view

**Figure 23–22** The anterior leading edge of the tibia is beveled with the saw as shown. (From Wheelock, F. C., Jr.: Surgical Techniques Illustrated. Little, Brown, Boston, Vol. 3, No. 3, 1978.)

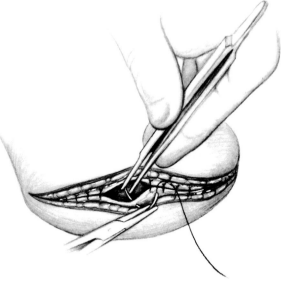

Figure 23–23 The circular incision with short anterior-posterior flaps is converted to a transverse incision. The fascia is closed with 2–0 or 3–0 chromic buried interrupted sutures. (From Wheelock, F. C., Jr.: Surgical Techniques Illustrated. Little, Brown, Boston, Vol. 3, No. 3, 1978.)

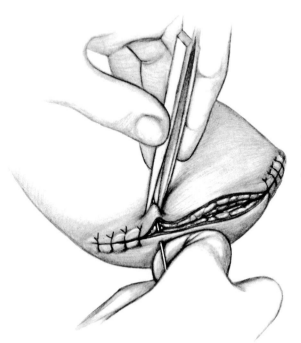

Figure 23–24 Interrupted 5–0 monofilament sutures are used in the skin. Mattress sutures and Steri-strips may be used to improve the closure. (From Wheelock, F. C., Jr.: Surgical Techniques Illustrated. Little, Brown, Boston, Vol. 3, No. 3, 1978.)

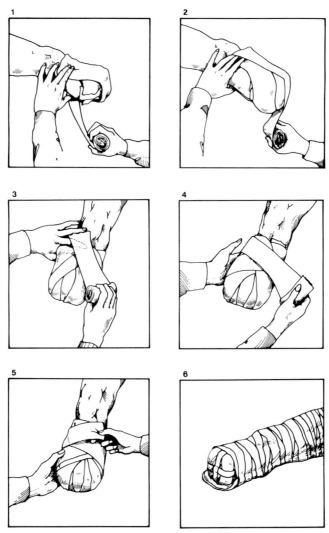

**Figure 23–25** A below-knee amputation stump dressing with splint to provide a snug, adequate dressing to a fresh below-knee amputation wound stump and to incorporate a wooden or plaster splint to prevent flexion contracture of the knee in the immediate postoperative days. Supplies: Sterile 4 × 8 dressing, sterile 4-inch soft roller gauze, a wooden padded arm board, and ½ inch adhesive tape. The end of the stump is covered with sterile 4 × 8's and these are held with a 4-inch roller bandage applied as illustrated (*1 through 6*). The padded splint is then put behind the leg, from stump to crease of buttocks, and held by wrapping in a circular fashion (*6*) with a 4-inch cotton roller gauze. *Elastic roller bandages may cause too much pressure and therefore should not be used.* (From Delaney, J. P., and Varco, R. L., (eds.): Controversies in Surgery II. Philadelphia, W. B. Saunders Co., 1983.)

If minor wound problems develop in the postoperative period, they should be carefully managed and will rarely require revision of the amputation. Fearon and Campbell et al. reviewed 100 consecutive below-knee amputations in 1983. None required conversion to above-knee amputation, and 85 per cent of patients were ambulatory at the time of discharge.

## Alternative Techniques

A surgeon should not be locked into any one particular method of performing an operation if certain circumstances indicate variation. In the case of the below-knee amputation, at times other techniques are appropriate. Not infrequently we do use a long posterior flap covering the end of the stump. On other occasions, medial and lateral flaps are useful, although this requires better circulation than might be present in the very

ischemic limb. Medial flaps and lateral flaps may be needed when there had been previous trauma to the skin of the anterior aspect of the lower leg. On other occasions straight circular incisions are made, with very small V's taken out at the corners. All of these procedures can be successful in the hands of trained surgeons.

## Results

The majority of the procedures we do are below-knee amputations, and relatively few above-knee procedures are carried out currently. This is because of the tremendous advantage provided by a knee joint in ambulation. Furthermore, it is important to realize that 25 per cent of patients who lose one leg will sooner or later lose the other. In our experience, the healing rate for below-knee amputations is above 90 per cent and the mortality rate is approximately 4 per cent (usually from cardiac complications).

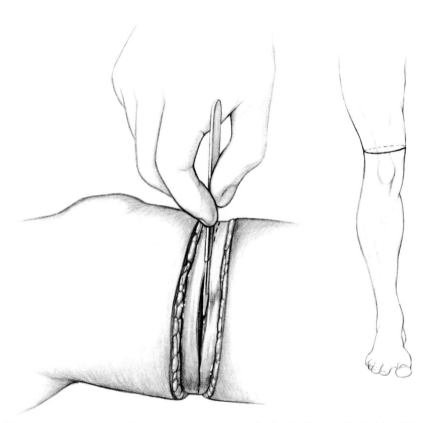

**Figure 23-26** The above-knee amputation is done at the suprapatellar level with a circular incision. (From Wheelock, F. C., Jr.: Surgical Techniques Illustrated. Little, Brown, Boston, Vol. 3, No. 3, 1978.)

## ABOVE-KNEE AMPUTATIONS

### Indications

An above-knee amputation is required if major problems in the foot demand amputation and if the requirements previously mentioned for below-knee amputation are not met.

### Technique (Figs. 23–26 to 23–31)

The above-knee amputation in most instances should be carried out at a level 2 cm above the patella. If it is done higher, the muscle mass is larger, the operation is much more difficult and healing is slower. In some

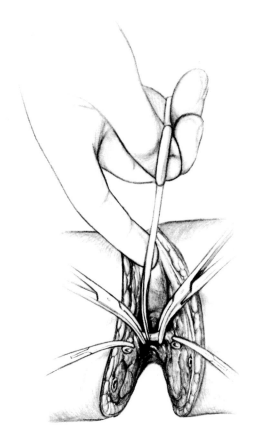

Medial view

**Figure 23–27** The saphenous vein, the popliteal artery, and the popliteal vein must be individually divided and ligated. (From Wheelock, F. C., Jr.: Surgical Techniques Illustrated. Little, Brown, Boston, Vol. 3, No. 3, 1978.)

cases there will be ischemia at the knee level, and then amputation must be higher for healing to take place. This circumstance, however, is very uncommon.

The above-knee amputation is carried out by use of extremely short anterior and posterior flaps, almost a circular incision with small V's pointed proximally at the medial and lateral corners. Care is taken to identify, locate, and ligate the saphenous vein. The fascia muscles are divided in line with the skin incisions without undermining until a level of the bone is reached. The major vessels are tied with 2–0 chromic catgut. The sciatic nerve is dissected well up among the muscles and ligated at a high level and then divided. It should be ligated securely with heavy catgut tie to avoid hematoma from a vessel in the nerve. The femur is then dissected up for a distance of approximately 5 cm from the point of original incision. The periosteum is removed with downward strokes using an appropriate instrument and the femur is divided squarely across with a straight saw. The incision is then carefully irrigated, and after a check for hemostasis, it is closed in a transverse fashion with interrupted 3–0 chromic fascial sutures and single-layer monofilament skin sutures. One point to remember is that if closure of the skin medially is difficult in a very obese patient, removal of a few of the medial fascial sutures will permit easy skin closure without tension. The medial closure of the fascia is not terribly important because the femur will drift laterally and put pressure away from the medial aspect of the incision.

### Postoperative Care

A simple dressing is applied without a splint, but the patient is carefully watched and reminded to avoid flexing the hip. Any significant period of hip flexion, which would be greatly enhanced by putting a pillow under the stump, creates a permanent hip contracture. Such a misfortune makes walking difficult if not impossible for the patient. Sutures are left in for approximately two weeks. A number of these patients find it impossible to walk because of pre-existing medical difficulties. Others are provided with a limb and taught to walk. The results of such training are disappointing in that it is extremely diffi-

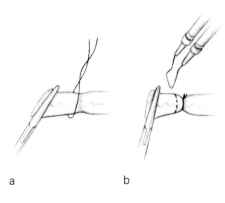

a                    b

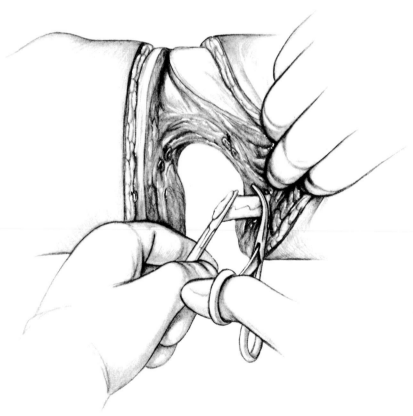

Medial view

**Figure 23–28** The sciatic nerve must be identified, pulled out a bit, crushed, and tied at the crush site before being divided 1 cm distal to the toe. (From Wheelock, F. C., Jr.: Surgical Techniques Illustrated. Little, Brown, Boston, Vol. 3, No. 3, 1978.)

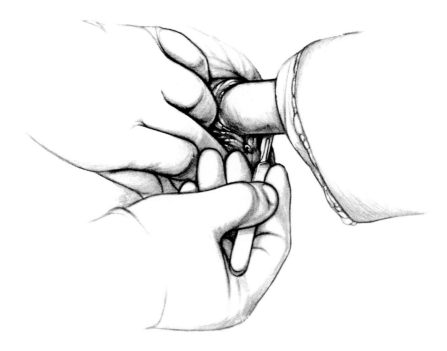

Lateral view

**Figure 23–29** The periosteum is stripped from the femur for a distance ot 5 to 6 cm higher than the original level of the skin incision. (From Wheelock, F. C., Jr.: Surgical Techniques Illustrated. Little, Brown, Boston, Vol. 3, No. 3, 1978.)

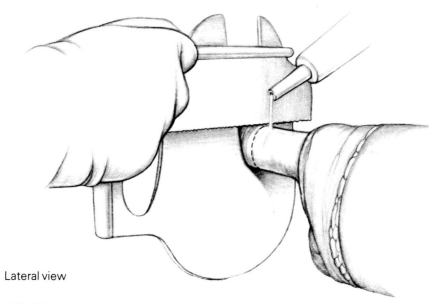

Lateral view

**Figure 23–30** The femur is divided as shown, 5 to 6 cm above the level of the skin incision. (From Wheelock, F. C., Jr.: Surgical Techniques Illustrated. Little, Brown, Boston, Vol. 3, No. 3, 1978.)

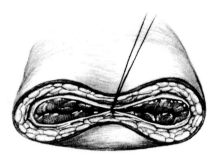

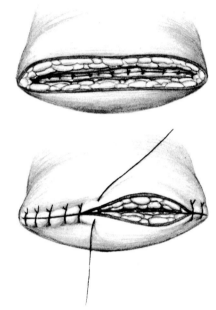

**Figure 23–31** The circular incision is closed transversely by suturing the fascia with 2–0 or 3–0 chromic catgut and fine monofilament nylon sutures in the skin. (From Wheelock, F. C., Jr.: Surgical Techniques Illustrated. Little, Brown, Boston, Vol. 3, No. 3, 1978.)

cult for a diabetic, usually elderly and often infirm with other medical problems, to walk effectively with this type of amputation. What may be accomplished, however, is to give them enough mobility to maneuver around the home with success.

## CONCLUSIONS

We hope that these comments will help the physician prevent amputations in diabetic patients, or at least to make as distal an amputation as possible a success. The decreased number of both minor and major amputations during the past decade is most encouraging and gratifying. Perhaps the most important principle deals with the fact that local amputations on an ischemic extremity must usually be closed completely. Careful consideration, lack of haste in making decisions, care in preparation, and the willingness to

take enough time in the operating room for meticulous surgery are important factors in achieving good outcome.

## SUGGESTED READING LIST

McKittrick, L. S., McKittrick, J. B., and Risley, T. S.: Transmetatarsal amputations for infections or gangrene in patients with diabetes. Ann. Surg. 130:826–842, 1949.

Wheelock, F. C.: Transmetatarsal amputations and arterial surgery in diabetic patients. N. Engl. J. Med. 264:316–320, 1961.

Fearon, J., Campbell, D. R., Hoar, C. S., et al.: Improved results with diabetic below knee amputations. Arch. Surg. 120:777–780, 1985.

Bunt, T. J.: Gangrene of the immediate postoperative above-knee amputation stump: role of emergency revascularization in preventing death. J. Vasc. Surg. 2:874–877, 1985.

Gibbons, G. W., Wheelock, F. C., Siembieda, C., et al.: Noninvasive prediction of amputation level in diabetic patients. Arch. Surg. 114:1253–1257, 1979.

Hoar, C. S., and Torres, J.: Evaluation of below the knee amputation in the treatment of diabetic gangrene. N. Engl. J. Med. 266:440–443, 1962.

# Chapter 24

# PLASTIC SURGICAL RECONSTRUCTION OF DIFFICULT DIABETIC FOOT WOUNDS

LEONARD MILLER, M.D., F.A.C.S.,
and BARRY ROSENBLUM, D.P.M.

The limb salvage rate in diabetic patients with difficult foot wounds has increased significantly over recent years as a result of a combination of improved plastic reconstructive techniques and more successful revascularization procedures. In addition to a better understanding of the blood supply in the foot with the development of various arterialized pedicle flaps, there has also been refinement in microsurgical techniques. Microvascular free tissue transfer procedures have permitted closure of wounds of any size and in any location. Because of the success of distal arterial bypass procedures, managing the severely ischemic ulcer does not present as formidable a problem.

In addition to limb salvage, a major task for the plastic surgeon is to provide stable wound coverage and bipedal ambulation as expeditiously as possible. This is made difficult because of the frequent presence of extensive vascular disease, neuropathy, and intractable infection. These all have major impact on wound healing, and there is a relatively high incidence of operative failures and early wound recurrence. Today, however, newer techniques in reconstructive surgery are helping achieve better long-term results. A more aggressive approach is therefore warranted in the management of difficult diabetic foot wounds.

## PREOPERATIVE MANAGEMENT

A multispecialty approach is essential in the management of difficult foot wound problems. A comprehensive, detailed analysis of factors such as the patient's general condition, peripheral circulation, and local wound status is initiated prior to the undertaking of any difficult reconstructive procedure. The ambulatory status and compliance of the patient must also be considered, as an amputation may be more favorable than involved revascularization and reconstructive procedures.

The podiatrist performs an essential role in assessing the function of the foot and altering its bony structure, alleviating pressure-bearing areas, and reducing the size of the defect. Foot x-rays are essential in most cases of difficult plantar wounds, mainly to detect underlying bony prominences. Magnetic resonance imaging and computed tomography are usually noncontributory, and the diagnosis of osteomyelitis in the presence of neuropathy remains primarily a clinical one.

Soft tissue infection and ischemia must be fully resolved prior to the undertaking of any closure procedure. Bed rest and leg elevation are essential to help resolve edema and local infection. Wound cultures are obtained and the appropriate antibiotic treatment initi-

252

ated, if necessary. In cases of invasive infection, wide drainage must be carried out immediately with extensive debridement of necrotic devitalized tissue. The wound is now managed with regular dressing changes, using a variety of antibacterial agents (Betadine, Silvadene, acetic acid). Previously infected wounds should be closed only when they are actively granulating and drainage is minimal. Cultures should show only sparse bacteria. Repeat debridement procedures may be necessary to achieve this state. Absence of granulation tissue usually indicates ongoing infection or severely compromised circulation.

Postoperative management is just as important as preoperative care. Podiatric involvement is essential in enhancing the success of the plastic reconstructive procedure. Incision lines must be kept dry as well as protected. Prolonged non-weight bearing (up to two months) is of critical importance. This is followed by partial weight bearing and gradual rehabilitation with special appliances and shoeing. Frequent follow-up and instruction by the podiatrist are essential.

The location and size of the wound usually determine the complexity of the reconstructive procedure. For example, a large wound on the dorsum or instep of the foot can often be treated with debridement and a skin graft. Unless the circulation is severely compromised, these wounds will granulate well, allowing a simple skin grafting technique. On the other hand, a small wound on the heel may require a distal arterial bypass procedure to the foot, followed by a complicated muscle or skin flap procedure.

Noninvasive studies are performed in the absence of peripheral pulses, giving some indication of the state of blood flow to the foot and the patency of the major vessels. Ankle/digital pressure recordings are not always accurate because of the frequent noncompressibility of the vessels. Ankle/brachial indices of less than 0.5 and monophasic Doppler wave forms usually are an indication for improving the circulation prior to a difficult wound closure. Other techniques helpful in assessing blood flow are transcutaneous oxygen tension measurements, directional Doppler studies, and various vessel-scanning techniques. However, noninvasive testing is not always helpful in planning specific pedicled and free flap techniques because of the segmental nature of the calcific arterial disease and the reverse flow patterns that develop through the plantar arch. Arteriography should therefore be considered before any flap procedure in the absence of palpable pulses.

Plantar heel ulceration due both to ischemia and neuropathy is frequently associated with occlusion of the posterior tibial artery near the ankle. Combined with this, there may be retrograde blood flow through the plantar arch from the dorsalis pedis artery. This affects the feasibility and design of a local flap procedure, which is usually proximally based. However, in the midfoot and forefoot, distally based flaps supplied from the dorsal circulation can be used for reconstructing wounds here. In those situations in which a revascularization procedure is necessary, distal in situ bypass grafts are performed into the dorsalis pedis vessels. For heel reconstruction a free microvascular flap can then be anastomosed to the bypass graft itself.

## SOFT TISSUE RECONSTRUCTION

Simple techniques such as direct closure and skin grafting are usually preferable but are not always possible because of the situation and extent of the wound. Closure of wounds under tension should be avoided as there are alternate methods to achieve primary healing. Skin grafting on weight-bearing surfaces may be initially successful, but breakdown frequently recurs. With the improved understanding of blood supply in the foot, refinements in flap techniques have been made. Available methods include island pedicle flaps, V-Y advancement flaps, rotation-advancement fasciocutaneous flaps, and free tissue transfer procedures.

The same surgical principles apply in almost all cases of wound closure, i.e. removal of infected and devitalized tissue, removal of bony prominences, avoidance of dead space, control of bleeding and drainage, and prolonged immobilization and protection of the healing site. Four different areas of the foot will be discussed relating to the various reconstructive procedures—dorsum, plantar aspect of the forefoot, midfoot, and the heel.

## DORSUM OF THE FOOT

Most wounds on the dorsum of the foot, large or small, can be closed with split-thickness skin grafts. Extensive wounds with exposure of bone and tendon usually occur in association with necrotizing infection. Sacrifice of tendon and bony cortex, if necessary, during the debridement procedure may not lead to alteration of function. Such wounds in the presence of adequate blood supply will granulate freely and can then be skin grafted. Rarely is a local flap indicated. However, with deeper and more proximal wounds where larger tendons, ligaments, and joints may be exposed, local muscle flap procedures can be performed (extensor digitorum brevis, abductor digiti minimi, and abductor hallucis). Other procedures include the dorsalis pedis skin island flap, turndown distally based fasciocutaneous flaps, and free tissue transfer.

## PLANTAR FOREFOOT

Difficult wounds on the plantar aspect of the forefoot are usually located over the metatarsal heads. Ulceration of the toes with exposed bone and tendon is frequently managed by digit amputation. An extensive wound proximal to the toe may necessitate a ray amputation or a toe filet flap procedure. Smaller wounds are usually chronic and may require alteration in the bony architecture (e.g. metatarsal head resection) before closure. By reducing the amount of bone in this area, these wounds may be closed primarily. However, if the soft tissue defect is too large, a number of reconstructive procedures can be performed (island neurovascular flaps, V-Y advancement flaps, and distally based muscle flaps). Skin grafts are usually unsuccessful as they are unable to withstand shearing and weight-bearing forces. This applies to all areas along the plantar aspect of the foot, except on the non-weight bearing instep portion. Free tissue microvascular transplantation is rarely necessary to close distal wounds, but has been used to salvage nonhealing transmetatarsal amputation stumps (Fig. 24–1).

## PLANTAR MIDFOOT

Most difficult wounds in this area are associated with Charcot's disease. Fracture-dislocations in the midfoot result in significant architectural changes, collapse of the arches, and alteration in the normal weight-bearing surface. Chronic ulceration results in scar tis-

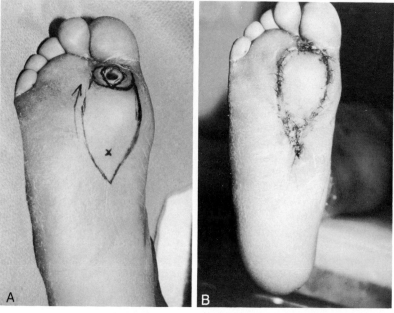

**Figure 24–1** *A,* Chronic nonhealing ulcer at base of great toe. *B,* Distally based V-Y advancement flap to close defect after excision.

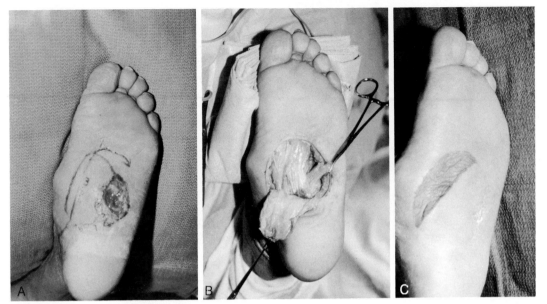

**Figure 24–2** Chronic neuropathic ulcer in Charcot foot. *B,* Elevation of instep fasciocutaneous flap and partial flexor digitorum brevis muscle flap to osteotomized defect. *C,* Two years after flap procedure.

sue buildup and bursa formation overlying an area of bony prominence, usually on the mid-lateral aspect of the foot (Fig. 24–5, 24–6).

Experience has shown that the most effective way to manage these difficult wounds is to do an extensive resection of the ulcer, including the scar tissue, bursal tissue, and underlying bony prominence. The enlarged defect is then closed with a combination of a local muscle flap to fill in the depths of the wound and a rotation advancement fasciocutaneous flap from the instep based on the medial plantar vessels. The muscle flap usually consists of a portion of the flexor digitorum brevis or abductor digiti minimi, depending on the position of the ulcer. Avoiding hematoma or seroma is essential to obtaining primary healing. In cases of diabetic neuro-osteoarthropathy, the circulation is invariably good, and flap compromise rarely if ever occurs. More extensive defects, especially when a large amount of bone has been resected, are best managed with a free tissue transfer procedure.

## HEEL

Primary closure of wounds in the posterior plantar area is difficult because of the lack of skin mobility and lack of vascularity of the heel pad tissue. Direct closure can, however, be facilitated by partial calcanectomy procedures, which may be indicated to remove bony prominences and prevent recurrence (Figs. 24–5 and 24–6).

Different reconstructive procedures are available to close wounds on both the plantar and posterior aspect of the heel. On the plantar aspect, techniques include local rotation or advancement heel pad tissue flaps, instep island pedicle flaps, turnover muscle flaps, and free tissue transfer. On the posterior aspect of the heel where the Achilles tendon is frequently exposed, wound closure is achieved by either skin grafts or local flaps (V-Y advancement, local rotation, and distally based vascularized pedicle flaps).

Situations may exist in nonhealing wounds in which the circulation is significantly compromised and the posterior tibial vessels are occluded. Even if the defect is small, a free tissue transfer may be necessary with anastomosis into the dorsalis pedis vessels or an in situ distal bypass graft (Figs. 24–7 to 24–9).

## CONCLUSIONS

Difficult cases of foot ulcers in the diabetic are often associated with multiple disease processes, e.g. neuropathy, ischemia, and infection. Each of these factors needs to be carefully addressed before definitive surgical management can be carried out. Careful

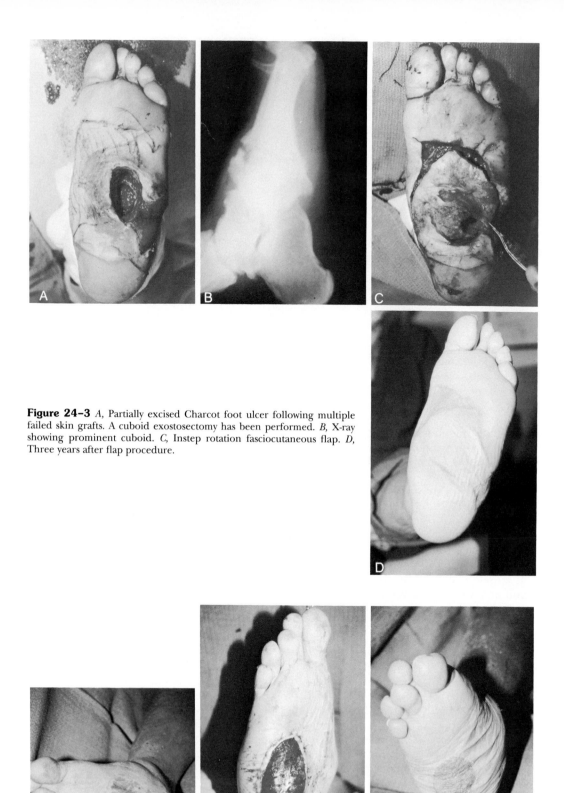

**Figure 24–3** *A,* Partially excised Charcot foot ulcer following multiple failed skin grafts. A cuboid exostosectomy has been performed. *B,* X-ray showing prominent cuboid. *C,* Instep rotation fasciocutaneous flap. *D,* Three years after flap procedure.

**Figure 24–4** *A,* Chronic ulceration and osteomyelitis in Charcot foot. *B,* Free microvascular transfer of rectus muscle flap to fill extensive midfoot defect. *C,* One year later with stable wound healing—skin-grafted muscle flap.

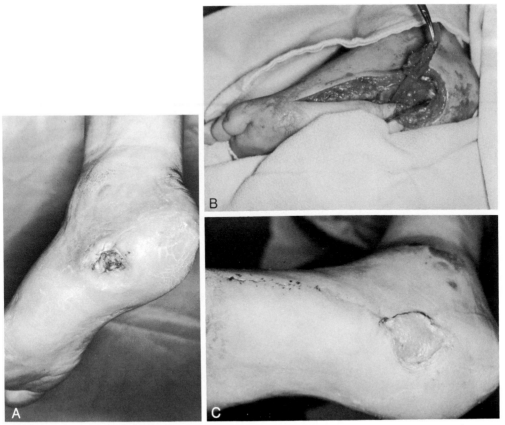

**Figure 24–5** *A*, Necrotic lateral heel ulcer in dialysis patient with severe neuropathy. *B*, Abductor digiti minimi muscle flap to debrided defect. *C*, Stable healing with skin-grafted muscle flap.

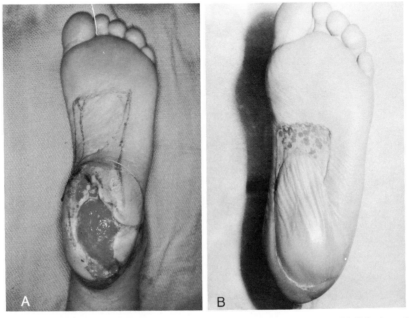

**Figure 24–6** *A*, Large posterior plantar heel ulcer with exposed calcaneus in 19-year-old diabetic patient. *B*, Medial plantar fasciocutaneous flap closure of defect.

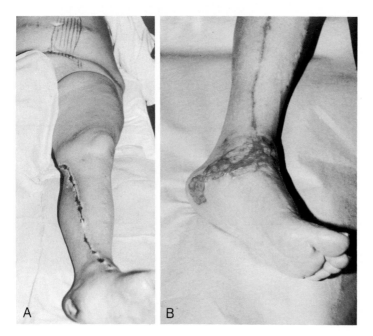

**Figure 24–7** *A,* Chronic ischemic ulcer in young diabetic woman. Distal in situ bypass graft procedure has been performed. A rectus muscle transfer is planned. *B,* One year after rectus muscle transfer with anastomosis into bypass graft.

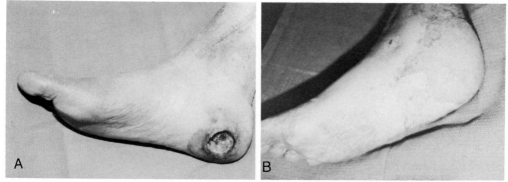

**Figure 24–8** *A,* Nonhealing ischemic heel ulcer in renal transplant patient despite distal bypass graft to dorsalis pedis artery. *B,* One year after rectus free flap reconstruction with anastomosis into graft.

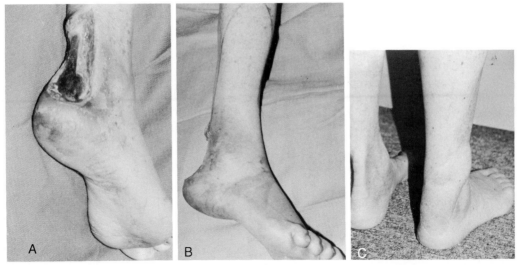

**Figure 24–9** *A,* Large necrotic ulcer with exposed calcaneus and Achilles tendon. *B,* Distally based fasciocutaneous flap on anterolateral aspect of lower leg. *C,* One year after turndown flap coverage and skin graft of donor defect.

work-up and preparation of the patient are essential before a plastic surgical procedure is undertaken.

Multiple procedures are available today to reconstruct almost any foot wound, and hence a more aggressive approach is warranted, e.g. wide debridement and immediate flap coverage. A multispecialty approach with increasing podiatric involvement has also resulted in more effective management of this challenging problem.

## SUGGESTED READING LIST

Baker, G. L., Newton, E. D., and Franklin, J. D.: Fasciocutaneous island flap based on the medial plantar artery: Applications for leg, ankle and forefoot. Plast. Reconstr. Surg. 85:1, 1990.

Bostwick, J., III: Reconstruction of the heel pad by muscle transposition and split skin grafts. Gynaecol. Surg. 64:295, 1979.

Chowdary, R. P., Celam, V. J., Goodreau, J. J., et al.: Free tissue transfers for limb salvage utilizing in situ saphenous vein bypass conduit as the inflow. Plast. Reconstr. Surg. 75:627, 1985.

Colen, L. B., and Cuncke, H. J.: Neurovascular island flaps from the plantar vessels and nerves for foot reconstruction. Ann. Plast. Surg. 12:27, 1984.

Colen, L. B., Replogle, S. L., and Mathes, S. J.: The V-Y plantar flap for reconstruction of the forefoot. Plast. Reconstr. Surg. 81:220, 1980.

Ger, R.: Newer concepts in surgical management of lesions of the foot in the patient with diabetes. Surg. Gynecol. Obstet. 100:213, 1984.

Grabb, W. C., Argenta, L. C.: The lateral calcaneal artery skin flap (the lateral calcaneal artery, lesser saphenous vein, sural nerve skin flap). Plast. Reconstr. Surg. 68:723, 1981.

Hidalgo, D. A., and Shaw, W. W.: Anatomic basis of plantar flap design: Clinical applications. Plast. Reconstr. Surg. 78:637, 1986.

Lai, C.-S., Lin, S.-D., Yang, C. C., et al.: Limb salvage of infected diabetic foot ulcers with microsurgical free tissue transfer. Ann. Plast. Surg. 26:212, 1991.

Marayama, Y., Iwahira, Y., and Ebihara, H.: V-Y advancement flaps in the reconstruction of skin defects of the posterior heel and ankle. Plast. Reconstr. Surg. 85:759, 1990

Masquelet, A. C., Beveridge, J., Romano, C., and Garber, C.: The lateral supramalleolar flap. Plast. Reconstr. Surg. 81:4, 1988.

May, J. W., Halls, M. J., and Simon, S. R.: Free microsurgical muscle flaps with skin graft reconstruction of extensive defects of the foot: A clinical gait analysis study. Plast. Reconstr. Surg. 75:627, 1985.

McCraw, J. B., and Arnold, P. G.: McCraw and Arnold's Atlas of Muscle and Musculocutaneous Flaps. Hampton Press Publishing, 1986.

McCraw, J. B., and Furlow, L. T., Jr.: The dorsalis pedis arterialized flap: A clinical study. Plast. Reconstr. Surg. 55:177, 1975.

Morrison, W. A., Crabb, D. M., O'Brien, B. M., and Jenkins, A.: The instep of the foot as a fasciocutaneous island and as a free flap for heel defects. Plast. Reconstr. Surg. 72:56, 1983.

Pomposelli, F. B., Jepsen, S. J., Gibbons, G. W., et al.: Efficacy of the dorsalis pedis bypass for limb salvage in the diabetic patients. J. Vasc. Surg. 11:745, 1990.

Reiffel, R. S., and McCarthy, J. G.: Coverage of the heel and sole defects. A new subfascial arterialized flap. Plast. Reconstr. Surg. 66:250, 1980.

Scheflan, M., Nahai, F., and Hartram, C. R. Surgical management of heel ulcers: A comprehensive approach. Ann. Plast. Surg. 7:385, 1981.

Shenaq, S. M., and Dinh, T. A.: Foot salvage in arteriosclerotic and diabetic patients by free flaps after vascular bypass: Report of two cases. Microsurgery 10:310, 1989.

Snyder, C. T. S., and Edgerton, M. T.: Principle island neurovascular flap in the management of ulcerated anesthetic weight bearing areas of the lower extremity. Plast. Reconstr. Surg. 35:518, 1965.

# Chapter 25

# PHYSICAL REHABILITATION OF THE DIABETIC FOOT

DANA BENNETT KARBASSI, M.S.P.T.

Rehabilitation for the diabetic foot is more than simply treating the most distal aspect of a patient's lower extremity. Diabetes mellitus is a systemic disease, often affecting many of the physiological systems in the body. Although our primary focus for rehabilitation at New England Deaconess Hospital may be the diabetic's foot, we feel it is of the utmost importance to take all diabetic manifestations into account, both physical and psychosocial.

The normal foot is a relatively complicated body part. Many principles of biomechanics, leverage, transmission of torque, and muscle pull must be kept in mind during its treatment. One of the major functions of the lower extremity is impact absorption, regulated primarily by eccentric muscle contraction, joint motion, and articular cartilage compression. It has been shown that in normal walking the compressive ankle force is five times body weight. In a diabetic patient who may have generalized weakness, decreased sensation in his feet and ankles, limited motion at many joints, and diffuse connective tissue changes, the principles of motion and force distribution are altered, often leading to ulcerations and joint deformities.

Physical therapy of the diabetic and the diabetic foot varies, depending on the type and degree of involvement of the neuromusculoskeletal system. While some authors report exercise is necessary only for non-insulin-dependent diabetics, most others feel it is quite important for all body systems (Table 25–1). In addition to the obvious benefits of improved strength and endurance, exercise can also help combat depression, improve the insulin sensitivity of exercising muscle,

bolster bone strength, and boost the hematocrit. Exercise also exerts a beneficial effect on blood cholesterol and lipoproteins, maximizes blood flow and increases vessel elasticity, increases aerobic metabolism, decreases blood glucose fluctuations, combats obesity, and lowers blood pressure.

In this chapter I will discuss the overall objectives of rehabilitation, factors that can affect its efficacy, and specific rehabilitation of various diabetic problems and operative procedures.

## OVERALL OBJECTIVES OF REHABILITATION

Physical therapy evaluation of a diabetic's rehabilitation potential follows a generalized format, which we use for all inpatients re-

### TABLE 25–1.  BENEFITS OF EXERCISE

**MUSCULOSKELETAL**
Improved strength
Improved endurance
Increased bone strength
**CARDIOVASCULAR**
Higher hematocrit
More regulated cholesterol levels
Better blood flow and blood vessel elasticity
Lower blood pressure
**METABOLIC**
Improved insulin sensitivity
Improved aerobic metabolism
Less blood sugar fluctuation
Reduced obesity
**PSYCHOLOGICAL**
Less depression
Less anxiety and stress
Overall sense of well-being

ferred to us. Therapists may specify particular diabetic problems within the general framework, exemplified in Figure 25–1.

General treatment objectives, as seen in Table 25–2, usually include the following:

*Increased—or prevention of decreased—range of motion, strength, and endurance.* Generalized or specific strengthening and stretching exercises, conditioning exercises, and aerobic activity are prescribed on an individual basis (Fig. 25–2).

*Optimal foot and/or leg support for maximal safety.* This goal is usually achieved via consultation with those in other disciplines, e.g. prosthetist, orthotist, and podiatry technician, for supportive and/or protective footwear or bracing.

*Decreased pain,* when present, if possible. Many of our patients have very little or no sensation, but others do have neuropathic or ischemic pain. Ischemic pain must be managed by physicians, but as physical therapists we encourage these patients to elevate their painful extremities (keeping in mind that prolonged elevation is contraindicated in cases of *severe* arterial insufficiency). We also teach gentle range-of-motion exercises to maximize blood flow and, it is hoped, decrease edema. If medically cleared, some sources advocate a regular walking program as treatment for intermittent claudication. For resistant neuropathic pain we have tried TENS (transcutaneous electric nerve stimulation) or occasionally biofeedback, but we have not had much success with these.

*Independence in bed mobility and transfers* while maintaining the proper weight-bearing status. Practice in rolling, scooting, and moving from bed to chair is provided, encouraging gradual progression to independence. In some instances, a trapeze over the bed or a sliding-board may be utilized.

## TABLE 25–2. GENERAL OBJECTIVES OF REHABILITATION

1. Increase range of motion, strength, endurance
2. Maximize safety of lower extremity
3. Minimize pain
4. Independent bed mobility and transfers
5. Independent ambulation on level
6. Independent on stairs—if necessary
7. Discharge planning
8. Maximize education

*Independence in functional mobility on level ground.* Many factors are involved here, including the patient's cardiovascular, motivational, and muscular ability to maintain the weight-bearing status indicated by physicians for proper healing. Patients who are full- or partial-weight bearing usually, with practice, can attain ambulatory independence with the appropriate assistive device, at least for short functional distances. On the other hand, patients who must be non-weight bearing (Fig. 25–3) often have a very difficult time maintaining it, for any or all of the aforementioned reasons. Geriatric diabetic patients, especially, often do not have the reserves for the necessary "hopping" gait. Therefore, to ensure patient safety, we may recommend that the patient *transfer only* to a wheelchair. Then he can elevate the affected extremity and still be in a safe position to get around independently at home.

*Independence on stairs,* with appropriate weight bearing—*only if necessary.* In Boston, we have large numbers of patients who live in family homes or old apartment buildings that have no elevators. For most of our patients who are elderly and/or have numerous diabetic complications, hopping up stairs (non-weight bearing) is impossible to do safely. Our first approach, then, is to encourage the patient who will be partial- or non-weight bearing for some time to have family members arrange his living quarters on one level (preferably street level). If this is not feasible, we assess the patient's balance and then instruct him on stairs with use of crutches, with use of a crutch and a railing, or sitting on the step and "bumping" up on his bottom. We then encourage the patient to negotiate stairs *only* when absolutely necessary.

*Overall assessment* of patient's condition and mobility status, *to recommend best discharge option* for the patient. Here we obviously work very closely with social workers and continuing-care nurses. The usual options are given in Table 25–3.

*Patient and family education.* This is easily the most important objective we have at New England Deaconess Hospital, and we share it with all members of the team—nurses, podiatrists, physicians, other therapists, nutritionists, social workers, prosthetist/orthotist, and others. Patients and families can never have too much education; unfortunately,

Addressograph

**NEW ENGLAND DEACONESS HOSPITAL**
**Inpatient Physical Therapy Consultation**

Primary Therapist: _____

Referring Physician: _____ Date: _11/1/93_

Diagnosis: _cellulitis, Charcot (R) foot_____

Treatment Request: (include precautions & WB status)

_walker amb NWB (R)_

Admission Date:

Age: _73_ Sex: _♀_

Assessment: _pleasant 73 y.o. ♀ referred for gait trng NWB (R) 2° Charcot foot. Pt presents c̄ ↓ability to maintain ↓WB, ↓vision & hearing, ↓endurance, ↓sensation, ↓coord., ↓ROM & strength, ↓'d Ⓘ c̄ transfers/standing balance/amb. Pt will benefit from P.T. for below goals - appears coop. but may have probs remembering ↓WB status - may need further rehab &/or ↑ services @ home. Pt agrees c̄ Rx plan._

Rehab Potential: _good_

| SHORT TERM GOALS | MET | LONG TERM GOALS | MET |
|---|---|---|---|
| ① pt able to amb ≥ 30 ft c̄ minimal SOB NWB (R) c̄ walker & min Ⓐ by 11/5 | | ① pt able to amb Ⓘ ≥ 50 ft NWB (R) c̄ walker c̄ minimal SOB by 11/8 | |
| ② Ⓘ transfers NWB (R) by 11/5 | | ② strength ≥ 4/5 by 11/8 | |
| ③ Ⓘ standing balance c̄ walker NWB(R) by 11/5 | | ③ pt knowledge of imp. of maint. ↓WB by 11/8 | |
| ④ ↑↓ 5 steps NWB (R) on bottom c̄ min Ⓐ by 11/5 | | ④ Ⓘ ↑↓ 10 steps NWB (R) on bottom by 11/8 | |

TREATMENT PLAN: _gait trng on level & stairs, pt ed_
_transfer trng_
_cond. exer_
_balance trng_

Frequency: _____  Duration: _7 days_

Date: _11/1/93_  Signature: _____

---

EVALUATION                                    HANDEDNESS:    Right         Left

| WNL | ABN | N/A | | WNL | ABN | N/A | |
|---|---|---|---|---|---|---|---|
| | ✓ | | Mental Status _↓ short-term memory_ | | ✓ | | Cardiac/Pulm _h/o CHF, s/p CABG x 3, ↓ EF - SOB c̄ min amb._ |
| ✓ | | | Communication | | ✓ | | Endurance _c/o SOB c̄ amb 20 ft NWB (R)_ |
| | ✓ | | Motivation/Affect _tends to be non-compliant_ | | ✓ | | Skin/Soft Tissue _ulcer (R) shin_ |
| | ✓ | | Vision _h/o hemorrhage, s/p laser Rx_ | | ✓ | | Pain (Intensity 0 - 10) _no c/o 2° neuropathy_ |
| | ✓ | | Hearing _sl. HOH_ | | ✓ | | Skeletal/Posture _kyphotic, Charcot deformity (R) foot_ |
| ✓ | | | Nutrition/Swallowing | | | | |
| | ✓ | | Bowel/Bladder _incont. urine_ | | ✓ | | Sensation _stocking (to mid-calf) ↓ to lt. touch, ↓ to proprio. (B)_ |

F920 Rev 3/91

**Figure 25-1** Evaluation form.

| WNL | ABN | N/A | |
|---|---|---|---|
| | ✓ | | Neurological Signs<br>st. ⊕ hemiparesis<br>↓ F→N ⊕ |
| | | ✓ | Reflexes |

*no c/o pain*

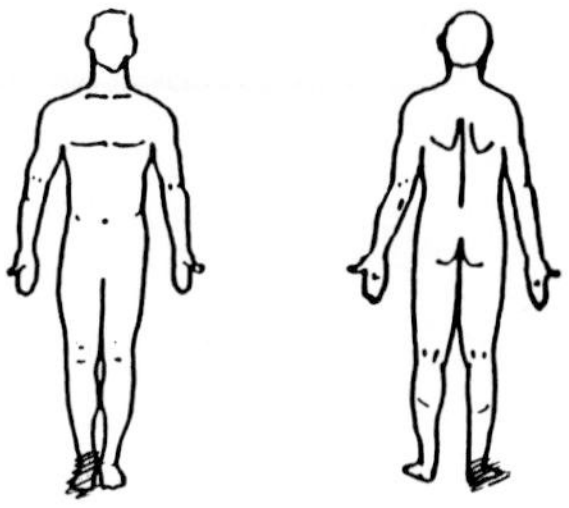

## ROM

**Upper Extrem.**

| | | ROM | R ROM | R Str | L ROM | L Str |
|---|---|---|---|---|---|---|
| Shld. | Flex | 0 - 180 | 0-150 | 4/5 | 0-150 | 4/5 |
| | Ext. | 0 - 50 | | | | |
| | Abd. | 0 - 180 | 0-130 | | 0-130 | |
| | Add. | | | | | |
| | I.R. | 0 - 90 | | | | |
| | E.R. | 0 - 90 | | | | |
| Elbow | Flex. | 0 - 145 | WFL | 4+/5 | WFL | 4+/5 |
| | Ext. | | | | | |
| Wrist | Flex. | 0 - 90 | | | | |
| | Ext. | 0 - 70 | | | | |
| | Pron. | 0 - 70 | | | | |
| | Sup. | 0 - 85 | | | | |
| Cx. | Flex. | | | | | |
| | Ext. | | | | | |
| Lat. | Flex. | | | | | |
| | Rotation | | | | | |

**Lower Extrem. & Trunk**

| | | ROM | R ROM | R Str | L ROM | L Str |
|---|---|---|---|---|---|---|
| Hip | Flex. | 0 - 120 | WFL | 4/5 | WFL | 4/5 |
| | Ext. | 0 - 10 | | | | |
| | Abd. | 0 - 45 | | | | |
| | Add. | 0 - 15 | | | | |
| | I.R. | 0 - 45 | | | | |
| | E.R. | 0 - 45 | | | | |
| Knee | Flex. | 0 - 125 | | 5/5 | | 5/5 |
| | Ext. | | -20° | | -15° | |
| Ankle | Dorsi | 0 - 20 | 0-5 | 3+/5 | 0-10 | 3+/5 |
| | Plant | 0 - 45 | 0-35 | | 0-30 | |
| | Inver. | 0 - 35 | 0-20 | | 0-20 | |
| | Ever. | 0 - 20 | 0-10 | | 0-5 | |
| Trunk | Flex. | | | | | |
| | Ext. | | | | | |
| Lat. | Flex. | | | | | |
| | Rota. | | | | | |

| Functional Ability | Indep. | Assist | Comments |
|---|---|---|---|
| Bed mobility | ✓ | | |
| balance: sitting | ✓ | | |
| standing | | ✓ | needs walker + min Ⓐ |
| transfers | | ✓ | sit ⇄ stand need walker + min Ⓐ  NWB Ⓟ |
| wheelchair mobility | NT | | |
| self care (dressing, food, bath) | ↓ | | |

Motor/Control/Tone: WFL c̄ atrophy Ⓑ hands

Gait: NWB Ⓟ c̄ walker & mod Ⓐ ~ 20 ft, c/o SOB

---

PATIENT HISTORY

PI:

Medications:

Lab Values:

PMH:

Test Findings:

Social History: (include D/C plans, equipment)
- Lives alone in 2nd floor walkup apt.
- has walker & w/c, has home health aide 2x/wk & Meals on Wheels qd

**Figure 25-1** *Continued*

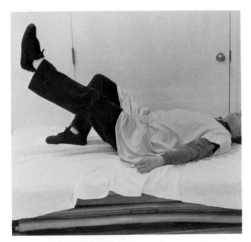

**Figure 25–2** Conditioning exercise.

### TABLE 25–3.  DISCHARGE OPTIONS

Short-term intensive inpatient rehabilitation hospital
Slower-paced long-term rehabilitation hospital
Skilled nursing facility with physical therapy available as needed
Home with various services (including physical therapy as needed)
Home independently or with family support

health care providers seldom take the time for it. It involves behavior modification, which takes time and needs much reinforcement. In physical therapy, our major concerns usually include:

1.  Skin and bilateral foot or stump inspection *every day*, to assess for breakdown. If the patient is unable to perform the inspection (because of retinopathy or joint stiffness), a responsible family member or home assistant must do it for him. He should use no foot soaks, home remedies, or self-pedicures and must contact his physician or podiatrist immediately if problems occur.

2.  Continuance of gentle but consistent prescribed exercise at home to maintain or increase strength, mobility, and endurance. Regular exercise can help decrease risk factors that lead to complications of diabetes. It can also decrease anxiety and stress and provide the patient with a sense of well-being.

3.  Cessation of smoking.

4.  Patient recognition of importance of blood glucose and blood pressure control, as well as control of blood cholesterol and fats.

5.  Patient recognition of importance of maintenance of prescribed weight-bearing status.

6.  Patient awareness and understanding of his individual complications, and of the adaptations necessary to ensure optimal health.

## CONCOMITANT FACTORS AFFECTING REHABILITATION

As mentioned previously and as seen in Table 25–4, there is a host of effects diabetes has on the body. Obviously the longer a person has diabetes, the more likely he is to develop diabetic complications. A rule of thumb is that a type I diabetic's physiological age is approximately his chronological age *plus* the number of years he has had diabetes mellitus. Many of our patients thus are ''elderly'' before their time. Here I will delineate these complications and the implications they may have on rehabilitation.

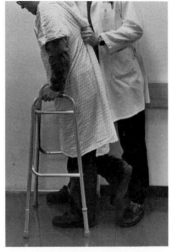

**Figure 25–3** Non-weight-bearing ambulation with walker.

### TABLE 25–4.  DIABETIC COMPLICATIONS WITH EFFECTS ON REHABILITATION

Retinopathy
Neuropathy
  Autonomic
  Peripheral
Nephropathy
Limited joint mobility
Atherosclerosis, peripheral vascular disease, and ischemia

## Retinopathy

As seen on the "typical" evaluation form in Figure 25–1, many of our patients have microvascular problems, which in the eye can lead to vessel rupture and hemorrhage, and/or blindness. Many patients are helped by laser treatments, which reduce chances of bleeding, but their eyes are still vulnerable. If one of our patients has a known history of intraocular hemorrhage or laser treatment, we keep this in mind and attempt to minimize activities that increase eye pressure. We avoid exercising the patient while he is completely supine, trying to keep the head of the bed at an angle of 30 degrees or more or having him sit up if possible. We also caution the patient to avoid any use of a Valsalva maneuver, which usually occurs with effort—e.g. using a trapeze, coughing, or straining, or non-weight-bearing ambulation. We use verbal and manual cues instead of visual if vision is severely compromised, and we give the patient minimal assistance or contact guard as needed for guidance while ambulating.

## Neuropathy

Entire books and articles have been written on the various diabetic neuropathies. Loss of thermal sensation is the most frequent abnormality in patients with long-term diabetes. Some of these neuropathies affect our treatment more than others. Briefly, we see two general types, autonomic and peripheral.

**Autonomic** (Table 25–5). While we cannot treat these disorders, they certainly impact on performance of the patient's activity, and we need to be aware of them. Usually the parasympathetic system is more involved than the sympathetic, leading to difficulty in re-

### TABLE 25–5.  COMMON PRESENTATIONS OF AUTONOMIC NEUROPATHY

Gastroparesis
Small-bowel malabsorption
Diabetic diarrhea
Atony—bladder, colon, esophagus
Orthostatic hypotension
Respiratory distress
Anhidrosis of feet/superhidrosis of trunk
Cardiac irregularities

gaining homeostasis once the body is "pumped up." We have seen orthostatic hypotension, anhidrosis of lower extremities accompanying superhidrosis of the upper extremities, and cardiac irregularities such as resting tachycardia and blunted heart rate and blood pressure responses to exertion. Patients with diabetes of long duration with autonomic involvement will have an abnormal response to exercise, which may be manifested as dyspnea, exaggerated fatigue, or vertigo. We are on the lookout for these symptoms, having our diabetic patients progress more slowly than nondiabetics, and always closely monitoring heart rate, respiratory rate, clammy skin, and feelings of dizziness. A diabetic reaction is also a possibility as a response to a change in activity level, so we try to differentiate it from an autonomic dysfunction and proceed accordingly. Vigilance is important, since it is possible for autonomic neuropathy to render a person unaware of his hypoglycemia. A patient using beta blockers for cardiovascular involvement is also watched closely, since these can mask a reaction as well as depress the liver's ability to produce replacement glucose for that used by exercising muscles.

**PERIPHERAL.** An autonomic nervous system disorder is almost always accompanied by distal symmetrical polyneuropathy. This is by far the most commonly seen form of peripheral neuropathy at New England Deaconess Hospital. The patient usually has a distal-to-proximal, progressive, stocking or glove distribution of one or more of the following: numbness, tingling, pain, a feeling of "heaviness," loss of proprioception, loss of muscle strength, or muscle atrophy. If the involvement is primarily sensory, we try to educate the patient to possible sequelae of this problem, advise him to be especially careful of balance (because of reduced proprioception and sensation), and to be cautious when handling hot or cold items. We emphasize the need for proper footwear (socks *and* shoes), daily foot inspection, and the need to rest the feet and legs every few hours. If the involvement is primarily motor, the typical patient may have weakness and atrophy of intrinsic foot muscles, which can produce toe deformity. When this is combined with decreased sensation, ulceration can result. We prescribe flexibility and strengthening exercises as indicated, and educate the patient to watch for early signs of skin breakdown.

Polyneuropathy may be accompanied by mononeuropathy simplex, involving the femoral or sciatic nerve, and often focuses on the peroneal portion, resulting in drop foot. This deficit is often permanent, and for safety reasons we consult our orthotist for a custom-made plastic ankle-foot orthosis (AFO) to provide dorsiflexion support to 90 degrees (Fig. 25–4). At New England Deaconess Hospital we prefer this type to the external brace given to "most" diabetics for the following reasons (Table 25–6):

1. It is internal to the shoe, and so is more cosmetic and appealing to the patient as well as convertible to many different shoes. This enhances patient compliance in wearing it.

2. The plastic is much lighter than the heavy metal upright and plantar bars of the external device. This is of particular importance here, when the foot and leg are already weakened. Many people will not prescribe the plastic AFO to diabetics, citing increased risk of breakdown with fragile skin. We, however, always tell our patients to wear a knee-high cotton or wool sock underneath the AFO and to continue regular daily foot inspections. So far we have heard of no breakdown related to AFO's, when used as instructed.

3. The plastic used is flexible, allowing the brace to move with the patient's foot and not restrict motion, thereby lessening the chance of friction and subsequent skin breakdown.

4. It is custom molded to the patient's foot, decreasing the chance for pressure and rubs leading to tissue breakdown.

5. It can be reshaped easily, if there is mi-

## TABLE 25–6. ADVANTAGES OF PLASTIC ANKLE-FOOT ORTHOSIS

More cosmetic
Light weight
Flexibility
Custom molding
Adaptability for body changes

nor weight loss or gain or biomechanical changes leading to differences in foot shape. This feature is very important, since many of our patients are susceptible to development of Charcot joints, and many also have renal disease with its accompanying fluctuations in peripheral edema.

We then train the patient in normal gait, provide him with any assistive device necessary, and prescribe gentle strengthening and stretching exercises. If the muscle involvement is extensive, we may also provide safety guidelines for exercising.

Interestingly, symmetrical peripheral neuropathy may be due to many factors other than diabetes mellitus, among them uremia. At New England Deaconess Hospital we have a very active renal treatment and transplant service as well, and often physical therapists are called upon to rehabilitate a person with uremic neuropathy due to poorly functioning kidneys. We follow the same procedures outlined above for diabetic peripheral neuropathy. It is different from diabetic neuropathy, however, in that when we see the patient after his renal status is balanced, we usually note the gratifying return of motor function to the feet. Often the patient may no longer need an AFO.

Another type of peripheral neuropathy is proximal amyotrophic neuropathy, which usually involves wasting of the iliopsoas and quadriceps muscles unilaterally and leads to falls due to instability. Its average course is about six months, with resolution within one to two years. Physical therapy here involves instruction in gentle active assistive range-of-motion exercise of the involved muscles, institution of a program of gentle stationary biking, and training with the appropriate assistive device (depending on severity of weakness). Again of crucial importance is patient and family education in what to expect and what to work on.

Charcot joints are another possible sequel of diabetic neuropathy. Owing to the altera-

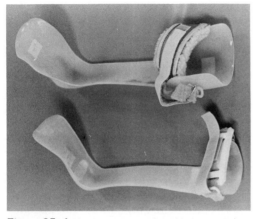

**Figure 25–4** Plastic custom-made ankle-foot orthoses.

tion in proprioception and pain perception in the weight-bearing joints, chronic micro-trauma and joint destruction occur. Although previous authors have theorized possible vascular contributions to the Charcot joint, the phenomenon is now felt to be almost purely neuropathic, since it usually occurs only in well-vascularized feet and ankles (infrequently in knees). Early Charcot joint dictates immobilization and strict non-weight bearing along with leg elevation for approximately two to six months. Physical therapy can assess the patient's overall mobility status and recommend the most appropriate means of maintaining non-weight bearing. We instruct the patient in wheelchair, crutch, or walker mobility and teach non-weight-bearing transfers. The patient is also instructed in general conditioning exercises (specific as needed), and foot care education is again reinforced.

When the lytic process in the bones stops, and coalescence starts, the patient can start to partially bear weight with adequate protection. This may include special extra-depth shoes, molded inserts, shoes with rocker-bottom soles, and bivalve cast bracing. The patient is instructed in partial weight bearing and is encouraged to be cognizant of any changes that take place in the contralateral foot or in the ipsilateral joints around the Charcot joint. This education is necessary since these joints will be taking up the slack for the affected one. Gentle passive range-of-motion exercises of unaffected joints are instituted to increase mobility and lessen further biomechanical changes.

Chronic Charcot joint is a slightly different situation. Patients will not have pain or acute lysis but will have biomechanical changes and bone displacements, which can lead to instability and gait deviations during ambulation and to ulceration. Physical therapists can instruct the patient in an individualized stretching and strengthening program to prevent further contracture and build up weakened muscles. We work with podiatrists and orthotists to determine the type and degree of external support needed—via shoe gear adaptations, bracing, and assistive devices—to maintain patient independence and prevent further deformity.

It should also be noted that patients with early-onset diabetes who have had a renal transplant are susceptible to development of Charcot joint and/or fractures of the hind-foot. This is due to osteopenia from immunosuppressive steroids, chronic uremia, and prolonged inactivity prior to or after transplant. Cyclosporine also contributes to avascular necrosis, and any peripheral neuropathy predisposes to fracture as well. Therefore, as we mobilize patients after transplant, physical therapists are in a position to detect insidious symptoms and report them to physicians. The best treatment is prevention.

## Nephropathy

Vascular changes can also lead to glomerulosclerosis or nephrosclerosis with resultant uremia. As noted previously, this can lead to bone weakness and fracture or can cause distal neuropathy. Patients also may demonstrate changes in mental status such as lethargy or apathy owing to the imbalance of electrolytes, as well as pruritus, anemia, changes in gastrointestinal or cardiac status, and changes in body metabolism. In patients with chronic or acute renal failure, physical therapists are usually consulted for general conditioning and maintenance or improvement of independent mobility.

Chronic renal failure can be managed first by either peritoneal dialysis or hemodialysis. These patients need an independent general exercise program to increase strength, endurance, and flexibility. If the renal failure progresses, the patient may opt for a transplant. At New England Deaconess Hospital both kidney and kidney-pancreas transplants are performed. In either case, patients will need instruction and training as outlined above, with extra emphasis on posture (counteracting surgical incisions) and on education. The patient will undergo immunotherapy for life and must be taught that regular exercise is imperative to minimize side effects of muscle atrophy and bone destruction. He must be given a nonaggressive yet regular exercise routine to carry out at home; individualization is important to ensure patient compliance. He must also be educated, if pain perception is diminished, to watch for skin or tissue changes that could signal foot fracture.

## Limited Joint Mobility

Many of our patients with chronic diabetes have decreases in range of motion, especially noticeable in the shoulder and hand in the upper extremity and in the foot and ankle in the lower extremity. In the foot, limited dorsiflexion and subtalar joint motion may restrict transverse rotation as well as the foot's ability to absorb shock, contributing to pathogenesis of plantar ulceration. The etiology of this progressive loss of mobility is unclear, although the loss may be due to increased collagen cross-linking, which may in turn be due to chronic hyperglycemia. This phenomenon may be equated with premature aging and may reflect the severity of internal complications of diabetes as well. Physical therapy for this entity usually includes various heating and cooling modalities to loosen tissues and decrease edema, as well as forms of strengthening, stretching, and mobilization. In resistant shoulder cases, orthopedic manipulation under anesthesia may be indicated.

## Atherosclerosis, Peripheral Vascular Disease, and Ischemia

Diabetics have a greater incidence than nondiabetics of coronary artery disease, cerebrovascular accident, and peripheral vascular disease—all secondary to large and small blood vessel abnormalities. In physical therapy we need to realize the extent of the patient's cardiovascular compromise, the history of previous transient ischemic attacks or cerebrovascular accidents, and the symptomatology of the presenting vascular problem. All of these can have significant impact on exercise tolerance and maintenance of the overall balance of health. We deal most directly with sequelae of peripheral vascular disease, which may or may not occur in conjunction with neuropathy. An in-depth look at rehabilitation of the patient hospitalized because of peripheral vascular disease follows.

A diabetic patient often initially has a foot ulcer that has been resistant to conservative measures. To avoid an amputation, the patient may be admitted for enforced bed rest, intravenous antibiotics, and incision/drainage. Strict bed rest, except for commode privileges, and an antibiotic course of ten days to two weeks may be required. In physical therapy, we institute a general bed exercise program (Fig. 25–5) to counteract deleterious effects of immobility. We also in-

struct the patient in safe non-weight bearing pivot-transfers from bed to commode. As the ulcer improves, we instruct the patient in progressive ambulation (non-weight bearing to partial weight bearing to full weight bearing), utilizing a walker, crutches, or cane as indicated. We determine the necessity of stair training, and teach it if necessary. Finally, we again educate the patient and family in the importance of proper footwear, daily foot inspection, rest of the lower extremities, avoidance of foot soaks, and maintenance of weight-bearing status and exercise program as instructed. Experimental padded hosiery to prevent ulceration is also available.

Our surgeons discourage the use of whirlpools at all costs. With our diabetic population at the Deaconess Hospital, a very conservative approach with all aspects of care is usually used. Whirlpools are felt to be contraindicated for the following reasons:

1. Increased maceration of tissues results, precluding rapid healing.
2. To increase warmth in an ischemic limb may heighten ischemia.
3. In a neuropathic limb with loss of sensation, accidental burns may result via chemical (iodine) or thermal means.
4. Probably the most significant reason is the increased risk of infection from anything less than ultrasterile equipment.

If an ulcer does not improve with conservative measures, surgical intervention is required. Options are as follows:

**LOWER EXTREMITY BYPASS GRAFT.** Deaconess surgeons may bypass any occluded lower extremity artery, utilizing the patient's own saphenous vein or cephalic or brachial artery, or using a synthetic graft. The length of the graft dictates the precautions given to the patient; if it extends over the hip or the knee, the patient is not to flex that joint past 90 degrees. This is especially true immediately post-surgery, and adaptive equipment may be required to maintain the restriction on motion. After a bypass site has healed, patients are still to avoid prolonged flexion of the affected joint. We reinforce this information, and work on progressive ambulation. Patients are usually permitted full weight bearing unless they have a plantar ulcer, in which case non-weight bearing or partial weight bearing is instructed. Patients may also progress slowly because of intolerance to pain and are encouraged to do conditioning exercises em-

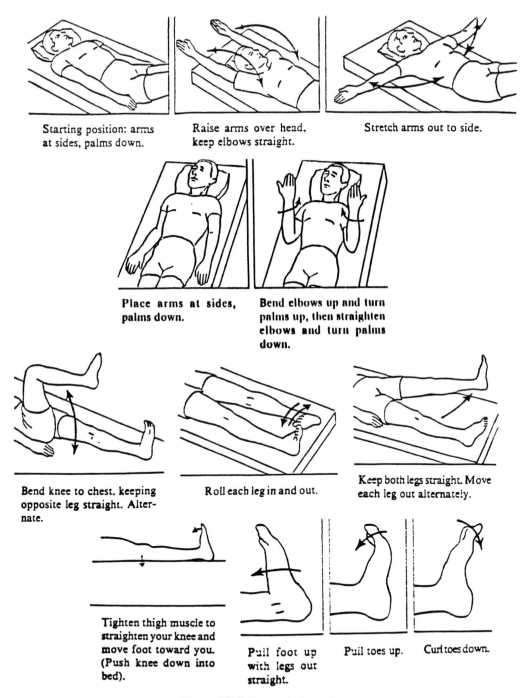

Starting position: arms at sides, palms down.

Raise arms over head, keep elbows straight.

Stretch arms out to side.

Place arms at sides, palms down.

Bend elbows up and turn palms up, then straighten elbows and turn palms down.

Bend knee to chest. keeping opposite leg straight. Alternate.

Roll each leg in and out.

Keep both legs straight. Move each leg out alternately.

Tighten thigh muscle to straighten your knee and move foot toward you. (Push knee down into bed).

Pull foot up with legs out straight.

Pull toes up.

Curl toes down.

**Figure 25–5** General bed exercises.

phasizing gentle range of motion to the affected joints, to increase flexibility and decrease edema and pain.

**TOE OR TRANSMETATARSAL AMPUTATION.** Depending on the extent of gangrene or ulceration, varying lengths of phalanges and metatarsals may be excised. The amputation site may be closed or may be left open to allow continued observation and treatment. The length of time a patient is non-weight bearing depends upon the site of the amputation, and whether it is open or closed. In general, a person with a closed small-toe amputation will be non-weight bearing for seven to ten days, whereas a person with a hallux amputation will be off his foot for two to three weeks, and a person with a transmetatarsal amputation will be non-weight bearing for four to six weeks. All of these patients need transfer training, gait training with a walker or crutches, and wheelchair training for long distances or if an assistive device is not an option. They are instructed in stair climbing and conditioning exercises as necessary and are given general education and training in the use of healing sandals and subsequent individualized footwear with lambs' wool fillers. They must be cautioned to be especially careful when resuming weight bearing, since the foot biomechanics will be altered, disrupting their balance. The importance of this caution is heightened if the patient has other diabetic complications that compromise balance. Physical therapists must work very closely with patients, their families, and social workers to ensure adequate support services and safe environments for non-weight bearing once the patient is home.

**BELOW-KNEE AMPUTATION.** When a patient's limb cannot be saved by bypass or digital amputations, a below-knee amputation is necessary. Our surgeons generally do not do any Syme's/ankle disarticulations, because of the subsequent instability and increased vulnerability to ulceration. Also, the ischemia usually extends above the ankle into the leg. For biomechanical advantage, a below-knee amputation with the longest possible stump (for leverage) is performed.

Our patients are measured for a temporary Boston prosthesis (Fig. 25–6) on postoperative day no. 1 to 3, depending on healing and resolution of symptoms. We then work with the patient on range-of-motion, strengthening, and conditioning exercises as seen in

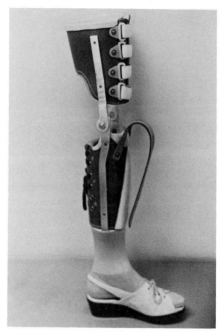

**Figure 25–6** Temporary below-knee Boston prosthesis.

Figure 25–7. The residual limb is dressed immediately postoperatively and is kept in a knee immobilizer to prevent knee flexion contracture. Use of an immediate postoperative prosthesis (IPOP), theoretically to minimize stump edema and maximize stump shaping, has not been espoused by our surgical team. The primary detractor to IPOP appears to be inability to check the incisional area daily. Some of our surgeons do not remove the initial dressing for three to four days postoperatively (unless there are symptoms warranting its removal); other prefer to keep a closer eye on the healing process. The same division of preference is felt with regard to "stump shrinkers" or Ace wraps to decrease stump edema. Some surgeons feel that it is appropriate, if the wrapping is done properly. Others feel that it is contraindicated because of pressure placed on fragile ischemic skin, increasing ischemia and thereby healing time, and unnecessary, since frequently there is not much edema secondary to overall limb malnutrition.

We also work on transfer training with the patient, bed to wheelchair and back. We instruct the patient in bed mobility and wheelchair mobility and educate him about care of his limb and prosthesis. "Hopping" is not

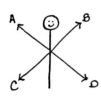

1. For opposite arm, hold tubing on right thigh with right hand. Pull against tubing with left arm (in direction of arrow B).

2. While left hand holds tubing securely by left shoulder, stretch right arm down and out (in direction of arrow C).

3. For opposite arm, hold tubing by right shoulder with right hand. Pull against tubing with left arm (in direction of arrow D).

4. Hold tubing with elbows straight and arms stretched out in front of you. Keeping elbows straight, spread arms out to the side and then slowly return to starting position.

5. Squeeze buttock muscles together, hold 6 counts, then relax.

6. TRAPEZE : HOLD TRAPEZE.
   RAISE YOURSELF OFF BED.
   HOLD FOR FOUR COUNTS.
   RELAX.

ABOVE KNEE

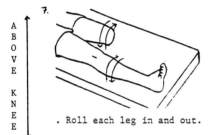

7. . Roll each leg in and out.

8. Keep both legs straight. Move each leg out alternately.

BELOW KNEE

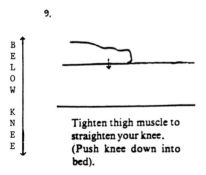

9. Tighten thigh muscle to straighten your knee. (Push knee down into bed).

WHILE IN SPLINT, DO ONLY
THIS FAR WITH SURGICAL LEG.

10. Pull foot up with legs out straight.      Pull toes up.      Curl toes down.

**Figure 25–7** Amputee exercise form.

*Illustration continued on following page*

FOR NON-SURGICAL LEG AND BELOW-KNEE AFTER SPLINT REMOVED

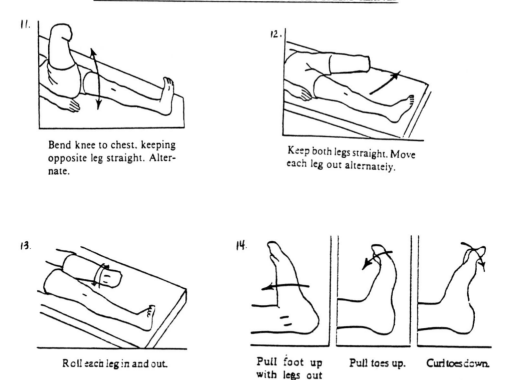

11. Bend knee to chest. keeping opposite leg straight. Alternate.

12. Keep both legs straight. Move each leg out alternately.

13. Roll each leg in and out.

14. Pull foot up with legs out straight. Pull toes up. Curl toes down.

**Figure 25-7** *Continued*

allowed for amputees at New England Deaconess Hospital because of the risk of injury to the healing stump in case of a fall; many of our patients also have many of the other previously discussed diabetic complications, which can mean a serious threat to their safety when combined with the imbalance problems of hopping. Therefore, we wait until the temporary prosthesis is finished and fitted to the patient before we work on gait training. Prosthesis fabrication takes three days on average.

Proper fit of the prosthesis is essential. The distal laces must be snugly and evenly tightened around the stump to promote edema reduction during wearing and ambulation. As edema is resorbed, the laces are tightened to accommodate the shrinking limb and to provide support. Both the proximal and distal corsets must be securely fitting to provide optimum leverage to the quadriceps muscles for ambulation and to prevent "pistoning," which in the diabetic can easily lead to ulceration. Correct alignment and height of the prosthesis are important as well. If they are off, the patient will have an abnormal, dysfunctional gait pattern, which can also contribute to ulceration.

After the prosthesis is fitted, the patient is instructed in putting it on and removing it, and we gradually increase the wearing time every day. We then begin gait training in parallel bars, and progress to a walker when indicated. Fortunately for the patients, but unfortunately for us as therapists, most patients are transferred to an inpatient program at a rehabilitation hospital as soon as their condition is medically stable and arrangements are made with the receiving facility. On average, our patients are transferred within a week after operation. In the exceptional case in which a patient may have problems with blood glucose regulation or infection control, we will be able to rehabilitate him further along his course than usual. However, in most instances, by the time the patients are fitted with their prostheses they are discharged.

The prosthetist follows up with the patient to make any necessary adjustments, and the patient is scheduled for Outpatient Amputee Clinic approximately one month after discharge from New England Deaconess Hospital. Together with the prosthetist, we evaluate for prosthetic fit (edema is usually markedly decreased), ease of activities of daily living, and possible progression of assistive device (e.g., walker to crutches or cane). The patient is then scheduled for Outpatient Amputee Clinic appointments only as needed and is fitted with a definitive prosthesis (Fig. 25–8) when edema reduction is complete, usually four to six months after amputation.

**ABOVE-KNEE AMPUTATION.** Obviously if ischemia or gangrene is extensive enough, an above-knee amputation is indicated. It is done only as a last resort because of the extremely high energy cost of ambulation with an above-knee prosthesis. Most of our diabetic patients, if an above-knee amputation is needed, are by that time elderly and with multiple complications, precluding ambulation.

With the patients who have had above-knee amputation, as for the below-knee amputees, we work on exercises (especially to prevent hip flexion contracture), bed and wheelchair mobility, transfers, and education. A pros-

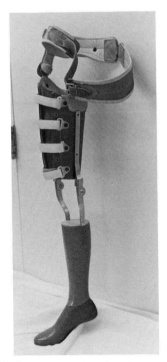

**Figure 25–9** Temporary above-knee Boston prosthesis.

thesis may be indicated for transfers (to maximize stability for safety) or for purely cosmetic reasons. If so, measurement and fitting of an above-knee Boston temporary prosthesis (Fig. 25–9) take place as for the below-knee prosthesis. The patient is also instructed in putting on and removing the prosthesis and in stand-pivot transfers. He may or may not be transferred to an intensive rehabilitation hospital, depending on his medical status and his goals. He may be discharged home, in which case collaboration with social service is necessary to ensure proper support services, including home physical therapy. The patient is eventually fitted with a definitive prosthesis as indicated (Fig. 25–10) and seen in Outpatient Amputee Clinic as discussed for the below-knee amputation.

**BILATERAL AMPUTATIONS.** The degree of therapy provided to these patients is ultimately very dependent on patient goals, medical status, and motivation. An elderly woman with an above-knee amputation and a below-knee amputation who also has cardiomyopathy and is legally blind should probably have a low-level rehabilitation program emphasizing overall conditioning and safe transfers to a wheelchair. However, a younger patient with two below-knee amputations who is very

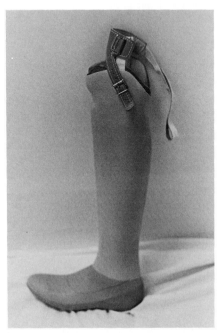

**Figure 25–8** Definitive below-knee prosthesis.

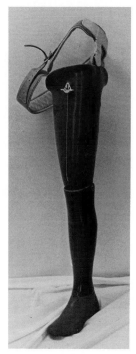

**Figure 25-10** Definitive above-knee prosthesis.

motivated and has few medical complications may well be a candidate for intensive rehabilitation, aiming toward top conditioning to permit ambulation with an assistive device.

## CONCLUSIONS

The foot/limb problems of diabetic patients can be very diverse and quite complicated. A team approach is necessary, even crucial, to care for all aspects of the problem. Discharge planning is essential, starting at the time of admission, to determine the physical and psychosocial needs of each patient and how best to meet them. Prevention and early detection of foot problems remain the most important components of good medical care to the diabetic foot, and all health professionals have an obligation to educate the patient and family as to *their* roles on the team. In one recent study, 81 per cent of amputations were attributed to initial minor trauma. In another, it was shown that a simple education program significantly reduced (by approximately threefold) the incidence of ulcer or foot and limb amputation in diabetic patients. Education and early treatment

are the keys to successful patient outcome; at New England Deaconess Hospital we see far fewer amputations now than we did even ten years ago. Physical therapists, as part of the team, do make a difference. Even though diabetes is an ongoing disease process, educating our patients to prevent complications *before* they occur can help them to lead a life of as much quality as possible.

I would like to express my thanks and appreciation to Jane Frasca, R.N., and Robert Easterbrooks, C.P.O., for their unreferenced contributions to this chapter as well as to our rehabilitation efforts.

## SUGGESTED READING LIST

Banks, A. S., and McGlamry, E. D.: Charcot foot. J. Am. Podiatr. Med. Assoc. 79:213, 1989.

Bild, D. E., Selby, J. V., and Sinnock, P.: Lower-extremity amputation in people with diabetes—epidemiology and prevention. Diabetes Care 12:24, 1989.

Clohisy, D. R., and Thompson, R. C.: Fractures associated with neuropathic arthropathy in adults who have juvenile-onset diabetes. J. Bone Joint Surg. 70A:1192, 1988.

Crausaz, F. M., Clavel, S., Liniger, C., et al.: Additional factors associated with plantar ulcers in diabetic neuropathy. Diabetic Med. 5:771, 1988.

Czerniecki, J. M.: Foot and ankle biomechanics in walking and running. A review. Am. J. Phys. Med. 67:246, 1988.

Frantz, S., Lawton, R., Schmagel, C., et al.: The physical therapist's role in the treatment of diabetes. Clin Management 7:30, 1987.

Greteman, B., and Dale, S.: Digital amputations in neuropathic feet. J. Am. Podiatr. Med. Assoc. 80:120, 1990.

Habershaw, G.: Notes from lecture to Massachusetts Podiatric Association, New England Deaconess Hospital, September 1990.

Kahn, J. K., Zola, B., Juni, J. E., et al.: Decreased exercise heart rate and blood pressure response in diabetic subjects with cardiac autonomic neuropathy. Diabetes Care 9:389, 1986.

Malone, J. M., Snyder, M., Anderson, G., et al.: Prevention of amputation by diabetic education. Am. J. Surg. 158:520, 1989.

Mueller, M. J., Diamond, J. E., Delitto, A., et al.: Insensitivity, limited joint mobility, and plantar ulcers in patients with diabetes mellitus. Phys. Ther. 69:453, 1989.

Mueller, M. J., Minor, S. D., Diamond, J. E., et al.: Relationship of foot deformity to ulcer location in patients with diabetes mellitus. Phys. Ther. 70:356, 362, 1990.

Pecoraro, R. E., Reiber, G. E., and Burgess, E. M.: Pathways to diabetic limb amputation—basis for prevention. Diabetes Care 13:513, 1990.

Schulte, L., Roberts, M.S., Zimmerman, C., et al.: A quantitative assessment of limited joint mobility in patients with diabetes—goniometric analysis of upper extremity passive range of motion. Arthritis Rheum. 36:1429, 1993.

Smith, L., Plehwe, W., McGill, M., et al.: Foot bearing pressure in patients with unilateral diabetic foot ulcers. Diabetic Med. 6:573, 1989.

Steinberg, F. U.: Rehabilitation of the diabetic amputee and neuropathic disabilities. In Levin, M. E. (ed.): The Diabetic Foot, St. Louis, C. V. Mosby, 1989.

Veves, A., Masson, E. A., Fernando, D. J., et al.: Studies of experimental hosiery in diabetic neuropathic patients with high foot pressures. Diabetic Med. 7:324, 1990.

Weber, G. A., and Cardile, M. A.: Diabetic neuropathies. Clin. Podiatr. Med. Surg. 7:1, 1990.

Young, J. R.: Foot problems in the diabetic patient. Cleve. Clin. J. Med. 55:458, 1988.

Ziegler, D., Mayer, P., Wiefels, K., et al.: Assessment of small and large fiber function in long-term type 1 (insulin-dependent) diabetic patients with and without painful neuropathy. Pain 34:1, 1988.

Zinman, B., and Vranic, M.: Diabetes and exercise. Med. Clin. North Am. 69:145, 1985.

# Appendix I
# YOUR FEET ARE IMPORTANT TO YOUR HEALTH

This information is intended to help you give your feet the good care that they deserve!

If you have diabetes, you may have *poor circulation* and a loss of sensation *(neuropathy)* in your feet and legs. *Poor circulation* and *neuropathy* mean that there is an increased risk for your feet to become infected. Proper foot care can prevent infection; therefore, we ask that you read and refer to this information until you have established a foot care regimen that you carry out faithfully on a daily basis. If you have any questions about the information in this booklet, ask your nurse to review it with you.

Remember . . . these are the only feet you will ever have—they deserve proper care and attention!

## GET TO KNOW YOUR FEET

As living parts of your body, your feet need a constant supply of food and energy. Your circulatory system (arteries and veins) brings freshly oxygenated blood to your feet and returns the "used" blood to your heart and lungs: The arteries bring the fresh blood carrying the food and energy to your feet; the veins carry out the used blood along with the waste materials.

If your circulatory system is not working properly, you may have *poor circulation*. Some of the signs and symptoms of poor circulation are:

- Dry and scaly or shiny skin
- Absence of hair growth over the legs
- Pale or bluish colored feet
- A tendency for the development of cracks in the skin or heels and between the toes
- Cramp-like discomfort in the legs when walking or at rest
- Numbness of the feet

The nerves in your legs and feet may also be affected; this is called *neuropathy*. Signs and symptoms of *neuropathy* include:

- Tingling, pain, or numbness in legs or feet
- Development of calluses over pressure points (toe joints, ball of the foot, etc.)
- Loss of feeling or sensation
- Lack of awareness of the position of the foot

## A REGIMEN FOR FOOT CARE

*Poor circulation* and *neuropathy* put your feet at increased risk for infection. Therefore, it is essential that you develop and faithfully carry out a daily regimen for care and inspection of your feet.

**277**

**1. Check Your Feet Every Day.**

- Use a mirror if necessary to visualize the entire foot. Do this in an area where you have proper lighting.
- Check for any signs of pressure (redness, blisters, calluses), breaks in the skin, cuts or cracks between the toes, sores, or any change in the usual color of your feet.
- Be alert for any noticeable change in the skin temperature of your feet.

**2. Wash Your Feet Every Day.**

- Use a mild soap and *warm* (*never* hot) water.
- Pat your feet dry with a soft towel; do *not* rub the skin.
- Pay particular attention to drying the skin between your toes.
- *Do not soak your feet—ever!*

**3. Keep the Skin of Your Feet Soft and Pliable.**

- Apply lanolin or other mild lotion such as Eucerin cream on dry feet *except* between the toes or on any breaks or open sores.
- Do *not* apply powder to your feet because it can be too drying and may solidify into a hard irritating crust.

**4. Wear Clean Socks or Hosiery and Sturdy, Well-Fitting Shoes Every Day.**

**5. Pay Special Attention to Care of Your Nails.**

- If you file your toenails, always use an emery board and follow the shape of the nail.
- If you cut your toenails:
  - –Use proper lighting; if you are unable to see well, have someone cut your nails for you.
  - –Cut nails immediately after washing your feet when the nails are soft.
  - –Use blunt end scissors—*never* use a curved-end nail clipper.
  - –Follow the shape of the nail.
- Do *not* cut calluses or ingrown toenails; if you have calluses, ingrown toenails, or other problems with your nails, see a podiatrist.

## HELPFUL HINTS FOR HEALTHY FEET

- *Always* wear shoes and socks or hosiery—even at home. Sturdy slippers are fine when you are at home; be sure to take time to put them on as soon as you get out of bed. Wear lightweight sneakers at the beach and in the water; *never, never, never* go barefoot.
- Wear clean cotton socks; white seamless socks are the best. Avoid tight socks or pantyhose.
- Shake out your shoes before putting them on—you may be surprised at what you find!
- Shop for new shoes at the *end* of the day; if the shoes fit after you've been up and about all day, they will fit fine first thing in the morning. Have a shoe salesperson fit your shoes and say *no* to pointed toes or sandals.
- *Never* cross your legs when sitting or lying down; crossing the legs will impair your circulation.
- Get sufficient exercise; walking is good. If you must sit for long periods of time, bend your feet up and down and wiggle your toes frequently.

- If at all possible, raise your legs on a footstool or chair when you are sitting down.
- *Never* soak your feet in *anything*—and particularly *not* in boric acid, epsom salts, povidone iodine (Betadine), or similar solutions.
- Ask your doctor to check your feet as part of your regular check-ups.
- *Don't* walk around in the dark—put the lights on before entering a dark room or climbing the stairs.
- Be extra cautious when walking on icy or unevenly paved streets or sidewalks. Use your cane or walker or ask a friend to walk with you.
- *Don't* smoke! Smoking reduces blood circulation and for patients who have diabetes, this can lead to the loss of a limb.
- Avoid situations in which your feet may not be able to detect temperature changes. Exposure to sun, water of unknown temperature, heating pads, and direct heat from a fireplace, wood stove, or quartz heater can burn your feet. Exposure to cold can result in frostbitten feet. So . . . . . . . .

   –Avoid the direct sun for any extended length of time—stay in the shade!

   –*Always* check the water temperature before getting into the water.

   –Do *not* rest your feet close to a burning fire in the fireplace or wood stove or in front of a quartz heater.

   –Do *not* place an electric heating pad on or under your feet.

   –In cold weather, wear warm cotton or wool socks and insulated boots.

**If You Experience Any of the Following Signs or Symptoms, Notify Your Physician Right Away:**

- An open sore or blister on your feet.
- Numb, cold legs that are pale or blue in color.
- Cramp-like pains in your legs when walking.
- Athlete's foot (itching, blisters, scaly skin) between your toes or on the soles of your feet.
- Signs or symptoms of infection: fever, redness, increased swelling, pain, increase or change in the character of the drainage.

## Remember . . .

**Timely Reporting of Foot Problems Will Enable Prompt Treatment; If You Detect a Problem:**

- DO NOT DELAY NOTIFYING YOUR PHYSICIAN.
- DO *NOT* TRY TO TREAT EVEN WHAT MAY APPEAR TO BE A MINOR PROBLEM.

PROPER TREATMENT OF FOOT PROBLEMS REQUIRES EARLY DETECTION BY YOU AND TREATMENT BY YOUR DOCTOR.

---

Revised by Jane Frasca, R.N., Vascular Coordinator

# Appendix II
# PERIPHERAL VASCULAR DISEASE WOUND CARE GUIDELINES

| **DRESSING** | **WOUND** | | | | | |
|---|---|---|---|---|---|---|
| | | Ulcer/Wound (open) | | | Incision (closed) | |
| **Gauze Packing Moistened w/** | **Callus/Fissure** | *Necrotic* | *Granulating* | *Infected (Gram[−], Pseudo.)* | *Wet* | *Dry* |
| 0.25% Dakins | | X | | | | |
| 0.25% Betadine | | X | | | | |
| 0.25% acetic acid | | X | | X | | |
| Coly-mycin 75 mg/50 cc NS | | X | | X | | |
| Normal saline | | | X | | | |
| Bacitracin ointment | X | | | | | |
| Calcium alginate dressing | | | X | | | |
| Betadine swab | | | | | X | |
| Cover w/gauze | X | X | X | X | X | |
| Secure w/paper tape | X | X | X | X | X | |
| Change | BID | TID | QD/BID TID | BID/TID | BID/TID PRN | |

# *Appendix III*
# CHARACTERISTICS OF LILLY AND NOVO NORDISK INSULINS

| Type | Formulation | Concentration (units per cc or mL) | Species | Route of Administration* | Appearance | Zinc Content (mg/100 units) | pH/Buffer | Preservative | Modifying Protein Salt | Amount of Modifying Protein Salt (mg/100 units) |
|---|---|---|---|---|---|---|---|---|---|---|
| **R** REGULAR Insulin Injection | Humulin® R | U-100 |  | SQ | Clear Solution | 0.01-0.04 | Neutral | M-cresol | — | — |
| | Regular Iletin® I | U-100 | | SQ | Clear Solution | 0.01-0.04 | Neutral | M-cresol | — | — |
| | Regular Iletin II | U-100 U-500 | | SQ | Clear Solution | 0.01-0.04 | Neutral | M-cresol | — | — |
| **N** NPH Insulin Isophane Suspension | Humulin N | U-100 | | SQ | Cloudy Suspension | 0.01-0.04 | Neutral/ Phosphate | M-cresol Phenol | Protamine Sulfate | 0.32-0.44 |
| | NPH Iletin I | U-100 | | SQ | Turbid or Cloudy Suspension | 0.01-0.04 | Neutral/ Phosphate | M-cresol Phenol | Protamine Sulfate | 0.32-0.44 |
| | NPH Iletin II | U-100 | | SQ | Turbid or Cloudy Suspension | 0.01-0.04 | Neutral/ Phosphate | M-cresol Phenol | Protamine Sulfate | 0.32-0.44 |
| **L** LENTE® Insulin Zinc Suspension | Humulin L | U-100 | | SQ | Turbid or Cloudy Suspension | 0.12-0.25 | Neutral/ Acetate | Methyl-paraben | — | — |
| | Lente Iletin I | U-100 | | SQ | Turbid or Cloudy Suspension | 0.12-0.25 | Neutral/ Acetate | Methyl-paraben | — | — |
| | Lente Iletin II | U-100 | | SQ | Turbid or Cloudy Suspension | 0.12-0.25 | Neutral/ Acetate | Methyl-paraben | — | — |
| **U** ULTRALENTE® Extended Insulin Zinc Suspension | Humulin U | U-100 | | SQ | Turbid or Cloudy Suspension | 0.12-0.25 | Neutral/ Acetate | Methyl-paraben | — | — |
| **70/30** 70% Human Insulin Isophane Suspension 30% Human Insulin Injection | Humulin 70/30 | U-100 | | SQ | Cloudy Suspension | 0.01-0.04 | Neutral/ Phosphate | M-cresol Phenol | Protamine Sulfate | 0.22-0.26 |
| **50/50** 50% Human Insulin Isophane Suspension 50% Human Insulin Injection | Humulin 50/50 | U-100 | | SQ | Cloudy Suspension | 0.01-0.04 | Neutral/ Phosphate | M-cresol Phenol | Protamine Sulfate | 0.16-0.18 |

WARNING: Any change of insulin should be made cautiously and only under medical supervision. Changes in purity, strength, brand (manufacturer), type (Regular, NPH, Lente, etc), species (beef, pork, beef-pork, or human), and/or method of manufacture (recombinant DNA versus animal-source insulin) may result in the need for a change in dosage.

*Regular formulations may also be administered intravenously; this route affects onset, peak, and duration of action.

*Lilly*

**Eli Lilly and Company**
Indianapolis, Indiana
46285

60-HI-2782-3   PRINTED IN USA   300759-99320   ©1993, ELI LILLY AND COMPANY

Eli Lilly: 60-41-2782-3. Indianapolis, Eli Lilly and Co., 1993.

# Novo Nordisk Pharmaceuticals Inc.
## Product Reference Guide

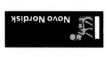

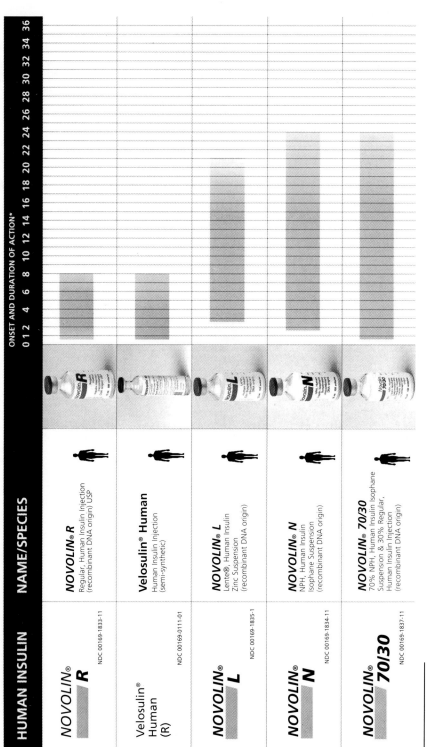

| HUMAN INSULIN | NAME/SPECIES | | ONSET AND DURATION OF ACTION* |
|---|---|---|---|
| | | | 0 1 2 4 6 8 10 12 14 16 18 20 22 24 26 28 30 32 34 36 |
| NOVOLIN® R    NDC 00169-1833-11 | NOVOLIN® R Regular, Human Insulin Injection (recombinant DNA origin) USP | | |
| Velosulin® Human (R)    NDC 00169-0111-01 | Velosulin® Human Human Insulin Injection (semi-synthetic) | | |
| NOVOLIN® L    NDC 00169-1835-1 | NOVOLIN® L Lente® Human Insulin Zinc Suspension (recombinant DNA origin) | | |
| NOVOLIN® N    NDC 00169-1834-11 | NOVOLIN® N NPH, Human Insulin Isophane Suspension (recombinant DNA origin) | | |
| NOVOLIN® 70/30    NDC 00169-1837-11 | NOVOLIN® 70/30 70% NPH, Human Insulin Isophane Suspension & 30% Regular, Human Insulin Injection (recombinant DNA origin) | | |

Novo Nordisk, Princeton, NJ.

Novo Nordisk

# INDEX

Note: Page numbers in *italics* refer to illustrations; page numbers followed by t refer to tables.